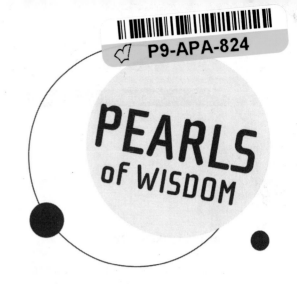

Nurse Anesthetist
EXAM REVIEW

Lisa J. Thiemann, CRNA, MNA

Kerri M. Robertson, M.D., F.R.C.P (C)

David A. Lubarsky, M.D., M.B.A.

Sudharma Ranasinghe, M.D., F.F.A.R.C.S.I.

McGraw-Hill
Medical Publishing Division

New York Chicago San Francisco Lisbon London
Madrid Mexico City Milan New Delhi
San Juan Seoul Singapore
Sydney Toronto

Nurse Anesthetist Review

1 2 3 4 5 6 7 8 9 0   CUS/CUS   0 9 8 7 6 5

ISBN 0-07-146436-0

Notice

Medicine is an ever-changing science. As new research and clinical experience broaden our knowledge, changes in treatment and drug therapy are required. The authors and the publisher of this work have checked with sources believed to be reliable in their efforts to provide information that is complete and generally in accord with the standards accepted at the time of publication. However, in view of the possibility of human error or changes in medical sciences, neither the authors nor the publisher nor any other party who has been involved in the preparation or publication of this work warrants that the information contained herein is in every respect accurate or complete, and they disclaim all responsibility for any errors or omissions or for the results obtained from use of the information contained in this work. Readers are encouraged to confirm the information contained herein with other sources. For example and in particular, readers are advised to check the product information sheet included in the package of each drug they plan to administer to be certain that the information contained in this work is accurate and that changes have not been made in the recommended dose or in the contraindications for administration. This recommendation is of particular importance in connection with new or infrequently used drugs.

The editors were Catherine A. Johnson and Marsha Loeb.
The production supervisor was Phil Galea.
The cover designer was Handel Low.
Von Hoffmann Graphics was printer and binder.

This book is printed on acid-free paper.

Cataloging-in-Publication data for this title is on file at the Library of Congress.

DEDICATION

To all my family, for their undying support and words of encouragement throughout the years; to Mary E. Shirk Marienau, Edward S. Thompson, and the faculty at the Duke University School of Nursing for their ongoing inspiration and advisement.

LJT

Dr. Jerry Reves

To a great man who has dedicated his career to creating a truly academic Department of Anesthesiology at Duke University.

Many thanks for your tireless efforts on behalf of the faculty and for your inspiration, guidance and support.

KMR and DAL

Dedicated to two great departments at the University of Miami and Duke University Medical Center who made this all possible.

DAL and SR

SPECIAL THANKS

To
Chris Keith
for his outstanding editorial assistance,
patience and humor.

To
my simply amazing children, Mitchel and Sasha,
my unconditional love, always.

Kerri Robertson, MD

EDITORS

Lisa J. Thiemann, CRNA, MNA
Assistant Clinical Professor
Associate Director
Duke University Nurse Anesthesia Program
Associate Director
Duke University Human Simulation and
Patient Safety Center
Durham, NC

Kerri M. Robertson, M.D., F.R.C.P. (C)
Associate Clinical Professor
Chief of GVTCCM Division
Chief Transplant Services
Department of Anesthesiology
Duke University Medical Center
Durham, NC

David Alan Lubarsky, M.D., M.B.A.
Emanuel M. Pappar Professor and Chair
Department of Anesthesiology, Perioperative
Medicine, and Pain Management
University of Miami/Jackson Memorial Hospital
Professor
Department of Management
University of Miami School of Business
Miami, FL

Sudharma Ranasinghe, M.D., F.F.A.R.C.S.I.
Associate Professor of Clinical Anesthesiology
Asst. Director of Obstetric Anesthesia
University of Miami/Jackson Memorial Hospital
Miami, FL

CONTRIBUTING AUTHORS

Joseph F. Answine, M.D.
Staff Anesthesiologist
Pinnacle Health System
Harrisburg, PA
Assistant Professor
Department of Anesthesia
Penn State Geisinger Health System
Hershey, PA

Sandralee A. Blosser, M.D.
Assistant Professor
Surgery, Anesthesia, & Medicine
Penn State Geisinger Health System
Hershey, PA

Christopher A. Bracken, M.D., Ph.D.
Associate Professor of Anesthesia
The University of Texas Health Science Center
San Antonio, TX

Richard Brenner, M.D.
Department of Anesthesiology
UCLA School of Medicine
Los Angeles, CA

Keith Candiotti, M.D.
Assistant Professor of Anesthesiology and
Internal Medicine
Director for Perioperative Services
University of Miami
Miami, FL

Susan M. Chan, M.D.
Assistant Clinical Professor
Department of Anesthesiology
UCLA School of Medicine
Los Angeles, CA

Biing-Jaw Chen, M.D.
Associate Professor
Co-Chief of OB Anesthesia
Department of Anesthesiology
Harbor-UCLA Medical Center
Torrance, CA

Jeffrey Chen, M.D.
Resident
Department of Anesthesia
Pennsylvania State University
Penn State Geisinger Health System
Hershey, PA

Susan Chlebowski, M.D.
Department of Anesthesiology
University of Rochester
Rochester, NY

Noel Lee Chun, M.D.
Assistant Clinical Professor
UCLA School of Medicine
Los Angeles, CA

Gerard DeSouza, M.D.
Assistant Professor of Anesthesiology
University of Miami School of Medicine
V.A. Medical Center
Miami, FL

Kathleen S. Donahue, D.O.
Associate Medical Director
Outpatient Surgical Unit
Assistant Professor of Anesthesia
Penn State Geisinger Health Systems
Hershey, PA

John B. Eck, M.D.
Assistant Professor
Department of Anesthesiology
Division of Pediatric Anesthesia and Critical
Care Medicine
Duke University Medical Center
Durham, NC

Tiberiu Ezri, M.D.
Kaplan Hospital
Rehovot, Israel

James Foster, M.D.
Department of Anesthesia
Children's Hospital
Buffalo, NY

David C. Frankenfield, M.S., R.D.
Department of Anesthesia
Penn State Geisinger Health System
Hershey, PA

Keith S. Getz, M.D.
Department of Anesthesia
Lakewood Medical Center
St. Joseph, MI

Howard B. Gutstein, M.D.
Research Investigator
Assistant Professor of Anesthesia
The University of Michigan
Mental Health Research Institute
Ann Arbor, MI

Christopher Heard, M.B., Ch.B.
Research Assistant Professor
Department of Anesthesiology and Division of
Pediatric Critical Care
Children's Hospital
Buffalo, NY

Eric Hsu, M.D.
Department of Anesthesiology
UCLA School of Medicine
Los Angeles, CA

Billy K. Huh, M.D.
Associate
Department of Anesthesiology
Duke University Medical Center
Durham, NC

Judi Hwang, M.D.
Department of Anesthesiology
UCLA School of Medicine
Los Angeles, CA

Alma N. Juels, M.D.
Assistant Clinical Professor
Department of Anesthesiology
UCLA School of Medicine
Los Angeles, CA

Gregory Juarez, M.D.
Department of Anesthesiology
UCLA Medical Center
Los Angeles, CA

John Knighton, M.D.
Anesthetic Specialist Registrar
Salisbury District Hospital NHS Trust
Salisbury, Wiltshire
United Kingdom
Assistant Professor of Anesthesia and Surgery
Co-Director of the Surgical Intensive Care Unit
Duke University Medical Center
Durham, NC

Atul Kshatri, M.D.
Fellow, Pain Medicine and Palliative Care
Clinical Instructor, Anesthesia
Penn State College of Medicine
Hershey, PA

Wing-Fai Kwan, M.D.
Associate Professor
Chief of OB Anesthesia
Department of Anesthesiology
Harbor-UCLA Medical Center
Torrance, CA

David Lindsay, M.D.
Clinical Associate
Department of Anesthesiology
Duke University Medical Center
Durham, NC

Michael C. Lewis, M.D.
Assistant Professor, Anesthesiology
University of Miami/Veterans Medical Center
Miami, FL

Stephen P. Long, M.D.
Co-Director
Pain Management Center
Medical College of Virginia
Virginia Commonwealth University
Richmond, VA

Stephen Longo, M.D.
Assistant Professor of Anesthesia
Director, Obstetrical Anesthesia
Penn State College of Medicine
The Milton S. Hershey Medical Center
Hershey, PA

David MacLeod, M.D., F.R.C.A.
Associate
Department of Anesthesiology
Duke University Medical Center
Durham, NC

Mary Mathai, M.D., B.S.
Clinical Assistant Professor
Department of Anesthesia
University of Michigan
Ann Arbor, MI

John Moore, M.D.
Resident
Department of Pediatric Anesthesia
Cardinal Glennon Children's Hospital
St. Louis University
St. Louis, MO

Eugene W. Moretti, M.D.
Associate
Department of Anesthesiology
Duke University Medical Center
Durham, NC

Gundappa Neelekanta, M.D.
Department of Anesthesiology
UCLA School of Medicine
Los Angeles, CA

Kirsten O'Neil, M.D.
Resident in Anesthesiology
University of Miami
Miami, FL

Gurpreet Singh Padda, M.D.
Assistant Professor
Department of Pediatric Anesthesia
Cardinal Glennon Children's Hospital
St. Louis University
St. Louis, MO

Lynnus Peng, M.D.
Fellow
Department of Anesthesia and Critical Care
Medicine
Johns Hopkins Hospital
Baltimore, MD

Scott D. Picker, M.D.
Assistant Clinical Professor of Anesthesia
UCLA Medical Center
Los Angeles, CA

Michael R. Pinsky, M.D.
Professor of Anesthesiology, Critical Care
Medicine and Medicine
University of Pittsburgh Medical Center
Oakland V.A. Medical Center
Pittsburgh, PA

Marcus Q. Polk, M.D.
Anesthesiology Resident
Emory University School of Medicine
Atlanta, GA

Juan Carlos Restrepo, M.D.
Diplomat of the American Board of
Anesthesiology
VA Medical Center
Jackson Memorial Hospital
University of Miami
Miami, FL

G. Chase Robinson, Jr., M.D.
Assistant Professor
Department of Anesthesiology
The University of Texas
Health Science Center at San Antonio
San Antonio, TX

Garfield B. Russell, M.D.
Acting Chair
Department of Anesthesia
Penn State Geisinger Health System
Hershey, PA

John Robert Schultz, M.D.
Associate
Department of Anesthesiology
Division of Women's Anesthesia
Duke University Medical Center
Durham, NC

Allan B. Shang, M.D.
Assistant Clinical Professor
Department of Anesthesiology
Division Chief of Offsite Anesthesia Services
Duke University Medical Center
Durham, NC

Jay R. Shayevitz, M.D., M.S.
Providence Hospital and Medical Centers
Southfield, MI

Jacques Somma, M.D., FRCP (C)
Director of the Human Pharmacology Laboratory
Assistant Professor
Department of Anesthesiology
Duke University Medical Center
Durham, NC

Timothy Stanley, M.D.
Associate
Department of Anesthesiology
Duke University Medical Center
Durham, NC

R. H. Steadman, M.D.
Department of Anesthesiology
UCLA School of Medicine
Los Angeles, CA

Yung-Fong Sung, M.D.
Professor of Anesthesiology
Emory University School of Medicine
Chief of Anesthesiology
Ambulatory Surgery Center
The Emory Clinic
Atlanta, GA

Kenneth M. Sutin, M.D.
Assistant Professor of Clinical Anesthesia and
Clinical Surgery
New York University
Director of Recovery Room and Associate
Director of Critical Care
Bellevue Hospital
New York, NY

Peter Szmuk, M.D.
Kaplan Hospital
Rehovot, Israel

James F. Szocik, M.D.
Clinical Assistant Professor
Department of Anesthesiology
University of Michigan Medical Center
Ann Arbor, MI

John Thomas, M.D.
Department of Anesthesiology
UCLA School of Medicine
Los Angeles, CA

Barbara Vineis, R.N., M.P.H., J.D.
Department of Anesthesiology
UCLA School of Medicine
Los Angeles, CA

Ian James Welsby, M.D., B.Sc., M.B.B.S.,
F.R.C.A.
Associate
Department of Anesthesiology
Duke University Medical Center
Durham, NC

Daniel P. Williams, D.O.
Clinical Instructor of Anesthesia
Penn State Geisinger Health System
Hershey, PA

David Wright, M.D., FRCA
Associate
Department of Anesthesiology
Duke University Medical Center
Durham, NC

Elaine Yang, M.D.
Associate Professor
Department of Anesthesiology
Harbor-UCLA Medical Center
Torrance, CA

Ahmed Zaki, M.D.
The University of Michigan
Mental Health Research Institute
Ann Arbor, MI

INTRODUCTION

1 and 3.
2 and 4.
1, 2, and 3.
4 alone.

If 1 is true, then 3 is true and vice-a-versa.
If 2 is true, so is at least one other choice.
We have it on good authority that the Marquis de Sade used "K-type" questions on those he wished to torture most. His minions, in the guise of academic test creators, have persevered over the centuries to make sure this unique form of torture is widely inflicted.

How many false answers will you read practicing "K-type" questions? 50%. How many false answers will you consider in the "one best answer" question type? 75%. We remember what we read. So, right before the exam, after you've practiced test-taking, and conquered the strategy for "K-type" questions, it's time to focus on correct answers. That way, what's freshest in your memory as you sit for the boards will always be a correct potential answer.

Hence, *Nurse Anesthetist Exam Review: Pearls of Wisdom*. One in a series of written board review texts created for many healthcare specialties, this format has proved itself as the best preparation immediately before the exam. Hundreds of questions garnered from across the nation and from multiple institutions. Questions that have only the correct answer. Read it, remember it, and score well!

As anyone will tell you, reading board review books doesn't make you smart, and just knowing the answers in this book does NOT guarantee a good board exam score. If you read something, and do not understand the answer, or are not sure about a related topic that pops into your mind, LOOK IT UP!

This book is *not* a substitute for Barash, Stoelting, Nagelhout, and Miller. Their textbooks are for the acquisition of knowledge; use their books when you need a more complete understanding. This book is a quick pre-boards review and was edited for that purpose.

If you would like to contribute questions for consideration into the next edition, please email them to thiem002@mc.duke.edu or lisajcrna@yahoo.com. To be considered a contributing author, please create a series of original questions with referenced answers based on board questions or requisite board topics.

LJT, KMR & DAL

TABLE OF CONTENTS

MACHINES

I Think That Anyone Who Comes Upon A Nautilus Machine Suddenly Will Agree With Me That Its Prototype Was Clearly Invented At Some Time In History When Torture Was Considered A Reasonable Alternative To Diplomacy.
Anna Quindlen

○ **If you are using a self-inflating resuscitation bag and mask to ventilate a patient, what will an increase in the minute ventilation do to the FiO_2 delivered?**

FiO_2 generally decreases. The exact change depends on the rate of oxygen delivery to the bag, the minute ventilation, and the specific method of oxygen delivery to the bag. The use of a reservoir combined with high oxygen flows allows 100% oxygen to be delivered irrespective of the minute ventilation. FiO_2 delivered is *directly proportional to O2 flow rate* (usually 100%- with 10L/ min of O2) and *inversely proportional to MV* . Use of a Venturi delivery system allows a constant FiO_2, although a lower maximal FiO_2 is achieved than with a reservoir and high flow oxygen.

○ **If you add an oxygen reservoir tube to a self-inflating resuscitation bag, what happens to the maximal FiO_2 that can be delivered?**

The addition of an oxygen reservoir tube to a self-inflating resuscitation bag increases the maximal FiO_2 that can be delivered.

○ **What are the primary components of soda lime?**

The primary components of "wet" or "high moisture" soda lime (the most common type in use today) are calcium hydroxide (76-81%), sodium hydroxide (4%), potassium hydroxide (1%), and water (14-19%).

○ **What are the primary components of Baralyme?**

Calcium hydroxide (80%), and barium hydroxide (20%). Moisture in Baralyme is incorporated into the structure of the barium hydroxide, which exists as an octahydrate.

○ **What are the basic reactions involved in CO_2 absorption by soda lime and Baralyme?**

In both cases, CO_2 first reacts with water to form carbonic acid. The carbonic acid then combines with the various hydroxides found in the absorber chemicals to form carbonates and heat.

○ **What is the optimum size for absorbent granules?**

The optimum size for absorbent granules is 4 to 8 mesh. Granules smaller than 8 mesh cause excess resistance and tend to cake, while granules larger than 4 mesh offer less surface area for absorption.

○ **What volume of intergranular air must be in the carbon dioxide canister to maximize carbon dioxide absorption?**

The intergranular air space must be at least as large as the maximal tidal volume in order to trap all the CO_2 that passes through the absorber.

○ **If the canister of Baralyme or soda lime doesn't feel warm, what should you suspect?**

The absorption of CO_2 by either Baralyme or soda lime is exothermic. If the canister is not warm, you should suspect that CO_2 is not being absorbed.

○   **What is the maximal absorbant capacity for Baralyme and soda lime?**

The maximal absorbant capacity for Baralyme is variously reported as 9-27.1 liters of CO_2/ 100g of absorbent. The maximal absorbant capacity for soda lime is generally reported as about 25 liters of CO_2/ 100g of absorbant. With either absorber, the color indicator may revert back to its pre-exhausted color if the absorbant is rested. This does not indicate a significant recovery of absorbant capacity and the color will quickly change to is exhausted state if the absorbant is re-used.

○   **What constitutes the dead space in a circle system?**

Everything distal to the partition in the Y-piece. Examples include the face mask, endotracheal tube, "artificial nose", etc.

○   **How much does the FiO_2 increase for each liter per minute increase in oxygen flow via nasal cannula?**

FiO_2 increases approximately 4% for each L/min increase in delivered O_2, up to 6 L/min. Flow rates beyond 6 L/min do not predictably increase FiO_2 above approximately 44% and are also poorly tolerated because of drying and crusting of the nasal mucosa.

○   **What is the main advantage of the Venturi (air-entrainment) face mask?**

The Venturi face mask provides a stable FiO_2 between 24-40%, irrespective of changes in minute ventilation and inspiratory flow rate.

○   **What is the purpose of using an isolation transformer in the electrical supply to the operating room?**

The isolation transformer converts the grounded electrical power from the utility company into ungrounded power in the OR. This decreases the risk of shock because there is no electrical potential between the wire and ground, only between the two wires. Thus, to receive a shock from an ungrounded power supply, a person must contact two wires. To receive a shock from a grounded system, however, a person must merely be in contact with ground and also touch the "hot" wire.

○   **What is the significance of the line isolation monitor sounding its alarm?**

The line isolation monitor measures the potential for current flow from the isolated operating room power supply to ground. It determines the amount of current that could flow if a second short circuit should develop and sounds the alarm if this current exceeds 2mA or 5mA, depending on the particular monitor used.

○   **Why is the line isolation monitor more useful for preventing macroshock than microshock?**

Macroshock is current delivered to the body surface and current up to 5 mA is accepted as harmless. The line isolation monitor alarms when there is potential for current flow of 2mA or 5mA. Microshock (current delivered directly to the heart) can cause ventricular fibrillation with current as low as 0.1 mA, well below the alarm point of a line isolation monitor.

○   **What is the purpose of the flow proportioning system?**

The flow proportioning system interlinks the oxygen and nitrous oxide flow controls such that a fresh gas mixture containing at least 25% oxygen is created at the level of the rotameters.

○   **What are the four major functions of the breathing bag in a circle system?**

1. Reservoir of exhaled gas which allows rebreathing.
2. Provides positive pressure ventilation.
3. Visual and tactile monitor of spontaneous ventilation.
4. Limits the maximum pressure that can develop in the system.

○   What equipment problems may contribute to a high end-tidal CO_2?

A high end-tidal CO_2 is indicative of hypercapnia usually due to inadequate alveolar ventilation. Predisposing causes may be due to increased CO_2 production or decreased carbon dioxide elimination.

Equipment problems include: inadequate minute ventilation (respiratory depression in the patient breathing spontaneously or inadequate tidal volume or respiratory rate if ventilation is controlled), depleted, faulty or bypassed carbon dioxide absorber and rebreathing (faulty unidirectional valves, inadequate flows with a semi-open circuit and any cause of increased dead space.) In a Mapleson circuit, significant rebreathing of CO_2 results from insufficient fresh gas flow. A hole in the inner tube of a coaxial circuit can allow significant rebreathing. Failure of the carbon dioxide waveform on the capnograph to return to baseline is diagnostic of rebreathing.

○   What safeguards are present to warn of airway disconnection?

A disconnect alarm which detects a drop in peak circuit pressure will be activated during controlled mechanical ventilation. A standing bellows (ascending) will fail to fill. Some machines offer an alarm that warns if insufficient expired gas is not returned. Failure of the reservoir bag to inflate will occur during spontaneous ventilation and the patient may show signs of insufficient depth of anesthesia. The capnograph will record no carbon dioxide waveform and the apnea alarm will sound. Clinical signs include failure of the chest to rise and loss of breath sounds if auscultating with a precordial stethoscope. A late sign is hypoxemia as measured by a reduction in SpO_2 with pulse oximetry.

○   What is the function of the fail-safe valve?

The fail-safe valve shuts off the flow of other gases and sounds an alarm in the event that oxygen supply pressure drops 50% below normal. It does not protect against other causes of hypoxia especially the problems downstream of the flow meters, therefore an oxygen analyzer is an essential monitor.

○   What are the two basic types of waste gas scavenging systems?

Passive and active.

A passive system is a simple direct line venting outside or into an air conditioning duct beyond any point of recirculation. An active system is connected to the hospital vacuum system. Components of the scavenging system include: a negative pressure relief valve (protects the patient from the suction effect of the vacuum system), a positive pressure relief valve (prevents barotrauma from back-pressure in the event of obstruction) and a reservoir (accommodates transient high flows).

○   What factors contribute to the generation of CO (carbon monoxide) through the interaction of the CO_2 absorbent and volatile anesthetic agents?

Physical properties of the absorbent, choice and concentration of volatile anesthetic agent.

The drier the absorbent, the more CO produced. At any given moisture content, Baralyme produces more CO than soda lime. Higher temperatures lead to greater production of CO. Increased concentration of the volatile anesthetic agent leads to greater CO production. The choice of inhaled agent influences the production rate; ranked in order of greatest to least CO production: desflurane $\geq$ enflurane > isoflurane >> halothane = sevoflurane.

O   **What are the consequences of an inspiratory valve malfunction?**

In the unlikely event that the inspiratory valve is stuck in the closed position and the expiratory valve is competent, it would be impossible to deliver a breath to the patient. The more common scenario is failure of the inspiratory valve to properly close allowing rebreathing of expired gas containing CO_2. Hypercapnia may be tolerated or the effect slightly ameliorated by increasing the fresh gas flow rates until the valve can be replaced or an alternate breathing system employed.

O   **What information is available from the analysis of the CO_2 waveform using capnography?**

Confirmation of tracheal placement of the endotracheal tube, adequacy of ventilation, detection of rebreathing of CO_2 (baseline > 0), evidence of obstructive lung disease or spontaneous breathing during mechanical ventilation and circuit disconnect or partial disconnection of the capnograph sampling hose. The capnometer gives a numerical value of the end-tidal CO_2 which can be used to approximate and follow the $PaCO_2$, although discrepancies exist between end-tidal and arterial CO_2. Early detection of increased CO_2 production from malignant hyperthermia, thyrotoxicosis or during carbon dioxide insufflation with laparoscopic procedures is possible.

O   **What surface lead is best for monitoring atrial activity?**

Lead II. It is the best surface lead for monitoring atrial activity as it displays the greatest P wave voltage.

O   **Name 5 different modes of mechanical ventilation.**

1: *Controlled Mechanical Ventilation (CMV)*: fixed tidal volume and a fixed rate.

2: *Assist-Control Ventilation (ACV)*: Senses the patient's inspiratory effort and delivers a set tidal volume when inspiratory effort is made. If no inspiratory effort is made, the ventilator functions as in control mode. Common problem associated with ACV is respiratory alkalosis in patients breathing at high respiratory rates.

3: *Intermittent Mandatory Ventilation (IMV)*: A fixed tidal volume and rate are delivered. In addition to this mandatory ventilation, the patient is able to take spontaneous breaths. The tidal volume and rate of the spontaneous breaths is determined by the patient's respiratory efforts. In SIMV mode, the machine creates timing windows around the scheduled mandatory breaths in order to synchronize each machine's breath with the patient's inspiratory effort, which might vary the machine cycle times slightly. If no inspiratory effort is detected within the time window, the machine delivers a mandatory breath at the scheduled time.

4: *Pressure Support Ventilation (PS)*: Maintains a predetermined positive pressure throughout inspiration. This helps overcome increased resistance from the mechanical components of the breathing system (ETT, tubing, etc). It is often combined with Intermittent Mandatory Ventilation.

5: *Inverse Ratio Ventilation*: This is ventilation in which the inspiratory time is greater than the expiratory time, the opposite of normal breathing.

O   **What are the OSHA standards for acceptable levels of anesthetic exposure?**

OSHA sets the maximum acceptable level of nitrous oxide at 25 parts per million (ppm). The maximum acceptable level for halogenated agents is 0.5 ppm when used in combination with nitrous oxide, 2 ppm if used alone.

O   **What are some advantages of a circle system versus a Bain (coaxial) circuit?**

The circle system allows for use a CO_2 absorber. The absorber allows CO_2 to be scrubbed from rebreathed gas. This in turn allows rebreathing of gas without hypercapnia. Rebreathing of gas allows conservation of heat and humidity and the use of lower fresh gas flow. Lower fresh gas flow allows for reduced pollution and reduced use of agent with resultant lower cost. The downside of the circle system is that it is bigger, less portable, more complex, has more components which can disconnect or fail, and has greater resistance.

○   **How does the anesthesia ventilator generate positive airway pressure?**

The bellows in an anesthesia machine ventilator takes the place of the breathing bag. A breathing bag is compressed by hand, while the bellows is compressed by pressurized oxygen delivered to the space between the bellows and the bellows enclosure. Oxygen used to power the ventilator is used at a rate at least equal to the minute ventilation.

○   **What is the preferred order of components in a circle system?**

The unidirectional valves should be as close to the patient as possible, but not in the Y-piece as that may lead to improper orientation of the valves. Practically speaking, since the valves are not disposable , they are closer to the machine rather than closer to the patient in the flexible breathing tubes. The fresh gas inlet should be between the CO_2 absorber and the inspiratory valve, positioned upstream of the inspiratory valve. The pressure relief valve should be located immediately before the CO_2 absorber. The breathing bag should be located in the expiratory limb to reduce resistance to exhalation.

○   **What is the purpose of a low pressure circuit test?**

On machines equipped with a common gas outlet check valve, positive pressure is not transmitted upstream of the common gas outlet during a positive pressure check of the breathing circuit. Because of this, a leak upstream of the common gas outlet will not be detected by this test, and a negative pressure test is required. Leaks in vaporizers equipped with a check valve will go undetected by a positive pressure test only.

○   **How much oxygen is in a standard E cylinder when its pressure gauge reads 1000 psi?**

For a nonliquefied gas, the pressure decreases steadily as the cylinder is emptied. Therefore, an E cylinder containing 660 liters of oxygen at 2000 psi, will contain 330 liters if the pressure drops to 1000 psi.

With a liquefied gas, the pressure remains constant until all the liquid has turned to gas, then drops as the cylinder is emptied (nitrous oxide is ¾ empty before psi drops). Weighing the cylinder will determine the amount of liquid remaining.

○   **How does one know if a piece of OR equipment contains latex?**

Latex containing products must be labeled as such by the manufacturer.

○   **What is the significance of a circuit low pressure alarm?**

With an anesthesia machine, mechanical ventilation is achieved by generating positive pressure in the breathing circuit. A low pressure alarm sounds when sufficient pressure is not generated. This alarm is also referred to as a disconnect alarm. Low pressure alarm threshold should be set just below (< 7 cmH$_2$O) the minimum peak pressure expected in order to detect leaks and partial disconnections.

○   **How long can an E cylinder of oxygen supply 10 liters per minute oxygen flow?**

To determine how long an oxygen cylinder can supply a given flow, one must determine the amount of oxygen in the cylinder. A full E cylinder of oxygen contains 660 liters of oxygen at 2000 psi. This is expected to last 66 minutes at 10 lpm.

○   **What factors can cause errors in measuring SpO_2?**

Carboxyhemoglobin and methemoglobin, intravenous dyes, nail polish, electrical interference and pulsatile veins.

Because the pulse oximeter measures light absorbance at two wavelengths, it can only accurately measure two solutes (ie: oxyhemoglobin and deoxygenated hemoglobin). Carboxyhemoglobin is interpreted as oxyhemoglobin and the SpO_2 is artifactually raised toward 100%. Methemoglobin causes the SpO_2 to trend toward 85%. Fetal and sickle hemoglobins have little effect. Intravenous dyes can cause artifacts in the SpO_2: methylene blue a large decrease, indigo carmine a small decrease and indocyanine green an intermediate effect. Certain nail polishes can cause falsely low SpO_2 readings. Electrical interference can occur from the electrosurgical unit. Pulsatile veins (ie: tricuspid regurgitation) can not be distinguished from pulsatile arteries and can cause falsely low SpO_2 readings.

○ **What fresh gas flow is required to prevent significant rebreathing of CO_2 with a Mapleson A circuit?**

For spontaneous ventilation, a fresh gas flow equal to the minute ventilation is sufficient. Mapleson A design is the most effective Mapleson Circuit for spontaneous ventilation. For controlled ventilation, a very high and unpredictable fresh gas flow is required to prevent significant rebreathing of CO_2.

○ **What fresh gas flow is required to prevent significant rebreathing of CO_2 with a Mapleson D circuit?**

For spontaneous ventilation, 2 to 3 times the minute ventilation is required. For controlled ventilation, fresh gas flow of 1 to 2 times the minute ventilation is sufficient to prevent rebreathing of CO_2.

○ **What methods are available to add or maintain humidity of inspiratory gases?**

- Addition of moisture to the inside of the breathing tubes
- Heat and moisture exchangers (artificial noses)
- Heated humidifiers
- Nebulizers
- Rebreathing circuits with low fresh gas flows
- CO_2 absorber

○ **What effect does changing fresh gas from 100% O_2 to 70% nitrous oxide have on vaporizer output?**

This change will transiently lower the volatile anesthetic concentration coming out of a variable bypass vaporizer.

○ **What effect does increased altitude have on an anesthetic vaporizer?**

Contemporary variable bypass vaporizers, such as isoflurane, sevoflurane vaporizers deliver a constant partial pressure of anesthetic. Decreased barometric pressure such as found at high altitude will increase the vaporizer output because high resistance path through vapor chamber offers less resistance. Therefore may require decrease dial settings at high altitude. When vaporizer delivery is measured as volume percent (not partial pressure), such as desflurane vaporizer Tec 6, it requires increase dial settings at high altitudes.

○ **When does rebreathing occur in a circle system?**

Rebreathing occurs with low fresh gas flow rates and requires use of a CO_2 absorber to remove carbon dioxide from the exhaled gas. Increasing fresh gas flow to greater than 5 liters per minute minimizes rebreathing.

○ **What factors may cause an elevated inspired CO_2?**

Rebreathing of CO_2 results in elevated inspired CO_2. Rebreathing may be caused by a depleted, faulty or bypassed carbon dioxide absorber, faulty unidirectional valves, and any cause of increased dead space. In a Mapleson circuit, significant rebreathing of CO_2 results from insufficient fresh gas flow. A hole in the inner tube of a coaxial circuit can allow significant rebreathing.

In some countries, anesthesia machines are equipped with CO_2 tanks and flowmeters. Delivery of CO_2 from such a tank, a misfilled tank, or an incorrect connection would cause the inspired CO_2 to be elevated.

○   What is the effect of a ventilator bellows leak?

In an anesthesia machine with an oxygen-powered ventilator, a leak in the bellows will allow oxygen to enter the breathing circuit and may raise the FiO_2. It may also cause barotrauma (high pressure driving gas can enter patient circuit), and even awareness by diluting anesthetic gases with high O_2.

○   What is the theoretical basis for infrared (IR) gas analysis?

Molecules containing at least two dissimilar atoms have unique IR absorption spectra. For this reason, IR analysis can be used for nitrous oxide and the halogenated agents, but not for oxygen as it does not absorb IR light.

○   What is the significance of plateau pressure during mechanical ventilation?

Plateau pressure is measured during a time of no gas flow (inspiratory pause) and reflects static compliance.

○   What is the significance of peak inspiratory pressure?

Peak inspiratory pressure is the highest pressure generated and reflects dynamic compliance. Increase in PIP (peak inspiratory pressure) without any change in PP (plateau pressure) Signals an increase in airway resistance (bronchospasm, secretions) or inspiratory gas flow rate. Increase in both PIP and PP implies an increase in tidal volume or decrease in pulmonary compliance (i.e. pulmonary edema, pleural effusion, tension pneumothorax, ascites).

○   What safety features does an anesthesia machine have to reduce the chance of delivering a hypoxic gas mixture?

Oxygen, nitrous oxide, and other anesthetic gases use the Pin Index Safety System to reduce the chance of connecting the wrong tank to a gas line. Line oxygen supply uses the Diameter Index Safety System for the same purpose. Tanks and lines are color coded. The fail-safe valve reduces or cuts off nitrous oxide flow in the event of decreased oxygen supply pressure. An oxygen supply failure alarm sounds when oxygen pressure falls below a certain level. The flowmeters are sequenced so that the oxygen meter is closest to the patient. This reduces the chances that a leak in one flowmeter will cause a hypoxic mixture. The oxygen flowmeter knob has a distinct feel compared with the other flowmeter knobs. Some machines have a minimum oxygen flow that can be delivered even if the O_2 flowmeter is off. Various methods are used to ensure at least a minimum oxygen ratio is delivered. O_2 ratio control monitor links N_2O flow to O_2 flow. Low pressure alarms signals leaks and disconnections.

An oxygen analyzer measures the FiO_2. Using oxygen as a driving gas to power the ventilator ensures that a bellows leak leads to increased rather than decreased FiO_2.

○   How is liquid oxygen stored?

Although banks of compressed gas cylinders or oxygen concentrators may be used for the hospitals central O_2 supply, storing O_2 as a liquid is more economical. It is stored in insulated tanks at or below its boiling point of 297˚C.

○   What is the significance of the "standard" sequencing of flowmeters?

The oxygen flowmeter is always positioned to the right, furthest downstream, and nearest the outlet of the common manifold. The reasoning is that if a leak develops from a crack in the glass tubing of the flowmeter, gas delivered upstream of the leak is lost before gas delivered downstream. This avoids the delivery of a potentially hypoxemic gas mixture.

○   **What causes the low O_2 pressure alarm to sound?**

Low O_2 pipeline pressure, a disconnected O_2 supply hose, or a depleted or closed tank will cause this alarm to sound. This is an oxygen fail safe valve and anything upstream of the flow meter causing low O_2 pressure will be detected by this system (except in the case of cross over in pipeline system).

○   **Describe the function of a temperature compensated variable bypass vaporizer.**

The variable bypass vaporizer divides incoming gas into two streams. First, 20% or less of the gas goes through the vaporizing chamber and becomes saturated with agent. The reamining portion of gas flow goes through the bypass chamber. Finally, The two streams are combined to make the output of the vaporizer. Both the bimetallic strip (temperature compensation device) and the concentration dial are situated in the bypass channel and compensate for temperature changes and desired final concentration.

○   **Describe the function of a desflurane (Tec6) vaporizer.**

Tec 6 vaporizer is an electrically heated, pressurized,electro-mechanically coupled, dual-circuit, constant-temperature, gas-vapor blender. None of the fresh gas passes through the vaporization chamber. Rather, desflurane is heated to 39°C (well above its boiling point) and creates a source of pure desflurane vapor. This vapor is blended with the fresh gas to create the vaporizer output. The vaporizer has an electronic display that indicates an initial warm-up period with an amber LED and when the operating temperature reached is a green LED is lit. A red LED flashes and an audible alarm sounds if the vaporizer cannot deliver vapor. There is an LCD desflurane liquid level meter.

○   **What significance is the anesthetic vapor pressure?**

Anesthetic vapor pressure determines the concentration of anesthetic vapor coming out of the vaporizing chamber of a variable-bypass vaporizer. Filling a vaporizer with an anesthetic agent with a lower vapor pressure than the agent it was meant to be used with will cause a lower concentration than is selected on the dial to be delivered. Filling a vaporizer with an anesthetic agent with a higher vapor pressure than the agent it was meant to be used with will cause a higher concentration than is selected on the dial to be delivered.

○   **Of what significance is desiccation of CO_2 absorbent?**

Desiccated absorbent makes the formation of compound A from sevoflurane more likely. It also increases the heat produced and the use of sevoflurane with desiccated absorbent has been associated with fires. Desflurane is degraded into potentially significant amounts of carbon monoxide by desiccated CO_2 absorbent.

○   **What triggers the ventilator to deliver a breath in pressure support ventilation?**

Patient inspiratory effort. The ventilator delivers the gas flow required to maintain a selected positive pressure during inspiration.

ACID BASE, FLUIDS AND ELECTROLYTES

For A Long Time It Seemed To Me That Life Was About To Begin-Real Life. But There Was Always Some Obstacle In The Way, Something To Be Gotten Through First, Some Unfinished Business, Time Still To Be Served, A Debt To Be Paid. At Last It Dawned On Me That These Obstacles Were My Life. This Perspective Has Helped Me To See There Is No Way To Happiness. Happiness Is The Way. So Treasure Every Moment You Have And Remember That Time Waits For No One. Happiness Is A Journey, Not A Destination.
Souza

○   **What causes a right shift in the oxygen hemoglobin dissociation curve?**

A right shift in the oxygen hemoglobin dissociation curve means oxygen is more easily released from hemoglobin to tissues (increase P_{50}). Some causes include: acidosis, increased carbon dioxide, increased temperature and increased 2,3-DPG.

○   **What causes a left shift in the oxygen hemoglobin dissociation curve?**

A left shift means oxygen is less easily released to tissues. Some causes include: alkalosis, decreased temperature, decreased 2,3-DPG and abnormal forms of hemoglobin (fetal hemoglobin, methemoglobin, carboxyhemoglobin and hemoglobin S).

○   **What acid base disturbance is seen in severe pyloric stenosis?**

Hyponatremic, hypokalemic and hypochloremic metabolic alkalosis.

○   **What happens to the $PaCO_2$ and the PaO_2 in a patient with a high fever?**

In general, increases in temperature will cause the $PaCO_2$ and PaO_2 to increase. As the temperature of a solution increases, more molecules will enter the gas phase, the partial pressure of each gas thus increasing. Gas solubility is inversely proportional to temperature.

○   **What are two common and clinically relevant causes of metabolic alkalosis?**

Loss of gastric fluid (vomiting and nasogastric suctioning) and loss of acidic urine secondary to diuretic therapy (thiazides, furosemide and ethacrynic acid). Both are associated with NaCl deficiency and extracellular fluid depletion, and are often described as chloride-sensitive.

○   **What is the acute respiratory compensatory response to metabolic alkalosis?**

Reflex alveolar hypoventilation. $PaCO_2$ increases 0.4-0.9 per mEq increase in bicarbonate. Eventually, the kidneys will tend to excrete more bicarbonate (chronic compensatory response).

○   **What happens to the PaO_2 and $PaCO_2$ in an arterial blood gas sample that has an air bubble trapped in the syringe?**

In general, the blood values move to equilibrate with the air bubble values. This means blood PaO_2 will tend to move towards 150mm Hg (value in air at atmospheric pressure), increasing or decreasing to achieve that. The $PaCO_2$ will tend to decrease moving towards 0. Air has negligible CO_2 and the typical blood gas sample has some value higher than this for $PaCO_2$, so with equilibration the $PaCO_2$ in the sample will tend to decrease.

○   **What information is necessary for the accurate interpretation of a blood gas sample?**

Source (arterial versus venous), temperature of the sample (body, room or room air temperature or stored on ice), ventilator settings, the FiO_2 at which the sample was drawn and age of the patient. Also, consider when the sample was drawn.

○   **Where must you sample blood to measure mixed venous oxygen saturation?**

Pulmonary artery. A true mixed venous blood sample measures venous drainage from the inferior vena cava, superior vena cava and heart.

○   **Why is mixed venous oxygen sampling so important?**

It represents the overall balance between oxygen consumption and oxygen delivery and therefore provides a critical assessment of tissue oxygen metabolism.

○   **What is the normal mixed venous oxygen tension ($P\bar{v}O_2$) and saturation?**

Normal mixed venous oxygen tension ($P\bar{v}CO_2$) is 35-45 mm Hg, corresponding to a mixed venous oxygen saturation of 65-75%. It is higher under general anesthesia.

○   **What factors determine mixed venous oxygen?**

Oxygen delivery (cardiac output, hemoglobin concentration, saturation and a very minor component of dissolved plasma oxygen determined by FiO_2) minus oxygen consumption (temperature and activity).

○   **What factors cause a low mixed venous oxygen?**

Increased oxygen consumption and decreased O_2 delivery (hypoxia, low cardiac output and decreased hemoglobin concentration). Lowering of hemoglobin saturation and a right shift of the oxygen hemoglobin dissociation curve will also tend to decrease mixed venous oxygen tension.

○   **What causes a high mixed venous oxygen?**

Increased cardiac output, decreased oxygen consumption (hypothermia), impaired tissue uptake (cyanide poisoning), or a severe left shift of the oxygen hemoglobin dissociation curve all cause increased mixed venous oxygen saturation. A sampling error from a wedged PA catheter, left-to-right intracardiac shunt or sepsis should be considered.

○   **What effect does alkalosis have on serum potassium, serum calcium and shifting of the oxygen hemoglobin dissociation curve?**

Alkalosis causes a decrease in serum potassium and ionized calcium and a left shift in the oxygen hemoglobin dissociation curve.

○   **How does acetazolamide work in ophthalmology?**

It inhibits carbonic anhydrase, an enzyme important in aqueous humor synthesis in the ciliary processes. As such, it decreases the production of aqueous humor and lowers the intraocular pressure.

○   **What effect does acetazolamide have on acid base status?**

It causes a mild hyperchloremic metabolic acidosis. Acetazolamide causes alkalinization of urine by significantly interfering with hydrogen ion secretion in the proximal tubule and impairing bicarbonate reabsorption. In exchange for this filtered bicarbonate, more chloride is absorbed in the kidney. Because of this, acetazolamide results in diuresis of alkaline urine, causing hyperchloremic metabolic acidosis.

○   **How does apnea affect $PaCO_2$?**

$PaCO_2$ increases by 6 mm Hg in the first minute of apnea and then increases by 3 mm Hg for each minute thereafter.

○   **What happens to PaO_2 and $PaCO_2$ as the dead space to tidal volume ratio increases?**

Remember dead space areas are ventilated but not perfused. As dead space increases, PaO_2 falls and $PaCO_2$ rises.

○   **What fetal scalp blood gas values indicate that the fetus is in trouble?**

In general, there will be a low pH and a low PaO_2 with high $PaCO_2$ for the fetus. Considering the normal fetal scalp blood gas values, you could expect a pH less than 7.20, a PaO_2 less than 25 and $PaCO_2$ greater than 60 mm Hg, in a troubled fetus.

○   **What is the normal $A\text{-}aDO_2$ gradient?**

The normal alveolar-arterial oxygen gradient is < 20 mm Hg, for patients less than 50 years of age breathing room air.

○   **What is the most common cause of a widened A-a gradient for oxygen?**

Right-to-left shunt.

○   **At what level of shunt fraction does oxygen administration cease to be of value in raising the PaO_2?**

If the shunt is 30% or greater. If the shunt fraction is in the range of 10-20%, oxygen administration may raise the PaO_2.

○   **What are causes of shunt?**

Right to left intracardiac shunt (absolute shunt where V/Q=0), pneumonia, bronchospasm, and pneumothorax (relative shunt in an area of lung with low V/Q). V/Q = ventilation/perfusion ratio.

○   **Given that TBW (total body water) is about 60% of body weight, what percentage of body weight is intracellular, extracellular, interstitial and intravascular?**

Intracellular water is 35% of body weight.
Extracellular water is 22 to 25% of body weight, with interstitial water about 15-18% of body weight.
Intravascular volume is about 7% of body weight.

○   **What effect does mannitol have on serum sodium concentration?**

Acutely, mannitol causes transient hyponatremia due to acute hemodilution. Mannitol is then filtered at the glomerulus but not reabsorbed creating an osmotic gradient into tubules promoting excretion of water in excess of sodium. If fluid and electrolyte losses are not replaced, hypernatremia and hypovolemia result.

○   **What acid base abnormality does spironolactone cause?**

Metabolic acidosis and hyperkalemia.

O   **What acid base abnormality do both thiazide-type diuretics and furosemide cause?**

Metabolic acidosis and hypokalemia.

O   **Metabolic alkalosis is frequently associated with what volume status change?**

Hypovolemia from marked loss of sodium.

O   **Should total body water estimates be increased or decreased in obese patients?**

Decreased by 20-30% on a per kg basis. Estimates are lower as a result of decreased lean body mass.

O   **Extracellular and intracellular fluid volumes comprise what percentage of total body water?**

ECF = 34-40%.
ICF = 60-66%.

O   **Describe the EKG changes frequently associated with hyperkalemia and hypokalemia.**

Hyperkalemia: peaked T waves to widened QRS and PR intervals, flattened P waves, loss of R waves and deep S waves progressing to ventricular fibrillation or asystole.
Hypokalemia: flattened T wave, prominent U wave, increased P wave amplitude, prolongation PR interval, ST depression, cardiac arrhythmia in the presence of digitalis toxicity and AV block.

O   **A patient admitted after one week of persistent vomiting from gastric outlet obstruction is expected to have what acid base disturbance?**

Hypokalemic, hypochloremic metabolic alkalosis. Loss of gastric secretions results in ECF depletion and avid sodium reabsorption by the kidney. Ionic neutrality is maintained by hydrogen secretion and reabsorption of bicarbonate in the face of insufficient chloride availability.

O   **What is the most common underlying disorder in respiratory acidosis?**

Alveolar hypoventilation.

O   **Compensation for persistent hypoventilation occurs by what mechanism?**

The respiratory acidosis caused by hypoventilation is compensated fully by reabsorption of bicarbonate in the kidney, causing a metabolic alkalosis.

O   **What is the emergent treatment for severe hyperkalemia?**

1. Promote cellular uptake (insulin 10 to 20 units and glucose 30 to 50 g; hyperventilation; sodium bicarbonate).
2. Treat hypotension (10% calcium chloride or calcium gluconate; epinephrine infusion)
3. Increase elimination (diuresis with furosemide; cation exchange resin with Kayexalate; dialysis).

Therapeutic goals are to lower serum potassium concentration, correct hypotension and prevent arrhythmia.

O   **In the surgical patient, metabolic acidosis is frequently caused by circulatory failure and accumulation of lactic acid. What is the appropriate treatment?**

Adequate tissue perfusion and oxygenation. Volume resuscitation with fluid or blood and maintenance of cardiac output should be the initial therapy. If the arterial pH is less than 7.20, increasing controlled ventilation and administration of sodium bicarbonate to pH = 7.20 to 7.30 may be necessary. Impairment of liver function will compound the metabolic acidosis secondary to failure to metabolize lactate to bicarbonate.

○   **Describe the EKG abnormalities associated with hypercalcemia and hypocalcemia.**

Hypercalcemia: shortened Q-T interval (shortened ST segment)
Hypocalcemia: prolonged Q-T interval (prolongation of ST segment)

○   **Describe the medical therapy for severe hypercalcemia.**

Maximize renal calcium excretion with normal saline infusion containing 20-30 mEq/L K^+ and furosemide to promote a diuresis of 200-300 cc/hr. Careful monitoring of potassium and magnesium are required. Additional therapy options include pamidronate, calcitonin, steroids, mithramycin or dialysis.

○   **Describe the clinical manifestations of hyponatremia.**

Serious symptoms of hyponatremia seen at $Na^+ < 125$ meq/L are mainly CNS-related secondary to cellular water intoxication. Symptoms include weakness, fatigue, muscle cramps, confusion, anorexia, nausea, vomiting, headache, delirium, seizures and coma. Coma and seizures are frequently seen below Na+ levels <115 mEq/L. Hyponatremia with increased intravascular volume can cause pulmonary edema, hypertension and congestive heart failure, especially at $Na^+ < 100$ meq/L. Chronic changes are partially compensated; acute changes are much more dramatic.

○   **Describe the consequences of excessively rapid sodium replacement in hyponatremia.**

Central pontine myelinolysis consisting of quadriplegia, dysarthria and dysphasia. In general, one should not replete the sodium much faster than it was lost.

○   **Urine sodium levels below what value may distinguish extrarenal from renal sodium losses contributing to hyponatremia?**

Urinary sodium concentration less than 20 mEq/L imply extrarenal sodium loss.

○   **Diabetes insipidus (DI) implies what tonicity of urine and plasma (hyper or hypotonic)?**

DI is characterized by dilute urine with hypertonic plasma osmolality. This condition may be caused by decreased synthesis or secretion of ADH (central DI) or renal organ unresponsiveness (nephrogenic DI).

○   **A diagnosis of diabetes insipidus may be confirmed by what test?**

Failure of urine osmolality to increase more than 30 mOsm/L in the first hours of complete fluid restriction is diagnostic with confirmation by increased plasma ADH levels. Aqueous vasopressin will test the responsiveness of renal tubules.

○   **Characterize urine sodium level and plasma osmolality in SIADH.**

SIADH features elevated urinary sodium (>20 mEq/L) with hypotonic plasma (< 270-280 mOsm/L) and low serum sodium <130 mEq/L.

○   **Would a patient with metabolic alkalosis be expected to have hyper- or hypokalemia?**

Hypokalemia. Metabolic alkalosis promotes transcellular shift of potassium into the cells in exchange for hydrogen ions. Alkalosis also promotes potassium excretion in the distal convoluted tubule.

○   **What is the major cause of extrarenal potassium depletion?**

Decreased potassium levels are always either renal or gastrointestinal. The most common cause of renal potassium depletion is related to diuretic therapy or enhanced mineralocorticoid activity. GI losses are secondary to vomiting, nasogastric suctioning or diarrhea.

O   **What is carcinoid crisis?**

A stress-induced condition exacerbating carcinoid syndrome (enterochromaffin tumor secreting vasoactive substances ie: serotonin, kallikrein, histamine) in which there are markedly increased serotonin levels with pronounced symptoms. Requires urgent pharmacological control with octreotide, invasive monitoring and hemodynamic support.

O   **What is the sodium concentration of the following frequently used intravenous fluids?**

Normal saline (0.9% NS) – 154 mEq/L
Half normal saline (0.45% NS) - 77 mEq/L
3% saline – 513 mEq/L
Lactated Ringers (LR) – 130 mEq/L
5% dextrose (D5W) – 0

O   **How is plasma osmolality calculated?**

Plasma osmolality (mOsm/kg) = Na^+ (mEq/L) x 2 + glucose (mg/dL)/18 + BUN (mg/dL)/2.8 + any solute (mg/dL)/(molecular weight of the solute/10).

O   **What is the relationship between serum sodium concentration and water balance?**

Generally, due to renal mechanisms: hypernatremia means "too little free water" rather than "too much sodium"; hyponatremia means "too much free water" rather than "too little sodium."

O   **How is plasma sodium concentration interpreted in the presence of hyperglycemia?**

High glucose concentration draws water out of cells and dilutes sodium in plasma. For every 100 mg/dL of glucose above 200 mg/dL, serum sodium is decreased by 1.8 mEq/L.

O   **What is "pseudohyponatremia?"**

Pseudohyponatremia, also called isotonic hyponatremia, is a laboratory artifact in the presence of severe hyperproteinemia or hyperlipidemia. Plasma sodium concentration is normal. Dilution of the measurement sample produces an artificially low sodium measurement by flame photometry. Hyperosmolality resulting from non-sodium molecules (glucose, mannitol) results in water shifting from the intracellular space to dilute the extracellular sodium concentration.

O   **What are frequent causes of SIADH?**

1. Malignancies producing ADH-like compounds.
2. Pulmonary disease (tumor, tuberculosis, pneumonia and asthma).
3. CNS disorders (meningitis, tremor, tumors, subarachnoid hemorrhage, and acute intracranial hypertension).
4. Drugs (chlorpropamide, oxytocin, vincristine, cytoxan, nicotine, narcotics, clofibrate, vinblastine, cyclophosphamide).
5. Pain in the postoperative period.
6. Hypothyroidism.
7. Adrenal insufficiency.

O   **What findings are diagnostic of Diabetes Insipidus?**

Large volumes (usually greater than 3 L/day) of dilute urine (osmolality <300 mOsm/L; specific gravity <1.010) and hypernatremia.

○   **How is Diabetes Insipidus treated?**

Aqueous pitressin 5-10 units q 4-6 hourly intravenously or DDAVP 10-20 units q 12-24 hourly intranasally. Chronic therapy with chlorpropamide (stimulates ADH release) and thiazide diuretics have been used successfully.

○   **How fast should hyponatremia be corrected?**

No faster than 0.5-1.0 mEq of Na^+/L/hour using normal saline in patients with decreased total body sodium content. Initial goal is to correct the plasma sodium to 130 mEq/L. Water restriction is the treatment in hyponatremic patients with normal or increased total body sodium. If the patient is symptomatic (coma, seizures) the sodium level is corrected with a combination of hypertonic saline 3%, fluid restriction, and/or furosemide, until symptoms resolve, then slowly thereafter.

○   **If hypertonic saline 3% is used for correction of hyponatremia, how is the replacement volume calculated?**

Na^+ deficit = total body weight x (desired $[Na^+]$ - present $[Na^+]$)

Total body water = weight (kg) X 0.60 (for women replace 0.60, with 0.50))
Salt replacement = (130 – actual serum sodium) x total body water
Volume of hypertonic saline (L) = salt replacement / sodium content of 3% saline

Sodium content of 3% saline is 513 mEq/L.
For the calculation of salt replacement 130 mEq/L or the lowest serum sodium level reached until the patient becomes asymptomatic may be used. Goal rate of correction = 0.6 to 1 mEq/L/hr to a sodium concentration of 130 mEq/L. Half the deficit should be replaced over the first 8 hours and the remainder over 1-3 days, if symptoms remit.

○   **How is urine osmolality calculated?**

Urine osmolality (mOsm/kg) = 2 x (urinary sodium-mEq/L + urinary potassium-mEq/L) + urine urea nitrogen-mg/dL / 2.8.

○   **Loss of free water may cause hypernatremia. What are normal insensible losses? How does temperature effect insensible losses?**

Insensible loss averages 700 cc/day of a total 2300cc daily loss of water. High temperature increases water loss as sweat - 100 cc to 1400 cc. Other insensible losses remain unchanged.

○   **What is the osmolality of sodium bicarbonate ($NaHCO_3$)?**

One ampule (50 mL) contains 50 mEq of sodium and 50 mEq of HCO_3. Sodium bicarbonate is hypertonic, about 1800 mOsm/L.

○   **What tests indicate that the kidney is conserving sodium?**

1.   Urine sodium (< 20 mEq/L).
2.   Fractional excretion of Na^+ < 1% of creatinine clearance.

○   **What is normal plasma osmolality?**

Normal plasma osmolality is 280-295 mOsm/kg.

○ **What are symptoms of hypernatremia?**

Dehydration of brain cells causes lethargy or mental status changes proceeding to coma, seizures and death. Acute and severe hypernatremia may precipitate intracranial hemorrhage. Additional signs and symptoms include thirst, shock, myoclonus, muscle tremor, rigidity and increased intravascular fluid volume, peripheral edema or pleural effusion.

○ **What are the major causes of hypernatremia?**

Diabetes insipidus (central and nephrogenic)
Insensible losses (burns, sweating)
Osmotic diuresis (mannitol, hyperglycemia)
Hypertonic fluid administration

○ **What is the mechanism by which hypovolemia results in metabolic alkalosis?**

The kidney will reabsorb sodium and secrete potassium and hydrogen ions (to restore extracellular fluid volume). This process is under the influence of aldosterone. Hypokalemia will augment hydrogen ion secretion and bicarbonate reabsorption, maintaining the metabolic alkalosis.

○ **What are the clinical manifestations of hyperkalemia?**

Hyperkalemia partially depolarizes the cell membrane. Patients present with weakness that may progress to flaccid paralysis and hypoventilation.

○ **What are the clinical manifestations of hypokalemia?**

Symptoms usually occur at potassium concentrations below 3.0 mEq/L. They include mental status changes, fatigue, muscle weakness and myalgias, hypoventilation (respiratory muscle weakness) and eventually complete paralysis. Smooth muscles may also be affected and present as paralytic ileus. Cardiovascular effects include dysrhythmias, hypotension and myocardial dysfunction.

○ **How do changes in pH affect serum potassium?**

Plasma potassium concentration changes 0.6 mEq/L per 0.1 change in arterial pH (range 0.2 – 1.2 mEq/L per 0.1 unit change). During alkalosis, plasma potassium concentration decreases. During acidosis, plasma potassium concentration increases.

○ **What factors produce intercompartmental shifts of potassium?**

Extracellular pH, insulin, catecholamines, plasma osmolality and possibly hypothermia.

○ **List medications that might cause hyperkalemia.**

1. Error, due to sample lysis
2. Internal potassium balance (intracellular shift) succinylcholine, digitalis, nonselective beta-blockers, antibiotics
   • External potassium balance (decreased renal excretion)
3. Non-steroidal anti-inflammatory drugs: impair renin and aldosterone secretion
   • Angiotensin converting enzyme inhibitors: block angiotensin II mediated aldosterone biosynthesis
   • Heparin: inhibits adrenal steroidogenesis
   • Spironolactone: blocks renal mineralocorticoid receptor
   • Triamterene, amiloride: aldosterone-independent defects in tubular potassium secretion

○ **How does magnesium depletion affect potassium?**

Magnesium depletion is associated with renal potassium wasting and hypocalcemia.

○   **How would you estimate the deficit in total body potassium in a patient with plasma potassium of 3 mEq/L? Or 2 mEq/L?**

A decrease in serum potassium from 4 to 3 mEq/L corresponds to a 100-200 mEq decrement in total body potassium in a normal adult. Each additional fall of 1 mEq/L in serum potassium represents an additional deficit of 200-400 mEq.

○   **What is the effect of non-depolarizing neuromuscular blocking agents on plasma potassium concentration?**

Non-depolarizing muscular blocking agents do not affect plasma potassium levels. However, when succinylcholine depolarizes muscle that has been previously traumatized or denervated, myoneural receptors proliferate over the cell membrane, and a depolarizing drug binding to the increased numbers of receptors can produce large increases in serum potassium. This can cause life-threatening arrhythmias and cardiac arrest.

○   **What are the options for handling total parenteral nutrition (TPN) during the intraoperative period?**

Continue the TPN as ordered, or replace TPN by 10% dextrose for the perioperative period. This prevents rebound hypoglycemia.

○   **During prolonged surgery, what laboratory tests should be monitored when a patient is receiving total parenteral nutrition (TPN)?**

Plasma glucose, potassium and pH.

○   **What are the factors affecting blood oxygen content?**

The amount of oxygen in blood depends mainly on the hemoglobin concentration (Hb) and hemoglobin saturation (SaO_2) at a given PaO_2, with a small contribution from dissolved O_2.

Oxygen content = CaO_2 = (Hb X SaO_2 X 1.34 mL/dL blood) + (0.003 mL O_2/dL blood/mm Hg) x PaO_2.

○   **How much oxygen is dissolved in blood and under what conditions is this significant?**

Only 0.003 ml of O_2 per mmHg PO_2 is dissolved in a 100 cc of plasma. At normal levels of hemoglobin this contribution is insignificant, but this situation changes in severely anemic patients. In a patient with Hg of 5.0 g/dL placed on supplemental O_2 with a PO_2 of 500 mmHg, 1.5 ml of O_2 is dissolved in each deciliter, accounting for 18 % of total oxygen content (normal 1.4-1.9%).

○   **What ABG results would you expect to see in acute respiratory acidosis?**

In respiratory disorders, pH and $PaCO_2$ are inversely related. The pH decreases 0.08 for each 10 mm Hg increase in PCO_2. In the acute stage, bicarbonate would increase in compensation only 1 mEq/ L for each 10 mm Hg increase in PCO_2.

○   **What is the blood: gas partition coefficient for a volatile anesthetic?**

The blood:gas partition coefficient describes the relative solubility of a volatile anesthetic agent in blood and air. For example: enflurane has a partition coefficient of 1.9 which means that at equilibrium there will be 1.9 times the concentration of inhaled agent in blood than in the gaseous (alveolar) phase.

○   **What are the differences between crystalloid and colloid solutions?**

Crystalloids are fluids that contain water and electrolytes which are grouped as balanced, hypertonic or hypotonic solutions. Colloids contain a high molecular weight solute (albumin or starch) that will not pass through an intact capillary membrane thus generating a colloid osmotic pressure (COP). Colloid solutions are 1:1 volume expanders, whereas the replacement requirement for crystalloids is 3- or 4-fold the volume of blood lost because crystalloid is distributed in a ratio 1:4 like extracellular fluid, leaving only 20% in the IV space.

The most common crystalloid solutions are normal saline, lactated Ringer solution, Normosol and Plasmalyte. The most common colloids are 5% and 25 % albumin, 6% hetastarch (Hextend or Hespan), pentastarch, and dextrans in 6% and 10% concentrations.

The choice of colloid or crystalloid for fluid resuscitation has been a contentious issue and is based on differences in price, availability, in-vivo capillary permeability (risk of pulmonary edema), and the possibility of adverse effects: coagulation disorders, nephrotoxicity, hyperchloremic metabolic acidosis, postoperative nausea and vomiting, incidence of mortality and allergic reactions.

○ **What is the oxygen-hemoglobin dissociation curve and P_{50}?**

The $Hb-O_2$ dissociation curve is the sigmoidal relationship of the partial pressure of oxygen and the saturation of hemoglobin. The P_{50} (26 mm Hg under normal physiological conditions) is the PO_2 that yields a hemoglobin saturation of 50% and defines the affinity of hemoglobin for oxygen.

○ **What is the effect of temperature on blood gas analysis?**

The PO_2 measurement performed with a blood gas electrode at 37 °C gives an overestimate if the patient is hypothermic and underestimate if the patient is febrile. The percentage of error is greatest for venous values (PO_2 values < 100 mm Hg) and if the patient's temperature is 20 °C. Conventionally, blood gas analysis is done at 37 °C. Warming a blood gas sample will decrease gas solubility (PO_2 and PCO_2) and elevate blood gas tension. The reverse is true for cooling a blood sample. Several algorithms exist for temperature correction (to the patient's temperature), such that the true partial pressure can be calculated. In hypothermic patients, the pH should be maintained close to 7.4, which would keep the corrected pH in the alkalotic range.

○ **What are the effects of infusion of lactated Ringer (LR) solution?**

LR is a balanced salt solution with electrolyte composition similar to extracellular fluid: Na 131 mmol/L, Cl 111 mmol/L, K 4-5 mmol/L, Ca 2 mmol/L, lactate 29 mmol/mL, 278 mOsmol/L, pH 6.5. Ringer's solution was developed by Sydney Ringer in 1880. In the 1930s Alexis Hartmann added lactate to act as a buffer, which hydrates to carbonic acid and finally CO_2. Lactated Ringer solution contains calcium and in a 1:1 ratio will clot blood at room temperature and 37 °C. LR is used to provide maintenance water and electrolytes and for IV resuscitation.

○ **What causes the metabolic acidosis seen with large volume IV infusion of normal saline?**

Saline solutions are non-physiologic due to: the level of chloride significantly greater than plasma (154 mmol, as compared to 98-102 mmol), lack of potassium, calcium and magnesium that are present in normal plasma, and the lack of bicarbonate buffer. The mechanism for the acid-base disturbance has been described as a "dilutional hyperchloremic acidosis" (plasma expansion and dilutional reduction of bicarbonate) or more recently Stewart's physicochemical theory where hyperchloremia reduces the strong-ion difference leading to acidosis through dissociation of water to maintain electrochemical neutrality.

The strong ion difference (SID) is the net charge balance of all strong cations (Na, K, Ca and Mg) and strong anions (Cl and lactate). The normal SID is 40-49 mEq/L. SID determines (along with CO_2 and weak acids) what the plasma hydrogen ion concentration will be. The electrochemical forces generating the SID determine water dissociation, and therefore the hydrogen ion concentration required to balance plasma ionic charges. The net result always has to be a plasma ionic charge equal to zero (electrochemical neutrality). An increase in plasma chloride ion concentration will result in a decrease in SID, leading to an increased hydrogen ion concentration, and acidosis.

○   **What are the possible adverse effects of hyperchloremia following normal saline infusion?**

Metabolic acidosis, derangement in coagulation and increased bleeding, renal vasoconstriction with a decrease in glomerular filtration rate and renal blood flow, and increased postoperative nausea and vomiting (gut hypoperfusion or splanchnic vasoconstriction).

○   **How do changes in the hematocrit affect oxygen transport?**

Total oxygen delivery is the product of arterial oxygen content and cardiac output: $DO_2 = CaO_2 \times CO$. The arterial oxygen content is dependent on P_AO_2 and hemoglobin concentration. Deficiencies in oxygen delivery may be due to a low P_AO_2 (V/Q mismatch, impaired diffusion of O_2 into blood), a low hemoglobin concentration, or reduced cardiac output (including distribution of blood to tissues and O_2 extraction). In patients with chronic severe anemia compensatory mechanisms to increase oxygen delivery include: increase in cardiac output (increase in heart rate and reduction in blood viscosity) and increased extraction (resulting in a lower mixed venous oxygen saturation).

○   **What are indicators of inadequate oxygen delivery to tissues?**

Although total oxygen delivery (DO_2) and oxygen uptake (VO_2) can be directly measured, they cannot be measured at the tissue or cellular level. Inadequate oxygen delivery to tissues produces hypoperfusion, ischemia and evidence of anaerobic metabolism. Clinical indicators are hypotension, decreased urine output and altered mental status, which are non-specific and late developing. Laboratory indicators include acidosis, worsening base deficit, anion gap and lactate levels. Gastric tonometry (measuring CO_2/pH) can be used as a measure of oxygen debt in the splanchnic circulation. The tongue has also been used as a site of measurement where elevations in sublingual CO_2 represent potential hypoperfusion.

○   **What acid-base disturbance would you expect to find in COPD?**

It will depend on whether the primary problem is bronchitis (blue bloater) or emphysema (pink puffer). Bronchitic patients have severely deranged matching of ventilation and perfusion which results in severe hypoxemia and hypercarbia. Under stable conditions the body will adjust to this respiratory acidosis with a compensatory metabolic alkalosis. The pH would decrease by 0.03 for each 10 mm Hg increase in PCO_2 due to the compensatory increase of serum bicarbonate by 3.5 mEq/L. Emphysematous patients are better able to maintain V/Q matching as lung tissue and vasculature are equally destroyed. ABG's typically show mild hypoxemia and minimal CO_2 retention, as patients are able to maintain a normal CO_2 by increasing their minute ventilation. As the disease progresses CO_2 will be retained and the ABG's will resemble those of a bronchitic patient.

○   **What is the effect of carboxyhemoglobin (HbCO) on ABG analysis and pulse oximeter reading?**

HbCO affects the O_2 saturation (true measured SaO_2 value) and O_2 content, but not PaO_2. The pH may be normal. Hypoxemia can be missed if the O_2 saturation is calculated in the laboratory based on the PaO_2 and standard O_2 dissociation curve. Pulse oximeters are not reliable. The oxygen saturation is read as *too high* as they do not differentiate hemoglobin bound to carbon monoxide from hemoglobin bound to oxygen; the machine reports oxygen saturation as the sum of both values. Blood co-oximeters use four wavelengths of light to separate out oxyhemoglobin from reduced Hb, metHb and HbCO, whereas pulse oximeters utilize only two wavelengths of light that do not detect hemoglobins that cannot bind oxygen.

○   **What are typical umbilical artery blood gases?**

In the fetus, the umbilical artery (UA) is traveling to the placenta. It therefore carries with it the metabolic waste products of the fetus. Hence, it has low PaO_2, SpO_2, and pH values, and high $PaCO_2$ values.

Conversely, the umbilical vein (UV) is returning blood from the placenta. It therefore has higher values for PO_2, SpO_2, and pH, and low values for pCO_2. See the table below.

	PO2	PCO2	SpO2	pH
UA	12-18	48-54	28%	7.24-7.29
UV	26-32	38-42	70%	7.30-7.35

PHYSICS, MATHEMATICS, AND ANESTHESIA

Get Your Facts First And Then You Can Distort Them As Much As You Wish.
Mark Twain

○ **Administration of 66% nitrous will increase a nitrogen filled space by how much?**

The space will increase in volume or pressure until equilibrium is achieved.
The maximum change in volume (%) = nitrous oxide in alveoli (%)/ (1- fractional % of nitrous oxide); 66% nitrous oxide increases volume in a compliant space by 200%.
Another way of saying the same thing: the total volume is 3 fold higher, and the formula for final volume is initial volume x 1/(1-Nitrous oxide %).

○ **What would happen if you filled an isoflurane vaporizer with halothane?**

Since the saturated vapor pressures (at 20°C) of halothane and isoflurane are almost the same, 243 mm Hg and 238 mm Hg respectively, the volume % outputs are almost the same. However, since halothane is more potent, a higher MAC value is being administered to the patient at the same % delivered.

○ **What does a line isolation monitor protect against?**

Macroshock hazards from undetected short circuits. The warning alarm sounds when the leakage current from a device is greater than 2 mA.

○ **What determines the difference between microshock and macroshock?**

Macroshock is 60-Hz current in excess of 1 mA (threshold of perception) which is applied to tissue at locations remote from the heart, whereas microshock refers to the application of small currents (100 ∫A will induce ventricular fibrillation) directly to the heart.

○ **What prevents a positive pressure check from detecting a leak in some anesthesia machines?**

A check valve, installed to prevent the pumping effect in vaporizers, also prevents back pressure from detecting a leak.

○ **What is the pressure at the O_2 flush valve?**

When the O_2 flush valve is activated, oxygen bypasses the flowmeters and vaporizers, and is delivered directly to the common gas outlet at 35 to 75 L/min at a line pressure of 45-55 psig.

○ **Where is the dead space in a properly functioning circle system?**

The dead space in a circle system with functioning unidirectional valves is limited to the area distal to the point of inspiratory and expiratory gas mixing at the Y-piece. The breathing-tube length of a circle system does not directly affect dead space.

○ **How can soda lime exhaustion be detected?**

A pH-sensitive dye (usually ethyl violet) added to the granules will change color (from white to purple) in the presence of carbonic acid. Dye indicator mimosa 2 will change from pink to white when the absorbent is exhausted. Additionally, baseline CO_2 on the capnogram will increase above zero if rebreathing occurs in the presence of exhausted soda lime.

O   Which is greater, the rate of rise of Fa/Fi for nitrous oxide or desflurane?

Fa/Fi is greater for nitrous oxide because of the concentration effect, although they both have nearly the same blood/gas partition coefficient.

O   Which patients are susceptible to microshock hazards?

Any patient having a low resistance pathway to the heart is at risk for microshock (pacing wire, saline filled central venous catheter or right ventricular ejection fraction pulmonary artery catheter).

Currents as low at 100 microamps can cause ventricular fibrillation. The source for such tiny currents can be the "leakage current" associated with any AC powered device. Recommended maximum allowable 60-Hz leakage current is 10 microamps.

O   What are the unique features of the desflurane vaporizer?

Desflurane has an extremely high vapor pressure (664 mm Hg at 20 °C) and low boiling point (23.5°C). Therefore a conventional vaporizer will not work. Several solutions to the problem have been applied (cooling the vaporizer, using liquid injection), but the Ohmeda Tec 6 vaporizer uses a heated sump. Unlike other vaporizers, it has a power supply which actively heats the liquid agent to 39°C. In addition, no fresh gas enters the vaporizing chamber, and it uses a special filling cap (desflurane boils at room temperature, so the bottle and vaporizer interlock to prevent the loss of agent while filling). Finally, there are electronic alarms for low agent level, no agent output and low battery.

O   Why are flowmeters (rotameters) not interchangeable?

Flowmeters are calibrated for specific gases. Flow rate across a constriction depends upon the gas's viscosity at low laminar flows and its density at high turbulent flows. Therefore, gases with similar viscosity (oxygen and helium) may read identically at low flows, while gases with similar densities (nitrous oxide and carbon dioxide) will read the same at high flows. Nitrous and oxygen rotameters would not read the same, having different density and viscosity.

O   How can you prevent a hypoxic gas mixture from being delivered to the patient, as determined by gas flowmeters settings?

There are two systems in use in U.S. anesthesia machines. Ohmeda machines use a Link-25 proportioning system which is a mechanical interlink. Dräger machines use a combined pneumatic and mechanical system (oxygen ratio monitor controller) which makes it impossible to deliver more than 75% N_2O, relative to the flow of oxygen. The alarm is disabled when the "all gases" mode switch is selected, which allows the addition of a third gas.

O   What factors alter delivered tidal volume on anesthesia ventilators?

Most anesthesia ventilators are volume preset ventilators. In a circle system, fresh gas flows continuously into the inspiratory limb of the breathing circuit. This additional volume is added to the gas delivered to the patient during the inspiratory phase of the breathing cycle from the ventilator. The positive pressure of the ventilator closes the pop-off valve, so any fresh gas delivered by the anesthesia machine while the ventilator is firing ends up going to the patient lungs. (This is also the reason why the flush valve should never be used when the ventilator is delivering a breath). The resulting increase in tidal volume depends on the respiratory rate (higher rate = less extra volume per breath), inspiratory-to-expiratory ratio (more inspiratory phase = more extra volume per breath) and fresh gas flow rate (higher = more extra volume per breath). Long circuits can also increase the distensible volume of the circuit and decrease delivered tidal volume. In addition, malfunctions (circuit leaks, bellows leaks, etc) can affect tidal volume.

○ How does "jet" ventilation work?

A small (16 gauge) cannula in the airway delivers a high-pressure jet of gas (usually oxygen). Additional air is entrained via the Venturi effect. A cone shaped wedge of gas actually reaches alveoli although total volume delivered per jet ventilation puff is less than anatomic dead space. Exhalation is passive.

○ Where should the transducer be located during intracranial surgery?

At the level of the head, preferably auditory meatus = circle of Willis.

A key concern during intracranial surgery is the cerebral perfusion pressure, which is mean arterial pressure minus central venous pressure or intracranial pressure, whichever is greater. Whenever the head is above the heart, the actual mean arterial pressure to the head is lower by the hydrostatic pressure of the column of blood. The simplest method to correct for this is to zero the arterial transducer at the level of the head, rather than the right atrium.

○ What are the implications of a right-to-left shunt for anesthetic uptake?

A slower inhalation induction with the least soluble volatile agents affected most.

In a right-to-left shunt, deoxygenated blood from the body moves to the left side of the heart, without passing through the pulmonary capillary bed. On the left side, it mixes with blood that has passed through the pulmonary vascular bed, decreasing the PaO_2 and slowing the rate of rise of the arterial concentration of anesthetic. However, because less blood has taken up agent from the lung, the alveolar concentration rises faster. Therefore, the patient may fall asleep more slowly, because of the slower rise in arterial concentration, yet the alveolar concentration may rise more quickly.

○ How does a doppler flow probe work?

The doppler technique utilizes the doppler effect, which is the reflection of sound waves off a moving object causing an apparent frequency shift.

A doppler probe emits an ultrasonic signal that is reflected by underlying tissue. A doppler frequency shift is caused by red blood cells moving through the artery. The difference between the transmitted and received frequency indicates blood flow, which is characterized by a swishing sound (systolic blood pressure). Use of a piezo-electric crystal will detect lateral arterial wall movement, measuring systolic and diastolic pressures.

○ Why are modern vaporizers temperature compensated?

Temperature compensation is required to maintain a constant concentration of gas output from the vaporizer over a wide range of ambient temperatures and gas flows.

Vapor pressure depends upon temperature. During vaporization the liquid anesthetic cools and the saturated vapor pressure decreases, as does the vaporizer output. Mechanisms of temperature compensation include: high thermal conductivity of the vaporizer (allowing rapid heat transfer to the liquid anesthetic as it cools) and a variable bypass mechanism (which directs more gas flow to the vaporizing chamber as the vaporizer cools to compensate for decreased saturated vapor pressure).

○ What is the ideal humidity in an anesthetic circuit?

The ideal humidity level is 28 to 32 mg H_2O/L gas (absolute humidity) or roughly 50 to 75% saturated at 37°C. Dry room temperature gases have a humidity level of < 10 mg H_2O/L.

Normal alveolar humidity is 44 mg H_2O/L at 37 °C. Inspiration of dry gases decreases relative humidity which can cause mucous plugging, loss of ciliary function, increased airway resistance, and atelectasis. Excessive humidity can also injure the lung, as well as serve as a source for bacteria.

○ **What safety features are incorporated into scavenging systems to prevent patient injury?**

Both positive and negative pressure relief valves (prevents suction effect in excess of 2.5 mm Hg or an occlusion from affecting the pressure in the breathing circuit) and a reservoir for the exhaust gas.

○ **What is the potential, in volts, between the ground wire in the OR and the "hot" wire?**

Electricity from a main power source is delivered to the OR through an isolation transformer. No wires are grounded, hence there is no potential created which would allow flow of current. If a wire does become grounded, then a potential of 117 volts is created, and current will flow to ground depending on the resistance to completing a circuit.

○ **Since isoflurane and enflurane are isomers, having the same charge to mass ratio, how does a mass spectrometer delineate between the two?**

The high energies involved in a mass spectrometer actually break the covalent bonds in the anesthetic molecules into components which have different charge to mass ratios. These fractions are the ones sampled to determine the percentage of gas present in the system.

○ **What is the capacity of an "E" cylinder for oxygen? Does this differ for air, nitrous oxide or nitrogen?**

A standard E-cylinder has the capacity for 625 to 700 L of oxygen, air, and nitrogen gas at 1800 to 2200 psi at 20°C. There is a linear relationship for gas and pressure in these. An E-cylinder of nitrous oxide contains 1590 L at 745 psi at 20°C. The cylinder is 75% empty before the "E" cylinder pressure changes.

○ **In what four ways does a patient lose heat in the operating room?**

By conduction, convection, evaporation and radiation.

○ **What is the difference between a thermistor, a resistance thermometer, and a thermocouple?**

A resistance thermometer uses increases in resistance of a metal (conductor) as temperature increases to measure temperature (the detector is part of a Wheatstone bridge). A thermistor is a semi-conductor which decreases its resistance as temperature increases. A thermocouple uses dissimilar metals, one junction is kept at a reference temperature, the other acts as a sensor and the voltage between the two is measured.

○ **Rank the Mapleson circuits in order of efficiency during spontaneous ventilation.**

A, D, E, C, B (All Doggi..Es Can Bite).

○ **Rank the Mapleson circuits in order of efficiency during controlled ventilation.**

D, E, B, C, A (DEad Bodies Can't Argue).

○ **Why can't a tank of liquid oxygen be used in the OR?**

At room temperature, oxygen is above its critical temperature, and therefore a gas. Above the critical temperature a gas cannot be condensed into a liquid however much pressure is applied.

○ **What is Poiseuille's law and how does it apply to IV catheters?**

For laminar gas flow, according to Poiseuille's law, resistance = $\dfrac{8NL}{\pi R^4}$

Where R= radius, N = viscosity of the fluid, and L = length of the tube. Therefore, if the radius is halved, the resistance within the tube increases 16-fold. If the length of the tube is doubled, the resistance is only doubled. The length of the tube minimally affects resistance; however, increasing the IV diameter makes a significant difference in resistance to laminar flow. (In practice, a short 16 gauge IV catheter will permit flow rates similar to a longer 14 gauge IV catheter. When you are in the middle of a tedious day in the OR, try it!).

○   **What is Reynolds' number?**

The Reynolds' number describes a value at which flow in a tube changes from laminar to turbulent. Laminar flow occurs at a Reynolds' number < 1000, and turbulent flow at > 1500.

Reynolds' number = 2rvd/N, r=radius, v=average velocity, d=density and N= viscosity.

○   **How does the oxygen analyzer on an anesthesia machine work?**

It uses an electrochemical sensor (galvanic or fuel cell). Oxygen reacts with the electrodes (anode: lead, cathode: silver or gold), generating a current that is proportional to the oxygen partial pressure in the sample gas. The polarographic method uses a Clark electrode (anode: silver and cathode: platinum or gold), battery power source and KCl electrolyte solution.

○   **What is the best estimate of anesthetic potency for inhaled agents?**

MAC.

○   **What is MAC?**

The minimum alveolar concentration (MAC) of an inhaled anesthetic required to abolish movement in 50 percent of patients, in response to a noxious stimulus.

○   **What is the stimulus used for determination of MAC in humans?**

Surgical incision.

○   **Using variations on the MAC concept, can you estimate the potency of anesthetic agents using other clinical end points?**

MAC awake, MAC skin incision, MAC intubation, MAC BAR .

MAC awake = the alveolar concentration of anesthetic at which a patient opens their eyes to command; (0.15 to 0.5 MAC).

MAC intubation = MAC of anesthetic that would inhibit movement and coughing during endotracheal intubation.

MAC-BAR = alveolar concentration of anesthetic that prevents adrenergic responses (BAR) to skin incision.

○   **What is the relationship between alveolar concentration (end-tidal concentration) and partial pressure of anesthetic in the CNS?**

After a short period of equilibration (8-10 minutes), alveolar concentration directly represents the partial pressure of anesthetic in the CNS (the site of anesthetic action).

First, arterial blood (Pa) equilibrates with the alveolar partial pressure (PA). Next, the brain equilibrates with the arterial blood, at which point the PA mirrors brain partial pressure (Pbr).

O   Does equilibration between two phases mean equal concentrations?

No. Equilibration means the same partial pressure exists in both phases (not concentration). It is the partial pressure gradient that propels the inhaled anesthetic across various barriers (alveoli, capillaries, cell membranes) until an equilibration is reached.

O   T/F: When the blood:gas partition coefficient of an anesthetic is 2.0, 1 ml of blood contains two times more anesthetic molecules than 1 ml of alveolar gas, at equilibrium.

True.

O   Two anesthetic agents are in equilibrium with blood. With agent A, there are 1050 volumes in the alveoli and 651 volumes in blood. With agent B, there are 355 volumes in the alveoli and 415 volumes in the blood. From this information can you predict that induction with agent A is faster than with agent B?

Yes. Since the two anesthetic agents have reached the equilibrium, it is possible to calculate the blood gas coefficient of these agents.
For the agent A, blood: gas coefficient = 651/1050 = 0.62
For the agent B, blood: gas coefficient = 415/355 = 1.16

Induction A has lower blood gas solubility than agent B and we can predict the induction (and recovery) with agent A will be faster than with agent B.

O   Two volatile agents are identical except that the blood:gas partition coefficient of anesthetic A is 0.75 and that of anesthetic B is 1.5. Can you conclude that at equilibrium, the partial pressure of anesthetic B in the blood will be twice that of anesthetic A?

Yes. At equilibrium, there will be twice the volume of anesthetic in blood with agent B compared to agent A.

O   What happens to MAC when body temperature decreases?

The MAC of volatile anesthetics decreases 5 to 7% per centigrade decrease in core body temperature. The speed of inhalational induction is not changed due to a decrease in cardiac output and increased blood solubility.

O   What is the effect of age on MAC?

MAC of volatile agents is maximal in infants at approximately 6 months of age and gradually decreases 4-5% per decade after age 40 years.

O   How do electrolyte abnormalities affect MAC?

Hypernatremia increases MAC, while hyponatremia decreases MAC.
Hyperkalemia or hypokalemia has no effect on MAC.

O   List some notable factors that do not alter MAC.

Duration of anesthesia, gender, type of surgical stimulation, hypo- or hypercarbia, metabolic acid-base status, hypertension, isovolemic anemia, and magnesium levels.

O   What is the importance of FA/FI ?

F_A is the alveolar gas concentration and F_I is the inspired gas concentration of inhaled anesthetic agent. Following the ratio of fractional concentration of alveolar anesthetic to inspired anesthetic over time (FA/FI) is a simple way to assess anesthetic uptake.

O   **What determines the FA/FI ?**

The FA/FI ratio is ultimately determined by the balance between the delivery of anesthetic by ventilation and its removal by uptake. Factors determining F_I include: fresh gas flow rate, volume of the breathing system and circuit absorption. Factors determining F_A include: uptake, ventilation and the concentration and second gas effects.

O   **What are the uptake factors that affect FA/FI?**

There are three factors: blood:gas solubility of anesthetic (B:G), cardiac output (Q), and alveolar to venous partial pressure difference (PA – PV).

O   **T/F: Uptake is a sum of those three factors.**

False. Uptake is the product of the three factors. This means that if any factor approaches zero, uptake must approach zero, and ventilation is free to rapidly drive the alveolar concentration upwards.
$$Uptake = (B:G) \times (Q) \times (PA - PV).$$

O   **What happens to FA/FI if cardiac output approaches zero (cardiac arrest)?**

Uptake would be minimal and FA/FI would quickly equal 1.

O   **What factors determine the input of anesthetic into alveoli (FA)?**

These factors include: (a) concentration of inspired anesthestic (FI), (b) alveolar ventilation, and (c) characteristics of the anesthetic delivery system.
In addition, the patient's functional residual capacity (FRC) influences the FA that is achieved.

O   **Name three ways to increase the inspired concentration (FI) and speed of inhalational induction.**

(a) Start with higher vaporizer setting
(b) Increase fresh gas flow
(c) Rebreathing bag can be collapsed prior to starting the FGF (capacity in the circuit is less)

O   **What is anesthetic overpressure?**

Overpressure is compensation for the uptake of anesthetic (especially the highly soluble ones) by delivering a higher concentration than we hope to achieve in the alveoli.
For example, on induction of anesthesia, one may use 4-5% of halothane to produce an alveolar concentration of 1%.

O   **Why is the concentration effect greater with nitrous oxide than with the volatile anesthetic?**

Because nitrous oxide can be used in much higher concentrations.

O   **List two effects of using nitrous oxide and oxygen for induction of anesthesia with sevoflurane versus 100% oxygen and sevoflurane.**

1.   *Concentration effect*- Nitrous oxide uptake increases alveolar sevoflurane concentration: Uptake of N_2O (first gas) reduces the total gas volume and therefore increases the concentration of sevoflurane (second gas) given concomitantly.

2.   *Second gas effect*- Tracheal inflow of sevoflurane is greater than it would be without nitrous oxide: The uptake of N_2O (the primary gas) increases the inspiratory volume, which in effect increases ventilation, and increases the alveolar concentration of sevoflurane (all inspired gases), regardless of the inspired concentration.

○   **Define vapor pressure of a volatile liquid.**

When a volatile liquid resides in a closed container, the molecules of the substance will equilibrate between the liquid and gas phases. At equilibrium, the pressure exerted by molecular collisions of the gas against the container walls is the vapor pressure.

○   **Is vapor pressure dependent on the volume of liquid in the container?**

No. As long as any liquid remains in the container, the vapor pressure is independent of the volume of that liquid. Vapor pressure is dependent on temperature and the physical characteristics of the liquid.

○   **Define partial pressure of gases in mixtures?**

When there is a mixture of gases in a closed container, each gas exerts a pressure proportional to its fractional volume (or mass). This is its partial pressure.

○   **What is Dalton's law of partial pressures?**

The total pressure of a gas mixture is the sum of the partial pressure of each gas.
P total $= P$ gas$_1 + P$ gas$_2 + \ldots\ldots + P$ gas$_N$
The entire mixture behaves just as if it were a single gas according to the ideal gas law.

○   **Explain how altitude influences vaporizer output.**

If the vaporizer delivers a constant partial pressure, like the contemporary variable-bypass vaporizer, adjustments are generally not necessary. There may be a slight change in the splitting ratio causing a slight increase in vaporizer output. This is due to the fact that high resistance pathway through the vaporizing chamber offers less resistance under hypobaric conditions. On the other hand, Tec 6 vaporizer requires manual adjustments of the concentration at high altitudes to maintain a constant partial pressure of anesthetic because Tec 6 delivers volume percent of desflurane. At high altitudes volume percent represents an absolute decrease in the partial pressure of the anesthetic.

○   **What is the primary mechanism for terminating the central effects of IV anesthetics administered for induction of anesthesia?**

Redistribution.

○   **Which monitors are based on Beer-Lambert Law?**

Pulse oximetry and infra-red analyzer.

○   **Based on the Beer-Lambert Law, how does pulse oximetry work?**

$A = \sum bc$ (A=absorbance value at specific wavelength, $\sum$=absorptivity coefficient of the material at that wavelength, b=pathlength through the sample, c=concentration of the compound in solution).

The first pulse oximeters manufactured in the early 1980s used the Beer-Lambert law to calculate the values of arterial SaO_2. Pulse oximeters measure the absorption of red (deoxy-hemoglobin) and infrared light (oxyhemoglobin). LEDs are used as a light source which passes through a patient's finger and is detected by light sensors. During an arterial pulse there is an increase in blood volume and this increase in absorption differentiate arterial from venous and other tissues. From this data the pulse oximeter determines the percent oxygen saturation of the arterial blood using the Beer-Lambert law. Measurements for SaO_2 values below 85% are often erroneous, as the effect of scattering of light by the red blood cell is not taken into consideration in this formula. Most pulse oximeters now use look-up tables derived from calibration studies of healthy volunteers whose oxygen saturation is measured invasively.

○   **How many wavelengths of light are required to distinguish HbO_2 from reduced Hb?**

Two different wavelengths, in the red (600-700 nm) and near infrared (800-940 nm) spectrum.

○   **What is the difference between the SpO_2 measured by pulse oximetry and the SaO_2 measured by the laboratory co-oximeter?**

Adult blood usually contains four species of hemoglobin: oxyhemoglobin (HbO_2), reduced hemoglobin (Hb), methemoglobin (metHb), and carboxyhemoglobin (COHb). Each of these hemoglobins has a different light absorption profile and therefore requires four wavelengths of light to measure them.
SpO_2 uses two wavelengths and measures the "functional saturation, which is given by the following equation: Functional $SaO_2 = O_2Hb / (O_2Hb + $ reduced Hb) x 100
Laboratory co-oximeters use multiple wavelengths and measures the "fractional" saturation, which is given by the following equation;

Fractional $SaO_2 = O_2Hb / (O_2 Hb + $ reduced Hb + COHb + MetHb) x 100

○   **What effect will COHb and MetHb have on the SpO_2 measurement?**

At 940 nm, COHb has an extremely low absorbance and does not contribute to total absorbance. However, at 660 nm, COHb has an absorbance very similar to that of O_2Hb, therefore, SpO_2 will read falsely high. In the presence of high MetHb, SpO_2 reads 85%, independent of the actual arterial oxygenation.

○   **How does the finger pulse oximeter differentiate arterial blood from venous blood to derive the arterial hemoglobin saturation?**

The pulse oximeter performs a plethysmographic analysis to differentiate the pulsatile "arterial" Hb saturation from the nonpulsatile signal from "venous" and other tissue absorption.

○   **What significant errors are seen with pulse oximetry?**

- Methylene blue IV results in a severe decrease in measured SpO_2.
- Blue, black, and green nail polish with absorbance near 660 nm may cause an artifactual decrease in SpO_2 reading.
- Ambient light, especially fluorescent light, can falsely elevate SpO_2 reading, especially if the flicker frequency of the light is close to the harmonic of the diode switching frequency.
- Vasoconstriction or hypotension can cause loss of SpO_2 signal.
- Delayed detection of hypoxic events may be seen due to a significant delay between a change in the alveolar oxygen tension and a change in the oximeter reading.
- Erratic performance with irregular rhythms, electrical interference and motion artifacts.

○   **What is meant by descriptive statistics? How does it differ from inferential statistics?**

There are two distinct steps in the process of analyzing study data.
The first step is to describe the study sample or data using standard methods to determine the average value, the range of data around the average, and other characteristics.
For example, if one reports that 55% of students in a class are female and that the class members' average height is 67 inches, they are describing the study sample and thus are engaging in descriptive statistics.

The second step in most studies is to derive a conclusion from facts or premises. Inferential statistics are used to draw conclusions about a population based on a random sample selected from that population.

○ List some basic rules and steps in the procedure of statistical inference.

1. (a) The starting point is almost always to assume that there is no difference between groups (null hypothesis -H_o).
    (b) They are all samples drawn at random from the same statistical population.
2. The next step is to determine the likelihood that the observed differences could be caused by chance variation alone.
3. If this probability is sufficiently small (< 1 in 20 or < 0.05), one "reject" the null hypothesis (accept "alternative hypothesis-H_1") and conclude that there is some true difference between the groups.

○ What is a Type I error?

Type I error (Alpha) is the probability of incorrectly rejecting the null hypothesis when the null is true. Most statistical analyses use an alpha level of 0.05 (5% significance level). This is the risk (out of 100 null hypotheses that we reject, 5 will be incorrectly rejected) you are willing to take in making a type I error. If the p-value is less than the risk you are willing to take ($p < 0.05$) then you reject the null and state that with a 95% level of confidence that the two parameters are not the same.

○ What is a Type II error?

Type II error (Beta) is the probability of failing to reject the null when the null is not true; it's the probability of saying there is no significant effect when there really is one. If you reject the null, you cannot make a Type II error.

○ What is "power"?

Power is the probability of rejecting the null hypothesis given that the null is incorrect (correctly rejecting the null). Some people also refer to power as precision or sensitivity. *Power is equal to 1-Beta*. To calculate the power you need: the population means under both the null and the alternative; the standard error; and alpha. Power is generally recommended at levels of at least 0.8 (therefore, Type II is 0.2).

○ List several factors that increase the statistical power of a study.

A larger alpha, directional hypotheses, one-tailed test, larger sample size, little measurement error, and a larger effect size.

○ What is the relationship between Type I, Type II and Power?

Decision	Truth of Null	
	True	Not True
Reject Null	Type I	Power
FTR Null	Correct	Type II

○ What is a biased sample?

A sample is biased if its characteristics differ systematically from those of the population about which one seeks to make inferences.

○ When would you be concerned about the possibility of bias?

Whenever nonrandom sampling methods have been used.

A famous case of what can go wrong when using a biased sample is found in the 1936 US presidential election polls. The *Literary Digest* used lists of telephone and automobile owners for their sample of two million registered voters. They predicted that Alfred E. Landon would defeat Franklin D. Roosevelt by 57% to 43%. The *Gallup poll* used a sample size of 300,000 and predicted Roosevelt would win, and they were right. So what went wrong? The wealthier citizens voted in majority for Landon, but the lower classes voted for Roosevelt. Because the *Literary Digest* sample was biased towards the middle and upper-class citizens purchasing luxury items, their result was incorrect.

○ **List two reasons for overshoot in the systolic upstroke of the invasive intra-arterial pressure waveform.**

1. If the monitoring system has a natural frequency that is too low, frequencies in the monitored pressure waveform will approach the natural frequency of the measurement system. This will cause the system to resonate and the pressure waveform will be exaggerated or amplified. This will be displayed as overshoot, ringing or resonance
2. The monitoring system should have an adequate damping coefficient for accurate reproduction of the arterial waveform. The underdamped pressure waveforms display systolic pressure overshoot.

○ **What does underdamping do to the systolic, mean, and diastolic pressures measured by direct arterial pressure monitoring?**

Underdamping will overestimate the systolic and underestimate the diastolic blood pressure, with little change in mean pressure. These changes are usually worse with tachycardia.

○ **T/F: Compared with central aortic pressure, peripheral arterial waveforms have higher systolic pressure, lower diastolic pressure, and wider pulse pressure.**

True. This is due to the physiologic amplification of the waveform from the aorta to the peripheral arteries.

○ **In aortic stenosis, the arterial pressure waveform appears overdamped. Why?**

In aortic stenosis, there is a fixed obstruction to left ventricular ejection. This results in a reduced stroke volume and a small amplitude arterial pressure waveform that rises slowly and peaks late in systole.

○ **Bisferiens pulse is diagnostic of which valvular cardiac lesion?**

Aortic regurgitation. Because of the large stroke volume ejected from the left ventricle, there is a wide pulse pressure and the pulse may have two systolic peaks.

○ **What is pulsus paradoxus?**

This is an exaggeration of the normal inspiratory decline in systolic arterial pressure, which exceeds 10-12 mm Hg during quiet breathing.

○ **When do you see pulsus paradoxus?**

Cardiac tamponade. Also in patients with airway obstruction, bronchospasm, dyspnea, or any condition in which there are large swings in intrathoracic pressure.

○ **List three characteristics of a nondepolarizing neuromuscular blockade.**

1. Tetanic fade at 50 Hz for 5 sec
2. Decreased train-of-four ratio
3. Post-tetanic facilitation

○ **T/F: Resistance to nondepolarizing neuromuscular blocking drugs occurs with nerve damage.**

True. This applies to peripheral nerve trauma, cord transection, and stroke. Monitoring of the involved limb tends to underestimate the degree of block, therefore, the uninvolved extremity should be used.

○ **Which muscles are most appropriate to monitor when assessing the quality of intubating conditions?**

The quality of intubating conditions depends chiefly on the state of relaxation of muscles of the jaw, pharynx, larynx and diaphragm. Facial nerve stimulation with visual observation of the response over the eyebrow (corrugator supercilii) gives better results because the response of the corrugator supercilii is close to that of the vocal cords.

○ **Muscles do not seem to respond in a uniform fashion to neuromuscular blocking drugs. What is the reason for this difference?**

Factors that modify access of the drug to and from the neuromuscular junction include: cardiac output, distance of the muscles from the heart, and muscle blood flow. The differences can be observed with respect to onset time, maximum blockade, and duration of action. For example, onset of action is faster in the muscles of the jaw, pharynx, larynx, and diaphragm, because they are closer to the central circulation and receive a greater blood flow.

○ **If profound surgical relaxation is required, what is the best place to monitor the neuromuscular blockade?**

Stimulation of the facial nerve with observation of the response over the eyebrow.
Among the central muscles, the diaphragm and especially the laryngeal adductors are the most resistant to nondepolarizing drugs; all the other muscles are most likely blocked if the resistant laryngeal muscles are blocked (the response of the corrugator supercilii is close to that of the laryngeal adductors).

○ **At the end of a case how do you determine the reversibility of paralysis with nondepolarizing blockers?**

Preferably, reversal agents should be given only when 4 twitches are visible using the nerve stimulator (first twitch recovery >25%); because the effectiveness of anticholinesterases depends directly on the degree of recovery present when they are administered.

○ **For the assessment of recovery, which muscle is preferable to monitor?**

The adductor pollicis. The geniohyoid (upper airway muscle that prevents airway obstruction after extubation) recovers approximately at the same time as the adductor pollicis.

○ **T/F: The presence of spontaneous respiration is a sign of adequate neuromuscular recovery.**

False. The diaphragm recovers earlier than the much more sensitive upper airway muscles, leaving the patient breathing spontaneously with an unprotected airway.

○ **List 4 factors that contribute to reversal of nondepolarizing muscle relaxants?**

1. Tissue redistribution
2. Metabolism
3. Excretion
4. Administration of cholinesterase inhibitors

○ **List three electrolyte disturbances that may augment a nondepolarizing block.**

Hypokalemia, hyponatremia, and hypocalcemia.

○   **List 4 conditions that change laminar flow to turbulent flow.**

1) high gas flows, 2) sharp angles within the tube, 3) branching in the tube, and 4) change in the diameter of the tube.

○   **During turbulent gas flow, what determines the driving pressure?**

Driving pressure is directly proportional to the square of the gas flow and gas density; inversely proportional to the fourth power of the radius of the tube.

○   **During laminar flow, the resistance is inversely proportional to gas flow rate. What happens to the resistance as the gas flow is increased during turbulent flow?**

During turbulent flow, resistance increases in proportion to the flow rate.

○   **What is the relevance of viscosity to turbulent flow?**

Turbulent flow is independent of viscosity. Viscosity is relevant under conditions of laminar flow.

○   **Will helium improve *laminar* gas flow?**

No. Helium has a low density, but its viscosity is close to that of air. Since density is directly proportional to driving pressure during turbulent flow, helium is useful when there is critical airway narrowing (subglottic edema, tracheal tumor) or abnormally high airway resistance (ventilating patients with small diameter ETTs).

○   **What is the density of mixtures of helium and oxygen compared to pure oxygen?**
The most popular mixtures of helium, 80/20 and 70/30 helium-oxygen, have densities that are 1.805 and 1.586 times less dense respectively, than pure oxygen.

○   **A patient is undergoing surgery with field block and sedation. List 2 ways of monitoring their sedation level.**

1.   Observer's Assessment of Alertness / Sedation Scale (OAA/S)
2.   BIS Index

○   **How does the BIS index correlate with OAA/S?**

In volunteers the BIS index has been shown to correlate with OAA/S scores during propofol-induced sedation. An increasing depth of sedation was associated with a predictable decrease in BIS index and absence of recall with BIS values below 80.

○   **Which monitoring method (BIS or OAA/S) appears to be superior?**

OAA/S involves patient stimulation at frequent intervals to determine the level of consciousness, requires patient cooperation, and is subject to testing fatigue.
Although the potential to titrate drugs more accurately using BIS values is appealing, conventional assessment of sedation is important to maintain continuous patient contact. Therefore, BIS monitoring should be employed as an adjunct to clinical evaluation rather than as the primary monitor of consciousness.

○   **List the two main factors that determine the central venous pressure.**

Intravascular blood volume and intrinsic vascular tone of the capacitance vessels.

○   **How does ventilation affect the CVP?**

There will be alterations in the intrathoracic pressure and juxtracardiac pressure during the respiratory cycle depending on whether the patient is breathing spontaneously or receiving positive pressure ventilation.

○   **What is the best time to monitor cardiac filling pressures?**

At the end of expiration, when intrathoracic and juxtracardiac pressures approach atmospheric pressures, whether the patient is breathing spontaneously or receiving positive pressure ventilation.

○   **What causes the sequence of waves seen in a typical CVP trace?**

Normal mechanical events of the cardiac cycle are responsible for the three peaks and two descents.
Waves: 'a' wave due to **a**trial kick
                'c' wave due to **c**ontraction of the ventricle (isovolemic)
                'v' wave with atrial filling
Descents: 'x' descent due to rela**x**ation of atrium
                'y' descent with ventricular filling

○   **The relationship between oxygen consumption, oxygen content and cardiac output is expressed by which equation?**

Fick equation: oxygen delivery = cardiac out put x $(CaO_2 - CvO_2)$.

With a normal oxygen consumption of 250 ml and a cardiac output of 5000 ml/min, the normal arteriovenous difference by this equation calculates to be about 5 ml O_2/dl blood.
Arteriovenous O_2 difference is a good measure of the overall oxygen delivery.

○   **List several factors that may cause measurement errors in the invasive pressure monitoring systems.**

1.   Miscalibrated or inappropriately zeroed transducers
2.   Damping with clot formation over the catheter tip
3.   Too low natural frequency of the measurement system causing the system to resonate (pressure waveforms recorded on the monitor will be exaggerated).
4.   Catheter location, alteration in airway pressure, etc, can markedly affect the data interpretation.

○   **How accurate is the thermodilution cardiac output measurement in the face of a large left-to-right or right-to-left shunt?**

The thermodilution technique measures right ventricular output and pulmonary artery blood flow. In those situations, right ventricular and left ventricular outputs will not be equal.

○   **What will happen if the constant entered in the cardiac output computer was 10 ml injectate, but only a 5 ml injectate was used, in determining cardiac output?**

The area under the thermodilution curve would be approximately one-half the expected value. The computed cardiac output would overestimate the true cardiac output by a factor of two.

○   **How does right-sided valvular regurgitation (severe tricuspid regurgitation) affect cardiac output as measured by thermodilution?**

In patients with tricuspid regurgitation, recirculation of the thermal signal occurs between the right atrium and right ventricle, resulting in an abnormally prolonged decay time and inaccurate measurement of cardiac output (usually underestimated, but may be overestimated depending on the severity of valvular regurgitation and the magnitude of the cardiac output).

○   **List four situations that will give rise to low-amplitude curves during the thermodilutional cardiac output measurements.**

1.   The injectate volume is too small (less than volume entered in the computer)
2.   The temperature differential between injectate and blood temperature is small
3.   When the thermistor is improperly positioned. If there is an undamped pulmonary artery waveform, one may assume acceptable thermistor position.
4.   Partly or completely wedged PAC will reduce flow past the thermistor. Therefore, the thermistor should be located in the center of the flowing blood.

○   **Why doesn't the pulmonary capillary wedge pressure (PCWP) always correlate with LV volume?**

Ideally, changes in LVEDP (hence, left ventricular volume) are reflected by all the proximal pressures (left atrial, pulmonary artery end diastolic pressure-PAEDP, and PCWP) because at end-diastole, there is cessation of forward blood flow, and a static fluid column is presumed to exist from the left ventricle to the PAC tip.

Factors that alter the premise that PAOP is a consistent accurate reflection of LVEDP/V are:
1.   Airway pressure
2.   Pulmonary hypertension
3.   Mitral stenosis
4.   Ventricular compliance

○   **Why is it important to position the pulmonary artery catheter (PAC) in West Zone III?**

Location in a low flow area of the lung exposes the tracing and PAOP to greater influences of airway pressure changes. Ideally the PAC should be in Zone III (Pa>Pv>PA) of the lung. This can be confirmed by X-ray, but typically occurs spontaneously since these are 'flow directed' catheters.

○   **List some characteristics that suggest the PAC tip is not in Zone III.**

a)   PCWP > PAEDP
b)   Nonphasic PCWP tracing
c)   Inability to aspirate blood from the distal port when the catheter is wedged.

○   **How does PEEP affect the PCWP reading?**

The effect of PEEP is minimal if the level of PEEP is low (<10 cm) or the PAC is located in Zone III. (When PEEP is above 10 cm H_2O, substracting 1-2 mm Hg from the displayed "wedge" pressure for each 5 cm H_2O of PEEP gives an estimate.)

○   **If a blood sample is obtained from a hypothermic patient for ABG analysis, is it important to correct for temperature?**

Yes. The PO_2 and PCO_2 derived from a 37°C electrode is overestimated in this hypothermic patient.

○   **If temperature correction is not applied, what is the percentage of error in PO_2 derived from a 37°C electrode?**

At high PO_2 values (> 400 mm Hg) the effect is small because hemoglobin is fully saturated in this region. However, at PO_2 values below 100 mm Hg, the degree of overestimation may be severe. For example, at a patient temperature of 30°C and PO_2 below 80 mm Hg, the true PO_2 is overestimated by about 60%.

○   **What is the difference between monopolar and bipolar electrosurgery?**

Electrosurgery is the standard method of "power" coagulating or cutting body tissue using radiofrequency electrical current. In both techniques, electrical current passes from an active electrode to heat or burn tissue, then through body tissue to a return inactive electrode. In the monopolar technique, the return electrode is a grounding pad placed on the patient's buttock or thigh, as far away from the heart as possible. The bipolar technique uses two closely spaced electrodes, often the two jaws of a surgical instrument (eg: forceps) with no return plate.

○   **What causes unintentional burns at the site of the ESU return plate or alternate return pathway?**

A properly applied ESU return plate does not cause burns because the surface area of the return plate over which the current diffuses is large (low current density) and the resistance to flow is low resulting in insignificant heating. If the ESU return plate is improperly applied or the cord connecting the return plate to the ESU is damaged, ESU will seek alternate return pathways. Anything attached to the patient, such as ECG leads or temperature probe, can provide this alternate pathway. The current density at these alternate sites will be considerably higher than that of the ESU return plate because its surface area is much smaller potentially resulting in serious burns.

○   **Most operating rooms have ungrounded electrical power supply. Why?**

Ungrounded power provides an extra measure of safety from gross electric shock (macroshock).

○   **What is an isolation transformer?**

An isolation transformer is required to provide ungrounded power. This device uses electromagnetic induction, and converts the grounded power on the primary side to an ungrounded power system on the secondary side of the transformer.

○   **How does a ground fault circuit interrupter (GFCI) prevent macroshock?**

GFCI prevents individuals from receiving macroshock in a grounded power system. GFCI interrupts the power when it detects a difference (5 mA) in the current flowing in hot and neutral wires due to short circuit.

○   **Compare and contrast line isolation monitor (LIM) versus GFCI.**

Both monitor macroshock hazard due to faulty equipment leakage current (short circuits).
LIM continuously monitors leakage current (5 mA) in an ungrounded system, and alarms, but the equipment can still be used. GFCI, which is used in a grounded power system, interrupts the power without warning if leakage current of more than 5 mA is detected; defective equipment could no longer be used.

○   **List two important factors that affect the success of defibrillation.**

1.   Energy output of the defibrillator
2.   Resistance to current flow during shock delivery

○   **What is the primary determinant of delivered energy?**

Transthoracic impedence. When transthoracic impedance is higher, the actual delivered energy will be lower.

○   **What factors affect transthoracic impedance?**

1.   Paddle size- resistance decreases with increasing electrode size. (common paddle size 8-10 cm in diameter)
2.   Use of gel or paste reduces impedance
3.   Transthoracic impedance decreases with successive shocks
4.   Impedance is slightly higher during inspiration than during exhalation. (air is a poor conductor)

5.   Firm pressure of at least 11 kg reduces resistance by improving paddle-skin contact

○   **What is the optimal energy for open-chest defibrillation?**

During cardiac surgery, internal paddles applied directly to the heart are used for direct defibrillation of the heart. Low energy levels, 5-25 J, are required since skin impedance is bypassed.

○   **A 57-year-old man is scheduled for a repeat total hip replacement under general anesthesia. He had a permanent endocardial VVIR pacemaker placed two years ago for complete heart block, and since arriving in the operating room he has paced continuously.   What is a VVIR pacemaker?**

In a pacemaker code the first letter refers to the chamber paced (V for ventricle), the second letter refers to the chamber sensed, and the third letter refers to the response to the sensed event (I for Inhibition), the fourth letter refers to the programmability (R:rate adaptive, designed to deliver a more physiologic response by changing the rate in response to exercise)

○   **In this patient, the pacer functioned normally during a recent evaluation by the cardiologist. What other preoperative evaluations are needed?**

Patients with permanent pacemakers are often elderly and have significant coexisting disease such as coronary artery disease, hypertension, insulin dependent diabetes or have received a heart transplant. These medical problems, medications, acid base status and electrolytes should be evaluated preoperatively.

○   **Surgeon is planning on using a unipolar electrosurgical cautery (ESU). What are your concerns?**

ESC, which emits radiofrequency energy has the potential to cause transient or permanent changes in pacemaker function. The most common problem is inhibition of the pacemaker. Patients with complete heart block are more likely to be pacemaker dependent and therefore are potentially at higher risk should a malfunction occur. If ESC is to be used extensively, then consideration should be given to reprogramming the generator to an asynchronous mode preoperatively, to avoid inhibition.

○   **Can you use a magnet to convert the generator to an asynchronous mode if intraoperatively the use of the electrocautery causes the pacemaker to malfunction intermittently?**

Although most devices respond to magnet application by a device-specific single or dual chamber asynchronous pacing mode, routine use of magnets without knowledge of the expected pacemaker response is not advocated. Applying the magnet to a programmable generator (VVIR) in the presence of electromagnetic interference (EMI) increases the risk of reprogramming and is discouraged. Unless the planned surgery is truly emergent or poses little risk of EMI from electrocautery, the pacemaker clinic, service or manufacturer should be contacted for advice.

○   **Is use of bipolar ESU safer than unipolar ESU in patients with a permanent pacemaker?**

Because the active and return electrodes are the two blades of the forceps in a bipolar ESU, current passes between the tips and not through the patient.   Exposure of the pacemaker generator to electrical interventions is minimal. However, bipolar ESU generates considerably less power than the unipolar and is mainly used for ophthalmic and neurologic surgery.

○   **What other measures should be taken to minimize susceptibility to electromagnetic interference from ESU?**

a)   Locate the ESU receiving plate as remote from the generator as possible
b)   The pulse generator and leads should not be between the operative site and the receiving plate (ensure the current flows away from the pacemaker system)
c)   Use the lowest current and short bursts only

d) Pacing function should be confirmed by monitoring heart sounds or the pulse waveform.

e) Stop all diathermy if arrythmia occurs

O What is AICD?

Automatic Implantable Cardioverter Defibrillator (AICD) is a device that is capable of sensing ventricular tachycardia (VT) and ventricular fibrillation (VF) and then automatically defibrillating the patient.

O How does external cardioversion or defibrillation affect AICD?

Shocks probably will cause at least temporary inhibition. Transient loss of capture or sensing should be anticipated. Pulse generator damage is determined by the distance of the external paddles from the pulse generator. Anteroposterior paddle configuration with the paddles located at least 10 cm from the pulse generator is recommended. Lowest possible energies should be used for cardioversion or defibrillation. After cardioversion or defibrillation the device must be interrogated to assure proper function. Reprogramming and/or lead replacement may be necessary.

O How does an AICD respond to magnet application?

Depending on the manufacturer and model of the ICD and how it is programmed (example, magnet switch inactivated), tachycardia sensing and delivery of therapy may be inactivated by magnet application. Therefore, interrogating the device and contacting the manufactures for advice remain the most reliable ways to determine magnet response.

O How should you manage the AICD device in the operating room?

The AICD should be disabled immediately prior to induction of anesthesia and reinstated in the postoperative recovery unit. The patient should be monitored continuously throughout. Provisions for immediate external cardioversion or defibrillation must be available in the OR.

INTUBATION

When You Reach The End Of Your Rope, Tie A Knot In It And Hang On.
Thomas Jefferson

❍ **What is the most common cause of upper airway obstruction?**

The tongue and jaw relaxation occluding the posterior oropharynx.

❍ **List important adjuncts often needed to help establish basic airway control.**

Suction equipment to remove secretions from mouth and throat, chin lift-jaw thrust maneuver, oral/nasal airway, bag-valve-mask device and mouth-to-mask ventilation device.

❍ **What are the main indications for endotracheal intubation?**

To address insufficient respiratory effort, inadequate airway patency, to protect the airway, or improve oxygenation.

Examples include: apnea or hypoventilation, burns, inhalational injury, acute airway obstruction, expanding neck hematomas, hemodynamic instability, loss of protective reflexes, severe head injuries, patients at risk of aspiration, inability to maintain or protect a patent airway, impending or potential compromise of the airway and tracheal toilet.

❍ **Does tracheal intubation prevent aspiration?**

Not absolutely. Microaspiration can still occur.

❍ **What are the possible deleterious effects of succinylcholine?**

Increased intraocular (no extrusion of eye contents ever reported) and intracranial pressure (debatable). Increase in intragastric pressure is offset by increase in lower esophageal sphincter (LES) tone. The patient is only at increased risk of aspiration if the LES is incompetent.

Hyperkalemia, particularly in patients with pre-existing hyperkalemia from renal failure, and after 24 hours in burns, neurologic injury, muscular dystrophies and trauma (proliferation of extrajunctional receptors).

Triggering masseter spasm and malignant hyperthermia.

Increased duration of action in patients with pseudocholinesterase deficiency (inherited pattern or liver disease, malignancies, pregnancy, and malnutrition).

Acetylcholine-like effects (esp. bradycardia and asystole) with multiple doses over a short time period or IV dose exceeding 3mg/kg in adult patients.

Anaphylaxis. Succinylcholine has a greater incidence than non-depolarizers.

Phase II or desensitization block at 7 to 10 mg/kg in adults.

❍ **What maneuver should be performed during tracheal intubation in a patient with a full stomach?**

Sellick's maneuver (firm pressure over the cricoid cartilage, which collapses the esophagus and prevents passively regurgitated gastric fluid from reaching the hypopharynx).

❍ **What is the correct position of the tip of the endotracheal tube?**

Approximately 4 cm above the carina.

○ **What are two contraindications to nasotracheal intubation?**

Maxillofacial trauma (basilar skull fracture) and coagulopathy.

○ **What is the most common complication of nasotracheal intubation?**

Epistaxis.

○ **How is transtracheal needle jet insufflation performed?**

A #14 or #16 gauge plastic cannula is inserted through the cricothyroid membrane and directed distally into the trachea. The cannula should be connected to a high-pressure oxygen source with a low compliance circuit (fresh gas outlet and oxygen flush valve) using a 5 mm ETT adaptor piece with oxygen tubing and a 3-way stopcock. Oxygen is delivered in intermittent bursts of one second on and four seconds off or to 40 to 50 psi if insufflation pressure is directly measured. Insertion of an oropharyngeal airway will allow passive exhalation of insufflated oxygen.

○ **How long can a patient be supported with needle jet insufflation until an airway can be secured?**

Approximately 45 to 60 minutes.

○ **What limits the use of needle jet insufflation as an airway?**

Hypercapnia, due to inadequate ventilation.

○ **When is an emergency cricothyroidotomy indicated?**

When a patient who can not be ventilated or intubated needs an emergent airway.

○ **When may emergency tracheostomy be performed instead of emergency cricothyroidotomy?**

In pediatric patients, where cricothyroidotomy is generally contraindicated. Because of the smaller size and greater soft-tissue compliance of the pediatric airway, the cricoid cartilage plays a major role in maintaining patency of the tracheal lumen. An injury to this structure could be disastrous.

○ **What is the narrowest part of the respiratory tract in children?**

The inferior ring portion of the cricoid cartilage

○ **Stridor is observed in what phase of respiration?**

Inspiratory.

○ **What is the most common type of tracheo-esophageal fistula?**

Blind esophageal pouch with a fistulous connection of the trachea to the distal esophagus.

○ **Why does a newborn with bilateral choanal atresia present with severe respiratory distress?**

The newborn is an obligatory nose breather.

○   According to Poiseuille's law, if the radius of the conducting airway is reduced from 4 mm to 3 mm, resistance to airflow will increase by how much?

Sixteen-fold.

○   The funnel-shaped narrowing of the glottis and subglottic airway commonly known as "steeple sign" is observed in what type of extrathoracic airway obstruction?

Croup or laryngotracheobronchitis.

○   A 12-year old with cerebral palsy and vegetative state was intubated for 10 days because of aspiration pneumonia. She is weaned from mechanical ventilation, extubated and 1 hour later develops stridor and severe retractions. She is appropriately suctioned and given 3 aerosol treatments of racemic epinephrine. Her arterial blood gas is pH 7.20, PCO_2 80 mm Hg, PO_2 80 mmHg on 100% oxygen. What should be done next?

Re-intubation.

○   Foreign body aspiration occurs most commonly in which age group?

Six months to 3 years of age.

○   Name the most common offender in foreign body aspiration.

Organic substances such as nuts, corn and cheerios. Coins and small pieces of toys are also common.

○   What will be the predominant symptom of a child who has aspirated a foreign body, which is lodged in his/her trachea?

Stridor will be seen acutely. Cough, wheezing and bloody sputum in the chronic stage.

○   What is the predominant auscultatory finding in a child with a foreign body lodged in the right mainstem bronchus?

Depending on the extent of the obstruction either expiratory wheezing or severely diminished airflow in the right lung.

○   An 11-month old male presents with rhinorrhea, cough and increased respiratory rate. Treatment with bronchodilators has produced equivocal results. He is now in obvious distress with retractions, grunting, prolonged expiratory time, inspiratory and expiratory wheezes. Chest x-ray shows a tracheal shift to the left and hyperexpansion of the right chest. The most likely diagnosis is:

Foreign body aspiration.

○   A neonate has Apgar scores of 8 and 8. He is pink when actively crying, but cyanosis and retractions appear when he is quiet. What is the most likely diagnosis?

Choanal atresia.

○   What is the mechanism of cor pulmonale resulting from chronic airway obstruction?

Chronic alveolar hypoventilation with an increase in pulmonary vascular resistance.

○   Which is the only abductor muscle of the vocal cords?

The posterior cricoarytenoid muscle.

O   **Which is the only muscle of the larynx supplied by the superior laryngeal nerve?**

The cricothyroid muscle.

O   **What is the average endotracheal tube length (measured at the lips) appropriate for a two and a five-year-old child?**

12 and 15 cm, respectively.

O   **What is the effective dose of intravenous lidocaine able to partially blunt the cardiovascular response to intubation?**

1.5 mg/kg.

O   **How long does it take for preoxygenation to achieve 96% denitrogenation of the lungs?**

In patients breathing 100% oxygen it will take 3-4 minutes. Preoxygenation will enable apnea without hypoxemia for 3 to 5 minutes in patients with a normal FRC.

O   **What is the minimal time required for preoxygenation before induction of general anesthesia for cesarean section?**

3 minutes.

O   **What is the minimal time required for four deep breaths of oxygen before induction of general anesthesia for cesarean section?**

About 30 seconds. These must be vital capacity breaths to effectively accomplish denitrogenation. Pregnant patients have a reduced FRC, and will desaturate very quickly, despite adequate preoxygenation.

O   **In which clinical situations are the use of retrograde intubation or a lightwand considered better choices than fiberoptic bronchoscopy for assisting endotracheal intubation?**

Bleeding in the oral cavity.

O   **What is the maximum safe dose of lidocaine for topical anesthesia of the airway?**

4.5 mg/kg, not to exceed a total of 300mg. Reduce dosage for children, elderly and acutely ill.

O   **Which approaches are useful for blocking the internal branch of the superior laryngeal nerve?**

Topical anesthesia of the pyriform fossae, inhalation of nebulized local anesthetic, nerve block through the thyrohyoid membrane.

O   **Is the use of a LMA contraindicated in a scenario of failed intubation and impossible mask ventilation if the patient is at increased risk for aspiration of gastric contents?**

No. The use of a LMA may be life saving in this situation. Hypoxemia and not aspiration is the major risk for this patient.

O   **What is the reported incidence of downfolding of the epiglottis during insertion of the LMA in adults?**

10%.

○ **Which are the only "fail safe" signs for the correct placement of an endotracheal tube?**

Persistence of appropriate levels of end-tidal carbon dioxide is the only one. In the unlikely situation where capnography is unavailable, visualization of the tube passing through the cords and fiberoptic confirmation of tracheal rings and the carina distal to the tip of the endotracheal tube. .

○ **Is fusion of the cervical spines a feature of Pierre-Robin syndrome?**

No. Pierre-Robin syndrome is characterized by small mouth, mandibular hypoplasia and large tongue.

○ **Is rapid sequence induction appropriate in a patient with a full stomach suffering from Ludwig's angina?**

No. Rapid sequence induction may lead to a catastrophic loss of the airway due to the inability to intubate and ventilate the patient. Safer options are an awake fiberoptic intubation, awake blind nasal intubation and elective tracheostomy.

○ **Which is the safest technique of intubation in children suffering from epiglottitis?**

Intubation in the OR after induction of anesthesia with an inhaled anesthetic agent (halothane or sevoflurane) in the semi-sitting position.

○ **Are there any differences in oxygenation and ventilation between endotracheal intubation and the Combitube?**

Yes. With the Combitube, the $PaCO_2$ is higher. The PaO_2 is also greater due to the physiologic "PEEP" maintained by the vocal cords.

○ **What should be done immediately after a failed intubation and inadequate two-handed mask ventilation?**

An LMA should be inserted immediately.

○ **What is the most effective external laryngeal maneuver that can achieve a better direct laryngoscopic view of the vocal cords?**

BURP - Backward, upward and rightward pressure on the cricoid cartilage.

○ **What is the failure rate of intubation using a lightwand?**

1 in 479 cases.

○ **What are the appropriate sizes of LMA and fiberoptic bronchoscope for patients weighing 10 to 20 kilograms?**

Number 2 LMA and 3.5 mm bronchoscope.

○ **What are the choices of LMA and fiberoptic bronchoscope for an average sized adult patient?**

Number 4 LMA and 5 mm bronchoscope.

○ **What is the incidence of malposition of double lumen tubes revealed by fiberoptic bronchoscopy?**

38 to 78%.

O   **Emergency cricothyroidotomy is performed with a #11 blade between which cartilages?**

Thyroid and cricoid cartilages.

O   **What is the cause of hoarseness after endotracheal intubation lasting more than 7 days?**

Pressure of the endotracheal tube on the recurrent laryngeal nerve between the thyroid lamina and arytenoid cartilage. Hoarseness lasting more than 7 days is rare.

O   **What is the first therapeutic strategy in treatment of airway fire?**

Discontinue oxygen, remove the endotracheal tube, reintubate the trachea and flush the pharynx with cold saline.

O   **Nitrous oxide and oxygen support combustion. What should the gas mixture be when using the CO_2 laser?**

No more than 30% oxygen in nitrogen or helium.

O   **What is the treatment of postextubation stridor?**

Warmed, humidified oxygen, nebulized racemic epinephrine and steroids.

O   **In an intubated patient; hypoxemia, bronchospasm, atelectasis and coughing are all signs of what?**

Right mainstem intubation.

O   **The first sign of negative pressure pulmonary edema following relief of upper airway obstruction is hypoxemia. What is the treatment?**

Diuresis, supplemental oxygen and possible reintubation - i.e. supportive therapy.

O   **How do you diagnose unilateral vocal cord paralysis?**

Flexible endoscopy in the awake patient with inspection of vocal cords.

O   **Superior laryngeal nerve palsy affects which areas of the larynx?**

The superior laryngeal nerve innervates the epiglottis, aryepiglottic folds and the laryngeal structures down to the false cord. Palsy would affect movement of the cricothyroid muscle and alter sensation above the vocal cords.

O   **What are the perioperative complications of laryngoscopy?**

Mechanical complications include possible trauma to eyes, neck, jaw, teeth, lips, mouth, tongue, pharyngeal and laryngeal structures. Others include: hypotension, hypertension, increased intracranial pressure, arrhythmias, bradycardia, laryngospasm, bronchospasm, aspiration, tube misplacement in the stomach or mainstem bronchus, as well as failed intubation.

O   **List the common causes of post-extubation stridor.**

Stridor results from an extrathoracic obstruction (laryngeal edema) and produces inspiratory wheezing. Common causes of post-extubation strider include; too large of an endotracheal tube, trauma from laryngoscopy and/or intubation, excessive coughing or bucking on the tube, neck manipulation during surgery and a current or recent upper respiratory infection. Bilateral recurrent laryngeal nerve injury due to excessive cuff pressure may also cause respiratory distress and obstruction.

○ What are the intubation criteria for patients with burns?

Four standard "P" criteria for intubation: patency of airway, protect against aspiration, pulmonary toilet, and positive-pressure ventilation.

Airway burns are most likely to occur in patients with severe facial burns, intraoral, nasal or pharyngeal burns, or burns suffered in an enclosed-space fire or explosion. Due to the risk of airway edema, hypoxemia, carbon monoxide and cyanide toxicity, early elective intubation should be strongly considered in all patients. Direct heat injury caused by inhalation of air heated to 150 °C or higher produces immediate injury to the airway mucosa resulting in edema, erythema and ulceration above the vocal cords. Edema causing upper airway obstruction may not occur for 12 to 18 hours. Deep face burns may cause edema with obstruction or distortion of the airway, decreased clearance of secretions and impaired protection of the airway from aspiration.

○ What is the incidence of pulmonary edema following laryngospasm?

0.05 to 0.1%.

PERIOPERATIVE EVALUATION

It Is No Measure Of Health To Be Well Adjusted To A Profoundly Sick Society.
Jiddu Krishnamurti

○ **What can be done to reduce the risk of acute alcohol withdrawal in surgical patients?**

Prophylactic benzodiazepines, haloperidol, carbamazepine, beta blockers, and/or clonidine may be useful for both prophylactic and acute treatment of alcohol withdrawal.

○ **What is the difference between hypertensive urgency and a hypertensive emergency?**

Both are defined as a BP > 180/120 mm Hg. A hypertensive *emergency* exists when this severe elevation of BP is associated *with* target organ dysfunction such as hypertensive encephalopathy, intracerebral hemorrhage, acute myocardial infarction, acute left ventricular failure with pulmonary edema, unstable angina pectoris, dissecting aortic aneurysm, or eclampsia. It requires immediate BP reduction (not necessarily to normal) to prevent or limit target organ damage.

Hypertensive *urgency* exists when there is severe elevation in BP *without* progressive target organ dysfunction. It should be treated with oral agents over days and follow up care. There is actually no evidence that failure to treat hypertensive urgency aggressively is associated with any increased short-term risk, while aggressive reduction of BP does have risks.

○ **Should elective surgery be postponed in the case of hypertensive urgency?**

Yes. While in many clinical practices the answer is no, the classic textbook answer is yes. The postponement of surgery is recommended for diastolic BP > 110 as, in a study decades old, that level of BP elevation was associated with severe cardiopulmonary perioperative complications. That exaggeration of poor outcomes occurred without the benefit of IV anti-hypertensive agents, which were not yet developed. While long standing hypertension is the commonest predictive risk factor for death, evidence for improved outcome with acute (for several days before surgery) treatment of very high BP is limited. The benefits of treatment (such as beta blockade) may be unrelated to the actual BP reduction.

○ **The American Heart Association/American College of Cardiology recommend preoperative cardiac investigation in which patients scheduled for noncardiac surgery?**

Those with major clinical indicators or the presence of two of the following: intermediate clinical predictors, high risk surgery, or poor functional capacity.

○ **What are the major clinical indicators?**

Decompensated congested heart failure (CHF), unstable coronary syndrome, significant arrhythmia, and severe valvular disease.

○ **What are the intermediate clinical predictors?**

History of CHF, history of MI, mild angina, diabetes, renal insufficiency.

○ **What surgical procedures are considered high risk?**

Vascular surgery, abdominal or thoracic surgery, prolonged surgery and surgery with significant blood loss.

○ **How is poor functional capacity defined?**

The inability to exercise at 4 METs (metabolic equivalents), which is equivalent to walking up one flight of stairs.

○ **In patients with Parkinson's disease, should levodopa/carbidopa be discontinued prior to surgery?**

No, except for neurosurgical procedures for tremor ablation. Even brief interruptions in scheduled Parkinson's medications may unmask tremors, dysphagia and/or ventilatory inadequacy secondary to chest wall rigidity. Levodopa/carbidopa should be given immediately prior to surgery. If a prolonged post-operative NPO course is anticipated, placement of a duodenal feeding tube should be considered. Prior to thalidotomy, pallidotomy, and placement of deep brain stimulators, Parkinson's medications are deliberately held in order to maximize tremor.

○ **What is the antiemetic of choice for patients with Parkinson's disease?**

Diphenhydramine, which has the additional benefit of reducing tremor by modifying a chemical imbalance of decreased dopamine relative to acetylcholine in the striatum. Propofol may unpredictably reduce tremor.

○ **The ASA practice parameter on preoperative fasting states that the minimum fasting period for drinking non-human milk is how many hours?**

6 hours

○ **Is the above practice parameter a standard, guideline, or advisory?**

A guideline.

○ **What is the difference between the following practice parameters: standards, guidelines, and advisories?**

Practice standards are rules or the minimum requirements for clinical practice. In general they represent accepted principles for sound patient management. They may be modified only under unusual circumstances. **Practice guidelines** describe a basic management strategy or a range of basic management strategies. Guideline recommendations are supported by analysis of the current literature and by a synthesis of expert opinion. They may be adopted, modified or rejected according to clinical needs and constraints. **Practice advisories** are intended to assist decision-making in areas of patient care where scientific evidence is insufficient. Advisories provide a synthesis and analysis of expert opinion. They may be adopted, modified or rejected according to clinical needs and constraints.

○ **Define *sensitivity* of a test.**

The percentage of patients with a disease who have a positive test (positivity in disease).
= True Positives/(True Positives and False Negatives); see table below

○ **Define *specificity*.**

The percentage of healthy patients with a normal test (negativity in health).
= True Negatives/(True Negatives + False Positives); see table below

○ **Define the *predictive value* of a positive test.**

The predictive value of a positive test is the percentage of positive results that are true positives.
= True Positives/(True Positives + False Positives); see table below

	Disease +	Disease -
Test +	a (TP)	b (FP)
Test -	c (FN)	d (TN)

TP = True Positive
FP = False Positive
FN = False Negative
TN = True Negative

Sensitivity = a / a + c
Specificity = d / b + d
Positive Predictive Value = a / a + b

○ Sildenafil (Viagra) is useful for what problem a nurse anesthetist might encounter (aside from the obvious one)?

Phosphodiesterase inhibitors such as sildenafil show promise in the management of pulmonary hypertension through pulmonary vasodilation.

○ What patient-specific risk factors are associated with an increased risk of postoperative nausea and vomiting (PONV)?

Female sex, nonsmoking status, and a history of PONV.

○ Is COPD a contraindication to prescribing beta blockers?

Generally not. A recent (2003) Cochrane analysis states that the use of long term cardioselective beta blockers in the treatment of patients with mild to moderate COPD results in no reduction in FEV_1.
Evidence of treatment of severe COPD is limited, and use of beta blockers in these patients should be done cautiously. Beta blockers should not be used during an acute exacerbation of obstructive airways disease.

○ What is the definition of moderate COPD?

The Global Initiative for Chronic Obstructive Lung Disease (GOLD) Workshop Summary defines COPD as *moderate* when airflow restriction of FEV_1 is < 80 % of predicted. A patient with FEV_1 < 30% of predicted is defined as having *severe* disease.

○ Is asthma a contraindication to the use of beta blockers?

Another recent (2002) Cochrane analysis on the use of cardioselective beta blockers in mild to moderate asthma came to the similar conclusion that the use of long term cardioselective beta blockers in the treatment of patients with mild to moderate asthma results in no reduction in FEV_1.

○ Beta blockers should be titrated to what heart rate in order to maximize protection from perioperative ischemia?

There is no one clear guideline. The four most recent studies on this issue have made the following recommendations: 50-60 beats/min; 55-65 beats/min; 20 % less than previously determined ischemic threshold, but no less than 60 beats/min; less than 80 beats/min. The definition of beta blockade is a resting heart rate of 50-60 bpm and not more than a 20% increase with stress or exercise. That is probably the best single answer to this question.

○ How long should metformin be discontinued prior to elective surgery?

Most clinicians discontinue metformin the day before surgery and restart it when the patient's renal function is stable. Older textbooks state that metformin needs to be discontinued several days before surgery, as metformin may cause metabolic acidosis in patients with hypovolemia or renal insufficiency.

A recent Cochrane meta-analysis of 37,000 patient-years showed no increase in lactic acidosis with metformin use. However, many of the these studies excluded patients with chronic renal insufficiency, liver function abnormalities, congestive heart failure, peripheral vascular disease, pulmonary disease, or age greater than 65. Therefore, these conditions continue to be relative contraindications to proceeding to surgery without discontinuation of metformin therapy.

○   **Why is a history of CHF considered important in a preoperative workup?**

All risk assessment schemes include CHF as a risk factor for increased post operative morbidity and mortality, with an odds ratio of 3.0.

○   **What is the association between smoking and postoperative complications?**

Increased risk of pulmonary, cardiac, and wound complications.

○   **How long does a patient need to stop smoking prior to elective surgery to reduce the risk of postoperative pulmonary complications?**

Smoking cessation results in improvement in some parameters such as a decrease in carboxyhemoglobin levels (with resultant increased tissue oxygen availability) within days. However, evidence on the optimal regime for preoperative smoking cessation is less clear. Limited prospective data suggest that cessation for at least 6 – 8 weeks preoperatively is necessary to decrease the incidence of pulmonary complication, improve ciliary function and pulmonary mechanics and reduce sputum production. There is some evidence to suggest that smoking cessation a few days prior to surgery may increase airway reactivity and anxiety.

○   **How long do nonsteroidal anti-inflammatory drugs inhibit platelet function?**

Aspirin *irreversibly* inhibits platelet function for the life-time of the platelet (about 7 days). Many other drugs such as indomethacin or ibuprofen cause *reversible* inhibition of platelet aggregation, but only at significant serum drug levels and only for 1-2 days.

○   **According to the American Society of Regional Anesthesia and Pain Medicine Consensus Statement, how long before neuraxial anesthesia do NSAIDs need to be stopped?**

NSAIDs do not need to be discontinued. The use of NSAIDs alone does not create a level of risk that will interfere with the performance of neuraxial blocks. There is little data concerning extremely high dose therapy however.

○   **How long before neuraxial anesthesia does clopidogrel (Plavix) need to be stopped?**

7 to 10 days.

○   **How long before neuraxial anesthesia does coumadin need to be stopped?**

4 - 5 days, with documented normalization of the PT.

○   **How long after placement of a coronary artery stent is it safe to perform surgery.**

Six weeks minimum, as surgical stress may precipitate occlusion of the stent. Generally, these patients should be on clopidogrel for three months to a year. Risk/benefit of individual cases may favor shorter periods. At the time of surgery, the patient will need to have discontinued clopidogrel for 7 days. No one has yet studied the newer drug eluting stents with decreased anticoagulant accompanying therapy.

O Are there any therapies that will reduce the perioperative pulmonary risk in a patient with COPD?

Yes. A decades old study showed addressing a reversible component of obstructive disease improved outcomes. There is some evidence that aggressive preoperative treatment of COPD may reduce the risk of perioperative pulmonary complications. This includes cessation of smoking, optimizing pharmacologic therapy (bronchodilators, steroids, antibiotics), detection and treatment of acute pulmonary infection and maximizing nutrition, hydration and chest physiotherapy.

O When should clinicians obtain preoperative spirometry in patients scheduled for non-thoracic surgery?

If a patient has poorly characterized dyspnea or exercise intolerance and diagnostic uncertainty exists between a cardiac or pulmonary limitation and simple deconditioning. In addition, spirometry might be useful in patients who have established obstructive lung disease if it is not clear from the clinical evaluation if patients' chronic therapy has maximally improved function.

O Should elective surgery be delayed in an asthmatic patient who is wheezing?

Yes, if the patient has not been absolutely optimized. History, physical examination, temperature, WBC, chest x-ray and response to aerosolized bronchodilator therapy should be assessed. Wheezing may be caused by bronchoconstriction, inspissated secretions, aspiration, vocal cord dysfunction, pulmonary edema or pneumothorax. If a patient with severe persistent asthma is compliant with optimal drug therapy and although still wheezing, is considered to be stable and optimized, it may be reasonable to proceed, employing minimal instrumentation of the airway, and maximizing drugs that are bronchodilating. If however, the etiology of the wheezing is not firmly established, or therapy could be improved, surgery should be delayed

O According to the ACLS protocol, what drugs are first choice to control the heart rate of a patient with atrial fibrillation and a rapid ventricular response?

Diltiazem (or other calcium channel blocker), or a beta blocker. Amiodarone is an alternative; but it may also convert the rhythm to sinus, which may be undesirable before anticoagulation. If the patient is unstable, electrical cardioversion should be considered rather than adding a second drug.

O What drugs can be harmful in the treatment of atrial fibrillation in a patient with WPW (Wolff-Parkinson-White)?

Adenosine, calcium channel blockers, digoxin, and possibly beta blockers slow conduction through the AV node, but not necessarily through the accessory pathway, which may increase the ventricular rate. Amiodarone or procainamide are the recommended drugs in this situation.

O Does a 50 yr old male with moderate mitral regurgitation, undergoing knee arthroplasty require SBE prophylaxis?

No. Although this patient has a valvular lesion, clean surgery through uninfected tissue does not require SBE prophylaxis.

O How is the creatinine level affected by age?

Serum creatinine levels slowly rise with age after 40 years.

O What is the death rate from general anesthesia in patients with an ASA class I or II?

Approximately 1 in 200,000 to 500,000.

○   **At what point should a patient be transfused?**

This is not a simple question. The use of a single hemoglobin "trigger" of 10 g/dL of hemoglobin for surgical transfusion is no longer recommended. One must consider all physiologic and surgical factors that place the patient at risk for complications of inadequate oxygenation. Transfusion is rarely indicated when the hemoglobin concentration is greater than 10 g/dL and is almost always indicated when it is less than 6 g/dL, especially when the anemia is acute. In clinical practice, most patients at risk for ischemia are transfused to a hematocrit of 27 to 30%, while those who are young and healthy may tolerate a hematocrit of 18 to 21% without detrimental effects. So, in summary, oxygen delivery is optimized with a Hgb of 10g/dl, and those with critical organs at risk (ischemic heart disease, chronic renal insufficiency, cerebrovascular disease) should probably be transfused to keep Hgb > 10 g/dl while those without compromised critical organ blood flow can be transfused at a Hgb of 6-7 gm/dl. Prolonged times with a Hgb < 5 g/dl is associated with poor outcomes.

○   **Is preoperative cardiac testing recommended for patients who have received doxorubicin (adriamycin) ?**

Female gender, age at treatment (younger is worse), cumulative dose, thorax radiation, and more time since treatment are risk factors for myocardial dysfunction after doxorubicin. These factors, and the type of surgery, must be taken into account when deciding whether to perform cardiac testing before anesthesia.

○   **Why would a pre-operative hematocrit in a pregnant woman be low?**

Pregnant women have a relative anemia. While the red blood cell volume increases 20%, the plasma volume increases 45%, resulting in a dilutional decrease in the hematocrit.

○   **Why are β-blockers not used alone for preoperative preparation of patients with pheochromocytoma?**

If β-receptors are blocked in these patients before the administration of phenoxybenzamine (alpha receptor antagonist), norepinephrine and epinephrine will produce unopposed alpha stimulation, resulting in a further increase in peripheral vascular resistance and worsening hypertension.

○   **A patient with symptomatic hyperthyroidism is scheduled for elective surgery the next day. What should you do for this patient?**

Cancel the case and refer the patient to an endocrinologist for preoperative assessment and preparation.

Treatment includes antithyroid drugs (propylthiouracil, iodine), radioactive iodine, and surgical subtotal thyroidectomy. If one must proceed, anesthetic risks include acute exacerbation of hyperthyroidism caused by surgical stress (thyroid storm) resulting in tachycardia, hyperthermia, hemodynamic instability and arrhythmia. Induction with volatile agents is slowed due to the increased cardiac output and the rate of drug metabolism is increased, with no change in MAC. Emergent cases should be treated intraoperatively with invasive monitoring, beta-adrenergic blockade, resuscitation with IV fluids and temperature control. Refractory hypotension from relative cortisol deficiency may respond to corticosteroids. The first dose of PTU can be administered down the nasogastric tube. Thyroid storm usually occurs 6 to 18 hours after surgery, so the patient should be monitored in a surgical critical care setting postoperatively.

○   **What is the most common significant cardiac valvular lesion found in the non-cardiac patient planned for surgery?**

Aortic stenosis. Mitral valve prolapse is the most common valvular disorder occurring in 5-10% of the general population, but it is often not significant.

○ **What are some causes of Q-T prolongation?**

Electrolyte imbalances: hypokalemia, hypomagnesemia, hypocalcemia.
Antiarrhythmic drugs: quinidine, procainamide, sotalol, amiodarone.
CNS disorders: subarachnoid or IC hemorrhage, closed head injury, tumor.
Cardiac: myocarditis, ischemia.
Drugs: phenothiazines, TCAs, lithium, droperidol.
Congenital form (Jervell and Lange-Nielson syndrome)

○ **What is SLUDGE syndrome?**

Signs and symptoms of muscarinic overstimulation in a patient with myasthenia gravis.

Salivation
Lacrimation
Urinary incontinence
Diarrhea
GI upset and hypermotility
Eyes: miosis and blurred vision (paralysis of accommodation)

○ **Do monoamine oxidase inhibitors (MAOI's) need to be stopped in a patient before surgery?**

No. However, indirect acting sympathomimetics and meperidine must be avoided in these patients to prevent an exaggerated response and hyperpyrexia, respectively.

○ **At what age would an otherwise healthy patient need a preoperative screening chest x-ray?**

In an otherwise healthy patient, unless indicated by the surgical procedure or by history, a CXR should be done in all patients over 75 years of age. This is based on the risk/benefits of a general group of patients. Some authors would suggest the cutoff at 60 years of age.

○ **An 18-year-old healthy white male is scheduled for knee surgery. What types of preoperative testing are mandatory for this type of patient and surgery?**

None. For male patients with no significant past medical history that are scheduled for minor surgical procedures there is no "mandatory" preoperative testing.

○ **Can the FEV_1 value on preoperative pulmonary function tests indicate whether or not a patient has obstructive lung disease?**

No. The FEV_1 may be reduced in both obstructive and restrictive lung disease. It is necessary to know the FVC as well to determine if the pattern is obstructive.

○ **What is the leading cause of postoperative morbidity in patients undergoing surgery for peripheral vascular disease?**

The major cause of postoperative death is cardiac, primarily myocardial infarction.

Patients between the fifth and eighth decades with peripheral vascular disease have multiple medical problems: coronary artery disease (65%), angina pectoris (15%), hypertension (35%), congestive heart failure (10-15%), history of myocardial infarction (25%), cerebrovascular disease, renal insufficiency, and diabetes mellitus. In addition, many are heavy smokers with COPD, chronic bronchitis and bronchospasm.

○ **What surgeries are considered high risk (>5%) for perioperative myocardial infarction?**

The highest risk non-cardiac procedure is aortic aneurysm repair.

• Emergent major operations, especially in the elderly
• Aortic and other major vascular surgeries
• Peripheral vascular surgery
• Prolonged surgical procedure with significant fluid shifts and/or blood loss (major abdominal and thoracic)

O   **Which two classes of hypertensive medications cause withdrawal hypertension and should not be stopped prior to a patient having surgery?**

β-blockers and clonidine.

Withdrawal of both is associated with rebound hypertension and myocardial ischemia. All anti-hypertensive medications should be continued until the day of surgery with the possible exception of diuretics (depletion of intravascular volume) and ACE inhibitors (hypotension with induction). Note that withdrawal hypertension may occur with many different anti-hypertensive drugs including reserpine, hydralazine, guanethidine, methyldopa and hydrochlorothiazide.

O   **What liver function tests are most predictive of outcome following surgery in patients with chronic liver disease?**

Laboratory evaluation of liver function is complicated by the liver's large functional reserve; routine laboratory values may be normal in the presence of significant underlying disease. Those that loosely reflect liver function include prothrombin time, albumin, bilirubin and serum ammonia level.

Child's scoring system is a predictive scoring index to stratify mortality risk in patients having hepatobiliary surgery.

Group	A	B	C
Serum bilirubin (mg/dl)	< 2	2 to 3	> 3
Serum albumin (g/dl)	> 3.5	3 to 3.5	< 3
Ascites	none	easily controlled	poorly controlled
Encephalopathy	none	minimal	advanced
Nutrition	excellent	good	poor

Using this method, mortality rate of 10%, 31% and 76% were identified in Child's class A, B, and C, respectively. The Pugh modification replaces nutrition with prothrombin time prolongation (A: 1-4 sec; B: 5-6 sec; C: > 6 sec). In patients with primary biliary cirrhosis, the bilirubin limits are increased in each category.

O   **At what diastolic blood pressure would it be reasonable to delay an elective surgical case?**

The answer to this question is dictated by the patient, surgical procedure, surgeon's, and anesthesia provider's preference. A reasonable cut-off would be a diastolic pressure of greater than 110 mm Hg, in a patient previously undiagnosed or not well medically managed. Old studies suggest an increased risk of severe cardiopulmonary complications.

If the patient is normally well controlled but suffering from "white coat anxiety", treatment may be as simple as IV anxiolytics and reevaluation. Checking several serial blood pressures is appropriate. Clonidine will reduce lability of intraoperative blood pressure and anesthetic requirements. Diastolic hypertension is associated with an increase in SVR and is thought to be the major contributor to hypertensive morbidity (coronary artery disease, intracranial hemorrhage and renal failure). Cardiac complications include: myocardial ischemia, congestive heart failure, intraoperative lability in blood pressure or death.

ANESTHESIA RISKS

Great deeds are usually wrought at great risks.
Herodotus

O   **What is the incidence of malignant hyperthermia (MH)?**

The incidence of malignant hyperthermia is about 1 in 50,000 when inhaled anesthetics and succinylcholine are considered. For reasons that are not well understood, MH is five to ten times more common in children than adults.

O   **Is cricoid pressure effective in the presence of a nasogastric tube?**

Yes.

O   **What is the recommended inflation pressure of endotracheal tube cuffs?**

The cuff pressure should be less than 25-35 mm Hg (capillary perfusion pressure of trachea mucosa), otherwise tracheal mucosal damage will occur, including possible necrosis.

O   **What is the incidence of "sore throat" after endotracheal intubation?**

Incidence 45-70%.

O   **If a patient becomes cyanotic, what is the likely hemoglobin saturation and PaO_2?**

The hemoglobin saturation is less than 70% and the PaO_2 is about 40 mm Hg, assuming arterial concentration of desaturated blood is 5 g/dL at hemoglobin of 16 g/dL.

O   **What is the recommended maximum duration of deep hypothermic cardiac arrest (DHCA)?**

The limit for "safe" circulatory arrest is a duration of 35-40 minutes.

O   **A patient complains of paresthesia in his left little finger after CABG. What is wrong?**

The incidence of postoperative brachial plexus injury is 5-30% in these patients.   These injuries are probably due to excessive chest retraction stretching the brachial plexus, hyperextension of the arms or direct nerve compression. Ischemic injury is compounded by a decrease in temperature and perfusion pressure during cardiopulmonary bypass.

O   **A patient with COPD complains of severe dyspnea after interscalene brachial plexus blockade. What is your differential diagnosis?**

Phrenic nerve block is almost guaranteed with interscalene anesthesia, and associated with a 25% reduction in pulmonary function. A pneumothorax may be a rare possibility. Also consider an epidural or intrathecal injection causing dyspnea with hypotension or local anesthetic toxicity.

O   **If you need to transfuse blood in an immunosuppressed patient, what are your instructions to Transfusion Services?**

Ask the blood bank for irradiated leuko-depleted blood. Removing leukocytes prevents graft versus host disease by suppressing lymphocytic mitotic activity and irradiation prevents the transmission of CMV.

○   **A patient tells you that he is allergic to penicillin. What is the reported incidence of penicillin allergy, and what is the true incidence of fatal anaphylactic reaction?**

Ten to 20% of hospitalized patients claim to be allergic to penicillin. The incidence of fatal reactions occur in 0.002% of penicillin treated cases, or 375 deaths per year in the U.S.

○   **What is the mortality of perioperative myocardial reinfarction?**

The reported mortality from reinfarction after noncardiac surgery is 50-70%, based on old studies.

○   **A patient had an MI two months ago. What is his cardiovascular risk with subsequent elective surgery?**

Traditionally, the rate of perioperative myocardial infarction rate in patients who have had an MI within three months is 30%, decreasing to 5% by six months. More recent studies suggest the risk is highly variable, depending on the amount of myocardium still at risk for ischemia, and the nature of the previous infarct (non-transmural with a higher reinfarction rate). According to recent studies, after an MI, 6 weeks is considered the time of high risk for a perioperative cardiac event, because it is the mean healing time of the infracted lesion. The period from 6 weeks to 3 months is of intermediate risk. More than 3 months is required for cases complicated with arrhythmias and ventricular dysfunction.

○   **A surgeon wishes to repair an inguinal hernia in a two month old baby as outpatient surgery. Is this appropriate?**

There is a concern that infants may develop apnea following general anesthesia. It is recommended that all former preterm infants younger than 55 weeks postconceptual age and all anemic former preterm infants be admitted to monitor their recovery.

○   **What factors predispose a patient to developing serious pneumonitis after aspiration?**

The factors of greatest concern in aspiration are gastric volume > 25 cc with a pH of less than 2.5, and aspiration of particulate matter.

○   **A surgeon is applying a 4% topical cocaine solution to the nasal mucosa in preparation for surgery. What is the recommended maximum dose of cocaine?**

The maximum recommended dose of intranasal cocaine is 3 mg/kg.

○   **A child is having outpatient strabismus surgery. What is the risk of postoperative nausea and vomiting?**

The incidence of significant postoperative nausea and vomiting is 50-80%.

○   **A trauma patient is being transfused with type O Rh-negative blood and has already been given eight units. Type-specific blood for the patient is now available. Should you switch?**

If more than two units of type O Rh-negative un-crossmatched whole blood have been administered, the blood bank must determine that transfused anti-A and anti-B antibodies have fallen to levels that permit transfusion of type-specific blood. There is a risk of a major transfusion reaction if the patient has received enough anti-A or anti-B antibodies in type-O blood to cause hemolysis if A, B or AB blood is subsequently given. It takes significantly more PRBC units to potentially transfuse enough plasma containing anti-A, anti-B antibodies to prevent switching to type specific blood.

O   **What are the risks of using tourniquets for extremity surgery?**

Neurologic injury resulting from inflation of a tourniquet is a function of tourniquet pressure and the duration of inflation. The recommended pressure is 100 mm Hg above systolic pressure or a tourniquet pressure of 250 mm Hg while maintaining the systolic pressure at 90-100 mm Hg. Tourniquet time should be less than two hours. (in the upper extremity and four hours in the lower extremity to avoid ischemic tissue damage.) delete red portion of sentence

O   **Are there any advantages of regional versus general anesthesia for total hip replacement?**

Blood loss is decreased about 30-50%. There is less risk of transfusion and a lower incidence of DVT. There may be less acute postoperative confusion. The quality of interface between bone and methylmethacrylate may be improved.

O   **Why is it recommended to administer a vagolytic drug prior to laryngoscopy in infants?**

Infants have a higher resting vagal tone, and laryngoscopy excites the vagal nerve, leading to potential vasovagal symptoms like complete heart block or sinus arrest. Intravenous atropine 10 μg/kg is given to prevent bradycardia and hypotension. The effect of atropine also helps with bradycardia and hypotension seen with the inhaled anesthetic halothane. Atropine increases cardiac output by increasing heart rate.

O   **What inhaled anesthetic agent is recommended for use in neurosurgery and why?**

Isoflurane. The level of CBF necessary to prevent ischemic changes in CNS tissue is least with isoflurane (critical cerebral blood flow is 10 ml/100gm/min) compared to enflurane (15 ml/100g/min) and halothane (20 ml/100 g/min). All volatile agents depress the cerebral metabolic rate for oxygen ($CMRO_2$) and cause cerebral vasodilation. This "uncoupling" of $CMRO_2$ and CBF is most marked with halothane and least with isoflurane. In addition, to prevent an increase in ICP, CO_2 reduction should be initiated just prior to the introduction of halothane. CO_2 reactivity is generally retained with isoflurane and sevoflurane.

O   **In premature babies or neonates, why is the pulse oximeter probe preferentially placed on the right hand or ear lobe?**

Placement of the probe on the right hand or ear lobe will accurately reflect preductal (coronary, cerebral) oxygenation. During the first several weeks of life these patients may develop persistent fetal circulation with stress (hypoxia, hypothermia, acidosis). In this case, if right atrial pressure exceeds left atrial pressure, there may be a right-to-left shunting of blood through the ductus arteriosus (and possibly foreman ovale).

O   **A three-year-old in the PACU shows signs of upper airway obstruction shortly after general anesthesia. The nurse suggests a nasal airway. Is this appropriate?**

No. Small children have abundant, friable lymphoid tissue in the nasopharynx which is a contraindication to nasal airways or blind nasal intubation.

O   **A patient is to have a hysterectomy for endometrial carcinoma. What are the implications of prior chemotherapy?**

Doxorubicin (Adriamycin) used in the treatment of endometrial carcinoma causes myelosuppression and has well-recognized cardiac side effects. The risk of irreversible cardiomyopathy increases with a cumulative dose greater than 550 mg/m^2, prior radiotherapy and concurrent cyclophosphamide treatment. Cisplatin causes acute renal failure, peripheral neuropathies and severe nausea.

O   **A patient develops brachial plexus nerve palsy after vaginal hysterectomy. What are the relevant positioning concerns?**

Typically the patient would be in lithotomy position with arms placed outstretched on arm boards. Care must be exercised to avoid arm adduction beyond 90 degrees, which may be exacerbated in steep Trendelenburg. The patient's head should be in a neutral position. Turning it to one side causes the brachial plexus on the contralateral side to be stretched. Flexion of the arms at the elbow will tend to relieve tension on the brachial plexus.

○ **During diagnostic laparoscopy for primary infertility, the patient suddenly develops hypotension, hypoxemia, and then arrests. What is the problem?**

There are many possible etiologies for the arrest. The most likely problem due to the described "sudden" nature of the problem is CO_2 embolus. Possibilities specific to this procedure include: CO_2 gas embolus, massive hemorrhage and pneumothorax or pneumomediastinum. One must attempt to diagnose the problem quickly and provide supportive care and resuscitation in the interim.

○ **A VBAC patient with a well functioning labor epidural infusion complains of persistent breakthrough pain. What are you concerned about?**

Uterine rupture. Always consider this possibility in patients with persistent breakthrough pain with epidural analgesia. Diaphragmatic irritation from uterine rupture may be referred to the shoulder. Abdominal ultrasound will confirm the diagnosis.

○ **Shortly after placing a pulmonary artery catheter (PAC), you notice bright red blood in the endotracheal tube. What is wrong?**

Your worst clinical nightmare…pulmonary artery rupture. The incidence is between 0.064% and 0.20% and mortality is high. Risk factors for PA rupture include advanced age, female sex, pulmonary hypertension and coagulopathy. Iatrogenic factors include inflation of the balloon when the catheter tip is positioned distally, overinflation of the balloon and prolonged wedging of the catheter. Treatment for PA rupture is initially to protect the patient from asphyxiation with bronchoscopy, suctioning, oxygen, positive pressure ventilation and lung isolation. Surgery may be necessary. Whether to deflate the balloon and pull the pulmonary artery catheter back or to leave it in place to retard bleeding and to provide a route for administration of fibrin glue is controversial.

○ **A patient's oxygen delivery is impaired by severe anemia. What are the compensatory mechanisms?**

Oxygen delivery is determined by arterial oxygen content and cardiac output (CO). Deficiencies in oxygen delivery may be due to a low alveolar O_2, a low hemoglobin concentration or inadequate cardiac output. In severe anemia, arterial oxygen content (normally 20 mL O_2/dL blood with hemoglobin 15 g/dL) is decreased. The compensatory mechanisms in anemia are to increase CO and tissue oxygen extraction.

○ **A patient complains of severe back pain after 2-chloroprocaine epidural anesthesia. Is this a significant problem?**

As many as 40% of patients will complain of back pain with 2-3% solutions of chloroprocaine. This pain is time limited and is not associated with neurologic deficits. The preservative disodium EDTA (ethylenediaminetetraacetic acid) is a high-affinity calcium chelator and may cause local muscle spasms by leaching calcium from paravertebral muscles. Chloroprocaine has become available in a preservative-free preparation.

○ **A patient with multiple sclerosis (MS) presents for left total knee replacement. What is your preference for choice of anesthesia?**

General anesthesia is usually preferred to regional anesthesia (RA). MS is not an absolute contraindication to RA, but postoperative exacerbation of the disease due to stress, pain or temperature elevation (an increase of 0.5 °C may completely block conduction in demyelinated nerve fibers) may be confused with presumed residual effects of RA. Epidural is recommended rather than spinal anesthesia, which has been reported to cause exacerbation of the disease. Epidural and other regional techniques appear to have no adverse effect.

○ **A patient arrests 10 minutes after induction of spinal anesthesia. What do you do?**

The most likely cause is a high spinal, and supportive therapy is the treatment including airway control and BP support. However, unexpected cardiac arrest during spinal anesthesia has been described. Sudden severe bradycardia and asystolic arrest can develop without evidence of high spinal respiratory depression or hypoxemia and hypercarbia. Immediate resuscitation along standard ACLS guidelines is indicated. For severe bradycardia or cardiac arrest, full resuscitation doses of epinephrine should be promptly administered Review drugs administered actions and therapeutic maneuvers performed prior to the arrest and correct any obvious underlying causes. The differential diagnosis includes profound sympathectomy, arrhythmia, oversedation, "high spinal", airway obstruction, hypo- or hyperkalemia.

○ **A patient is concerned about nerve damage with peripheral nerve block. What can you do to minimize these problems?**

Use preservative-free local anesthetic solutions, small short-beveled block needles, avoid the use of epinephrine and do not intentionally elicit paraesthesias, although this is not supported by available data. Avoid heavy sedation to make the presence of paresthesias evident, and prevent accidental injection into a nerve.

○ **A retrobulbar block is performed for cataract surgery. Shortly after injection, the patient has a respiratory arrest. What should you do?**

The optic nerve is usually a brain tract, and it is possible to have an intrathecal injection via the optic nerve sheath with this nerve block. Treatment is supportive and the patient usually recovers promptly. If the patient has good analgesia upon recovery, it is possible to proceed with surgery.

○ **You notice the anesthesia machine you are about to use does not have a functioning oxygen analyzer. What should you do?**

There are several possible equipment problems that could cause a hypoxic gas mixture to be delivered to the patient that can only be detected by an oxygen analyzer. AANA standard VIII for Nurse Anesthesia practice addresses proper inspection of the anesthesia machine and monitors.

○ **You need to use halothane for your next case. Your anesthesia technician says there is a full vaporizer sitting on the table behind the machine and you should just switch out the vaporizers. What are your concerns?**

Anesthetic vaporizers should always be secured in the upright position. It is possible someone may have tipped this vaporizer over, and liquid anesthetic may be in the bypass chamber, resulting in a high output concentration. It should not be used until it has been flushed for 20-30 minutes at high flow rates with the vaporizer set at a low concentration.

○ **A patient was prescribed "Hurricane spray ad lib" by the surgeons for nasogastric tube discomfort. The patient is cyanotic, agitated and tachycardic with frequent PVCs. What is wrong?**

Hurricane spray (Beutlich) is 20% Benzocaine. The patient has benzocaine-induced methemoglobinemia. Treatment is supplemental oxygen and intravenous methylene blue.

○ **A patient is receiving amiodarone for suppression of ventricular ectopy. What are your concerns for administering anesthesia for femoral-popliteal bypass surgery?**

Amiodarone causes a peripheral neuropathy and has been associated with intractable hypotension and bradyarrhythmias unresponsive to catecholamines under general anesthesia. Despite recommendations to discontinue 2 weeks prior to elective surgery, patients often require continuation for intractable arrhythmias.

○   **Norepinephrine (Levophed) is being infused through a peripheral IV, and extravasation is noted, with blanching of the skin. What should be done?**

The area should be infiltrated with phentolamine 5-10 mg in 10 cc saline to minimize the risk of skin necrosis. Phentolamine antagonizes undesirable alpha stimulation. Administration of norepinephrine should be restricted to central venous access.

○   **An otherwise healthy patient presents for knee arthroscopy. One gram of cefazolin is given preoperatively. General anesthesia is induced with midazolam, sodium thiopental, fentanyl and vecuronium. The patient unexpectedly arrests on induction. What is wrong?**

The most likely cause is an allergic reaction to intravenously administered drugs (antibiotics, muscle relaxants > thiobarbiturates > opiates). Other causes of hypotension (such as hypovolemia unmasked by thiopental) should be considered in the differential diagnosis. High doses of fentanyl and vecuronium have been associated with vagotonic bradycardic arrest.

○   **Following resection of a pheochromocytoma, the patient becomes hypoglycemic in the PACU. What is the cause?**

The high serum catecholamine levels in this disorder cause increased glycogenolysis, and gluconeogenesis and decreased insulin secretion. With removal of the tumor, rapid decrease in catecholamine levels can result in marked hypoglycemia.

○   **A thyroidectomy patient in the PACU is having respiratory distress. What is your differential diagnosis?**

Vocal cord dysfunction from recurrent laryngeal nerve damage, cervical hematoma with airway compression, tracheomalacia and pneumothorax.

○   **A patient is to have lower extremity revascularization surgery. What is the risk of coronary artery disease (CAD)?**

Less than 10% of vascular surgery patients have normal coronary arteries, and more than 50% have advanced or severe CAD.

○   **A patient with COPD is to have a right lung resection for carcinoma. How do you interpret preoperative pulmonary function tests (PFTs)?**

PFTs suggestive of increased operative risk for pneumonectomy and prolonged postoperative ventilatory support include: FVC< 50% predicted, FEV_1< 2L, FEV_1/FVC< 50%, MBC (maximum breathing capacity, or maximum minute ventilation)< 50% predicted, RV/TLC> 50%, diffusing capacity < 50% predicted, hypercapnia on room air, predicted postoperative FEV_1 < 0.85 L or > 70% blood flow to the diseased lung.

○   **Are patients with myasthenia gravis at increased risk for aspiration pneumonitis?**

Yes. Myasthenics are at increased risk for aspiration pneumonitis, as more than 60% will have a history of bulbar symptoms such as difficulty swallowing and clearing secretions during the course of their disease.

○   **You suggest the possibility of epidural narcotics after caesarean section to the surgeon, but he expresses concern about urinary retention. What can you tell him?**

Urinary retention occurs in up to 40% of patients receiving epidural narcotics. The incidence is probably lower with lipid soluble opioids than with morphine. If the plan is to have an indwelling urinary catheter, this is probably not an issue. The same side effects are observed with parenteral opioids (itching, nausea, urinary retention, sedation and ileus).

○ **In a patient with ischemic heart disease, why is tachycardia potentially more likely to precipitate ischemia than hypertension?**

Hypertension will increase myocardial oxygen demand, but it will also increase myocardial oxygen supply by increasing coronary perfusion pressure and perfusion time (if the heart rate reflexively slows). Tachycardia increases myocardial oxygen demand and decreases myocardial oxygen supply by decreasing diastolic coronary perfusion time.

○ **You are attempting to remove a pulmonary artery catheter in the PACU and encounter resistance. What should you do?**

Do not forcibly remove the catheter. Verify that the balloon is deflated. The catheter may be knotted, possibly around the cordae tendineae. Forcible removal could cause cardiac or vascular injury. Radiologic evaluation is necessary.

○ **A surgical patient is concerned about his risk of death due to anesthesia. What would you tell him?**

Numerous recent studies suggest that the risk of death from anesthesia is between one in 10,000 and one in 200,000. Far more important to perioperative morbidity and mortality are the patient's comorbidity and surgery risk factors.

○ **What are the most common causes of anesthesia-related death?**

Sixty percent of anesthesia-related deaths and 90% of anesthesia-related brain damage is caused by embarrassment of the respiratory system.

Ninety percent of cases are still deemed associated with operator error. The top five errors are overdose, wrong choice of anesthetic agent, inadequate preparation, inadequate crisis management and inadequate postoperative management.

○ **Why were sodium bicarbonate (NaHCO$_3$) and calcium chloride (CaCl$_2$) removed from cardiac resuscitation protocols?**

There is concern that NaHCO$_3$ may cause paradoxical intracellular acidosis (leading to myocardial depression), hyperosmolality and hypernatremia. Intracellular influx of calcium is intimately involved in the terminal stages of cell death, and this is a concern in the setting of resuscitation. CaCl$_2$ may also prevent reflow of blood into ischemic areas of the brain and heart, worsening outcome.

○ **Is it possible to cause ventricular fibrillation with electrocautery?**

No. Ventricular fibrillation is prevented by the use of alternating current of ultra-high frequency (0.5-3 million Hz) compared with line power (50-60 Hz).

○ **You are performing a general anesthetic and suddenly the power fails. After a few long moments, the lights come back on, but only some of the electrical equipment is working. What should you do?**

You are probably on emergency power. Electrical receptacles that are backed up on emergency power are red and all essential equipment should be plugged into these receptacles. You should finish the case expediently, and expect further power interruption. Do not start any elective cases on emergency power. You may consider changing your anesthetic technique to total intravenous anesthesia (hypnotic, narcotic, amnestic and muscle relaxant) and may need to manually ventilate the patient, preferably on 100% oxygen without using the anesthesia machine.

○   **A patient expresses concern about postoperative nausea and vomiting (PONV). What would be your advice?**

PONV is multifactorial in origin. The risk of PONV with general anesthesia is between 20% and 50%. It is much less common with regional anesthesia, approximately 15%, especially if one avoids narcotics. Propofol-based anesthetic regimens have an inherent anti-emetic effect. Prophylactic administration of 5 HT-3 blockers such as 12.5 mg dolasetron or 4 mg ondansetron work equally well as the much cheaper 1.25 mg of droperidol. In addition one may avoid nitrous oxide, administer antiemetics, adequately hydrate, remove gastric contents with suctioning, limit mask ventilation – especially avoiding high pressures or inexperienced operators, avoid opioid-based anesthesia and administer a bolus dose of steroids. Strabismus and laparoscopic surgery have more PONV, especially in young women during menstruation.

ALLERGIC REACTIONS

You See Things; And You Say "Why?" But I Dream Things That Never Were; And I Say "Why Not?"
George Bernard Shaw

○ **In general, prostaglandins produce what symptoms?**

Prostaglandins, produced from arachidonic acid via the cyclo-oxygenase pathway, are mediators of the inflammatory response, and the symptoms produced include: bronchoconstriction, systemic hypotension secondary to peripheral vasodilation, increased capillary permeability and coronary spasm. Prostaglandin E_1 and E_2, however, produce bronchodilation, inhibit histamine release and produce vasodilation of the peripheral, coronary and pulmonary circulations.

○ **What is the definition of *atopy* and what is the significance of this diagnosis?**

A patient has an *atopy* history if there are symptoms or signs of allergy including: asthma, allergic rhinitis, conjunctivitis, urticaria, eczema, multiple drug allergies, a history of anaphylaxis or a history of positive skin prick test or another test that signifies sensitivity to a substance. Patients with a history of allergy to non-drug allergens appear to have a much higher risk of having latex allergy or anaphylactic or anaphylactoid reactions during anesthesia.

○ **Early signs of anaphylaxis that can be seen in the awake patient include what?**

Flushing
Urticaria (hives)
Itching
Dizziness or decreased level of consciousness
Dyspnea and/or chest tightness

○ **Signs of anaphylaxis that may be seen in patients undergoing general anesthesia include what?**

Cardiac, respiratory or cutaneous manifestations including: tachycardia, hypotension, arrhythmia; bronchospasm, increase in peak airway pressures, hypoxemia, laryngeal or pulmonary edema; flushing, rash or hives.
Hypotension may be the only sign of anaphylaxis under general anesthesia.

○ **What is the most likely cause of death from anaphylaxis?**

Cardiovascular collapse. However, inability to intubate, ventilate or oxygenate secondary to upper airway edema, bronchospasm, pulmonary edema or a combination of any of the above also put the non-intubated patient at risk.

○ **What is the differential diagnosis following a suspected anaphylactic episode?**

In the awake patient, a vasovagal reaction can easily be confused with anaphylaxis because the patient becomes diaphoretic, nauseated and presyncopal. Itching, flushing, urticaria, wheezing or cyanosis, however, will not occur with a vasovagal reaction. With general anesthesia, the differential diagnosis includes: administration of anesthetic drugs with their associated hemodynamic effects, hypotension from other causes, bronchospasm, septic shock, cardiac arrhythmia, myocardial infarction, pneumothorax, fat embolism, pulmonary embolism or edema and venous air embolism.

○ **What is the mainstay of treatment for anaphylaxis?**

Epinephrine.

O   **What are the beneficial effects of epinephrine during anaphylaxis?**

It maintains myocardial and cerebral perfusion through peripheral vasoconstriction. It acts as a bronchodilator and decreases antigen-induced bronchospastic mediator release from mast cells.

Remember that the clinical effects of epinephrine are dose-dependent. *Beta-adrenergic* effects occur at lower dosages and *alpha-adrenergic* effects predominate at dosages greater than 10 µg/min.

O   **Describe the initial treatment protocol for intraoperative anaphylaxis?**

Stop the administration of the expected allergen. If the allergen has been given IM or SQ, place a tourniquet above the injection site and consider injecting a small dose (0.2 mg) of epinephrine at the site to reduce uptake of the allergen into the intravascular space.

Maintain the airway and administer 100% oxygen. Support oxygenation and ventilation.

Intubate the patient if an endotracheal tube is not already in place.

Discontinue all anesthetic agents because they are cardiovascular depressants. Remember that inhalation agents are not appropriate bronchodilators during anaphylaxis and that halothane also sensitizes the heart to catecholamines, leading to arrhythmias.

Rapid intravenous volume administration should be started. Liters of fluid may be needed because the patient can have large volume deficits secondary to massive losses due to the increased vascular permeability.

Epinephrine (the dose and route of administration depends on your clinical judgment). However, an infusion titrated to clinical effect is less dangerous than the typical CPR-like 1 mg bolus which can lead to unwanted side effects.

Inform the surgeons. Check for drugs injected or instilled into a body cavity. Prepare to terminate the surgery if there is no response to therapy.

O   **How much epinephrine should you give during anaphylaxis?**

Good clinical judgment is the key here!

If the blood pressure is normal, it is not necessary to give epinephrine intravenously.

If a patient is hypotensive and an intravenous line (IV) is in place, start with 5-10 micrograms (µg) IV boluses of epinephrine and gradually increase the dose by 5-10 micrograms every 30-60 seconds until the blood pressure improves.

With cardiovascular collapse, cardiopulmonary resuscitative doses of epinephrine should be given (0.5 to 1 mg IV and repeat as needed).

If an IV is not yet in place, 0.5 mL of 1:1000 epinephrine can be administered subcutaneously. *However, remember that the intramuscular and subcutaneous absorption of medications is unreliable when a patient is in shock.*

Epinephrine can be administered through the endotracheal tube in shock situations; however, the response is slower and somewhat delayed. If the patient has an epidural or spinal anesthetic in place, higher doses of epinephrine may be required because the patient may be partially sympathectomized.

Remember that epinephrine must be administered during an anaphylactic reaction even if tachycardia is present!

O   **Describe the secondary line of treatment of anaphylaxis.**

Administer H_1 antagonist diphenhydramine 50 mg iv; the use of H_2 blocking agents such as ranitidine or cimetidine is controversial.

Start a catecholamine infusion for persistent hypotension. Epinephrine 0.05 to 0.1 μg/kg/min (microgram per kilogram) is a good place to start

Place invasive arterial and venous catheters for monitoring, infusion of vasoactive drugs and blood sampling.

Give bronchodilators for bronchospasm. Epinephrine, aerosolized bronchodilators or as a last resort, aminophylline. Aminophylline may decrease mediator release by increasing intracellular cyclic AMP levels, but cardiac arrhythmias are a risk.

Re-evaluate the airway for persistent laryngeal edema.

Give corticosteroids now and over the next 24 hours to prevent delayed reactions; however, they likely have no acute effects. Hydrocortisone is the preferred steroid due to its rapid onset and response in alleviating respiratory symptoms.

Obtain an arterial blood gas and correct acidosis if present with sodium bicarbonate and/or increased ventilation. Reassess volume status.

In the absence of any identifiable causes, consider latex allergy and remove all latex products in contact with the patient.

Provide continuous observation for at least 24 hours and again re-evaluate the airway frequently prior to extubation.

○ **How long does it take for signs of anaphylaxis to occur after contact with an allergen?**

Usually, signs and symptoms of anaphylaxis occur within minutes, especially after an intravenous injection. The vast majority definitely occur within one hour of exposure. Symptoms may reappear six to eight hours after the initial anaphylactic manifestations have resolved.

○ **What medication is most commonly responsible for anaphylactic reactions?**

Penicillin antibiotics. (375 deaths per year in the U.S.). Anaphylactoid reactions are most commonly seen with intravenous contrast media (incidence of 5 to 8%).

○ **Is there really cross-reactivity between penicillins and cephalosporins?**

Yes, but the exact incidence is not known and is likely small, around 5%. Anaphylaxis to a cephalosporin can occur in a penicillin allergic patient.

○ **T/F: Does pre-medication prevent anaphylaxis?**

False! It may decrease the risk or the overall response, but anaphylaxis can still occur. Pretreatment with diphenhydramine, cimetidine (or ranitidine) and corticosteroids for 24 hours prior to exposure is common practice. Routine pre-medication with histamine receptor blocking agents is still being debated. High-risk patients who would likely benefit from prophylaxis with H_1 and H_2 receptor blocking agents include those with a history of adverse drug reactions and allergies, patients undergoing procedures with a higher incidence of histamine release (such as those involving extracorporeal circulation) and patients in poor physical condition (such as those with significant heart disease) who are at increased risk of complications from therapy, vigorous hydration and reduced response to drug therapies. It should be noted that pre-medication may mask and even delay a diagnosis of anaphylaxis if it occurs under general anesthesia.

○ **Which patients are at increased risk for latex allergy?**

Those with chronic exposure to latex-based products and a history of atopy.

Spina bifida patients.
Urologic reconstructive surgery.

Health care workers – especially with a history of atopy or hand eczema.
Patients allergic to bananas, avocados, chestnuts, kiwi or mangos.
Patients with multiple allergies or with a history of atopy.
Patients who have undergone multiple surgical procedures.
Rubber industry workers.
Spinal cord trauma patients.
History of intolerance to latex-based products (balloons, condoms).
History of intraoperative anaphylaxis of uncertain etiology.

O   What does "latex precautions" mean?

Special consideration exists for patients who are more susceptible to developing a latex allergy, such as children with spina bifida or GU anomalies necessitating multiple reconstructive surgeries or exposure to rubber urethral catheters. "Latex precautions" signifies that no obvious allergy exists but latex should be avoided.

O   Identify commonly used objects from the operating room that contain latex.

This is only a partial list: gloves, bite blocks, rebreathing circuit bags, nasal airways, red rubber endotracheal tubes, urinary catheters, IV injection ports, stoppers on medication vials, Penrose-type tourniquets, syringe plungers, BP cuff tubing, stethoscope tubing, elastic bandages and some tapes.

O   T/F: PVC tracheal tubes and laryngeal mask airways are safe to use in latex allergic patients.

True! These two types of airway management equipment do not contain latex.

O   What is the most effective way to manage a patient with a history of latex allergy?

A *detailed history* to identify those patients at an increased risk for latex allergy and *latex avoidance*. All latex containing materials should be identified and a *latex allergy kit* containing latex-free equipment for substitution should be created and available to use at a moment's notice when a latex allergy or latex precautions patient is identified. Prudence would dictate having epinephrine immediately available.

O   Who is at high risk for a protamine reaction?

Diabetics taking protamine insulin preparations, e.g., NPH insulin (*0.6% to 2% incidence*)
Vasectomized men (although reported, it appears to be rare)
Fish-allergic individuals (also appears to be rare)
Individuals with previous exposure to protamine for heparin reversal (an increasingly larger population)

O   Can you have an anaphylactic reaction to corticosteroids and antihistamines?

Although it is extremely rare, anaphylactic reactions to some of the commonly used corticosteroid preparations and antihistamines have occurred and positive skin tests were noted. As a rule, *any medication* can cause an anaphylactic reaction.

O   What is the etiology of a hemolytic transfusion reaction and how is it treated?

When ABO incompatible blood is transfused, anti-A or anti-B IgG or IgM antibodies from the recipient react with the donor red blood cells and the complement cascade is initiated, leading to the production of anaphylatoxins with their associated symptoms and donor red cell lysis. Symptoms often include: flushing, rigors, dyspnea, back pain, bleeding, hypotension and hemoglobinuria. Treatment involves stopping the blood administration and returning the remaining portion to the blood bank for compatibility testing, assessing the extent of the reaction and treating it as with any other allergic reaction. Coagulopathies are corrected with coagulation factors and a brisk diuresis is initiated with iv fluids and diuretics such as furosemide and/or mannitol to protect the kidneys from the hemoglobinuria, if the patient is otherwise hemodynamically stable.

O   **What is the etiology of a febrile transfusion reaction and transfusion-related acute lung injury?**

A *febrile reaction* occurs rather commonly and is secondary to antileukocyte antibodies (leukoagglutinins) from the recipient reacting with donor leukocytes. Leukocyte pyrogens are released leading to chills, rigors, tachycardia and fever.

Leukoagglutinins in the donor blood products can attack the recipient's leukocytes which are viable. These leukocytes are then activated and capable of aggregating in the pulmonary circulation and producing direct lung injury via the liberation of arachidonic acid metabolites, free radicals and lysosomal enzymes. Activation of the complement cascade is likely involved with this process. Clinically, hypoxemia, noncardiac pulmonary edema, pulmonary hypertension and respiratory failure can occur.

O   **How should a patient be monitored after an anaphylactic reaction?**

All patients should be observed for at least 24 hours, preferably in an intensive care unit. Recurrence of the symptoms of anaphylaxis can occur over that period of time. Medications used to support the blood pressure, such as catecholamine infusions, should be discontinued and weaned as tolerated. Frequent physical examinations should be performed looking for late appearing sequelae from shock and the resuscitation process.

O   **Describe the perioperative management of heredity angioneurotic edema.**

Prophylactic therapy includes; danazol, intravenous ε-aminocitric acid, plasma transfusion or C1-esterase inhibitor. Be gentle! Trauma can precipitate acute attacks resulting in edema involving the subcutaneous tissues and submucosa of the GI tract and airways. Treatment of an acute attack involves supportive therapy including epinephrine, antihistamines and corticosteroids, but indeed, the patient may be refractory.

O   **Which local anesthetics are more likely to cause allergic reactions- esters or amides**?

Esters are far more likely to cause allergic reactions, presumably because they are derivatives of para-aminobenzoic acid (PABA)

O   **What is the cause of "allergic reactions" to amide local anesthetics?**

Allergic reactions to amides may actually be caused by the preservative methylparaben (a chemical structure similar to aminobenzoic acid) that is found in multidose vials of amides.

O   **If a patient is allergic to novocaine, can they receive lidocaine?**

Yes. Novocaine is the trade name for procaine, an ester local anesthetic, and lidocaine is an amide. Cross sensitivity between esters and amides is very rare.

O   **What is the value of skin testing in determining the safety of a local anesthetic?**

It has limited value. Skin tests can actually cause anaphylactic reactions, so they are not entirely safe. In addition, even a normal skin test will not rule out a potential allergic reaction to a local anesthetic when administered.

O   **What are the main ester-type local anesthetics and how are they metabolized?**

Procaine (novocaine), tertracaine, chloroprocaine, and cocaine. They undergo hydrolysis by pseudocholinesterases in plasma.

O   **What are the main amide-type local anesthetics and how are they metabolized?**

Bupivacaine, lidocaine, etidocaine, mepivacaine, and ropivacaine. Amide local anesthetics contain and "i" in the drug name followed by "caine". Amides are metabolized in the liver by microsomal enzymes (hydroxylation, N-dealkylation, and hydrolysis)

O   **Which patients are at increased risk for systemic toxicity with lidocaine administration?**

Those with reduced drug metabolism due to impaired liver function, decreased liver blood flow (ie: cirrhosis or CHF), or markedly reduced plasma proteins (less bound, more free in plasma)

O   **What is the definition of an anaphylactoid reaction?**

An anaphylactoid reation is a reaction that occurs in the absence of prior antibody formation. It does not need an IgE Ab interaction with the antigen to occur. Anaphylaxis requires the antibody to crosslink with the antigen triggering histamine release from the mast cell. In anaphylactoid reactions, the triggering agent will result in direct activation of complement and histamine release leading to a serious allergic reaction.

O   **Can you differentiate between anaphylactic and anaphylactoid reactions clinically?**

No. They are clinically indistinguishable. Both are equally life threatening and can result in major cardiovascular, pulmonary, and dermatologic responses.

O   **What lab test can aid in making the diagnosis of allergic reaction in the OR?**

Serum tryptase. Tryptase is found in the mast cell along with histamine and has a half life of 2-3hrs aiding in diagnosis.

O   **Which classes of anesthetic drugs are most likely responsible for allergic reactions intraoperatively?**

Muscle relaxants, especially succinylcholine	69.2%
Latex	12.1%
Antibiotics	8%

O   **Why do muscle relaxants so frequently result in anaphylaxis and allergic reactions?**

Nondepolarizing muscle relaxants contain either quarternary or tertiary ammonium ions to which patients frequently develop IgE antibodies. The theory is that females, who more commonly have reactions to these medications, do so because of their prior exposure to the ammonium compounds in cosmetics and other products. The Benzylisoquinolinium compounds (atracurium, mivacurium) are more likely to cause anaphylactic reactions than their counterparts, the aminosteroids (vecuronium, rocuronium, pancuronium). Patients may develop cross reactivity between muscle relaxants so it is best to choose a relaxant from another group if there is a history. Also, patients may be sensitized for up to 30 yrs after exposure.

O   **What is the most common adverse effect of protamine administration?**

Of the patients receiving protamine, less than 1% develop some type of reaction. Hypotension is the most common reaction and it can be severe, especially if the medication is given too quickly or to a hypovolemic patient. These reactions are not always antibody mediated and can be due to complement activation.

O   **What are the proposed mechanisms for protamine reactions?**

Patients with previous exposures to protamine can develop IgE and IgG mediated reactions which result in severe hypotension and bronchospasm. Protamine is also known to cause nonimmunologic release of chemical mediators and complement activation. These anaphylactoid reactions to protamine administration can result in pulmonary vasoconstriction and right ventricular failure. Protamine has also been tentatively linked to noncardiogenic pulmonary edema post bypass.

PATIENT POSITIONING

Facts Do Not Cease To Exist Because They Are Ignored.
Aldous Huxley

○ **A patient develops foot drop following vaginal hysterectomy. Her ankles were placed in candy-cane stirrups to assume the classic lithotomy position. What happened?**

Injury to the common peroneal nerve due to improper positioning or padding.
Common peroneal nerve compression may occur where the nerve is most superficial and sweeps over the head of the fibula just below the lateral aspect of the knee. Compression against the leg support device or insufficient padding will cause nerve injury and weakness or paralysis in the dorsiflexion muscles of the foot and ankle.

○ **List the risks of lithotomy positioning.**

- Common peroneal nerve injury
- Venous stasis in the lower legs, with the risk of phlebitis
- Arterial vascular insufficiency
- Compartment syndrome
- Compression or stretching of sciatic (exaggerated hip flexion), femoral (kinked at the hip), saphenous (medial tibial condyle against the leg support), obturator (stretch) or posterior tibial nerve
- Back pain (especially with a history of herniated disc)
- Hip dislocation
- Lower extremity tendon and ligament injuries
- Crush injury to the fingers if they are caught when the leg section of the table is raised back to support a supine position

○ **Can median sternotomy and sternal retraction cause brachial plexus injuries?**

Yes. Excessive sternal retraction may result in fracture of the first rib and injury to the brachial neurovascular bundle.

○ **With supine positioning, what is the ideal placement of the arms?**

The goal is to avoid stretching the brachial plexus. The arms should be abducted less than 90 degrees, and pronated with palms down, and the head held in the neutral position (avoid rotation and flexion, especially to the contralateral side of the "out" arm, if the other is tucked). The arms should be properly secured and padded to prevent them from falling off the arm board, causing translocation of the humerus below the horizontal plane of the scapula. If the arms are suspended overhead, extreme abduction or anterior flexion must be avoided.

○ **What is the most likely mechanism of radial nerve injury?**

The most common site of entrapment of the radial nerve is in the middle of the arm seen with too frequent cycling of the NIBP cuff for long periods or too prolonged use of use of a tourniquet set at high pressure. In addition, resting the arm against a vertical bar (either screen or surgical retraction system) can also cause a compression injury. The radial nerve courses in the spiral groove on the lateral aspect of the humerus about three fingerbreadths above the lateral epicondyle.

○ **What are the signs of radial nerve injury?**

Injury occurring *proximal to the origin of the radial branches to the triceps muscle* (ie: "Saturday night palsy", with the arm thrown over the back of a chair to hold an intoxicated patient upright), results in no extension at the elbow joint.

With nerve injury *in the middle of the humerus* there is paralysis of the extensor muscles of the forearm and digits causing wrist drop, with normal strength of the triceps muscle. Sensory loss is variable, and usually limited to a patch on the dorsum of the hand between the first and second digits.

Selected injury of the *posterior interosseous nerve* on the dorsal aspect of the forearm from insufficient padding of the dependent arm with the patient positioned lateral will also cause wrist drop.

If the *deep branch of the radial nerve* is severed, the patient will be unable to extend the thumb and the metacarpophalangeal joints of the other digits. There is no loss of sensation.

Selective injury of the *superficial branch of the radial nerve* may result in loss of sensation on the posterior surface of the forearm, hand and proximal phalanges of the lateral three and one-half digits.

O   **Which of the three major nerves in the arm (radial, median and ulnar) is least likely to be damaged from improper positioning?**

Median nerve. Injury is usually due to entrapment (pronator syndrome due to compression between the two heads of the pronator teres) or laceration at the elbow or just proximal to the flexor retinaculum due to wrist slashing in an attempted suicide.

O   **What are the most common sites and signs of ulnar nerve injury?**

Ulnar nerve injury commonly occurs with nerve compression at the elbow where the nerve passes posterior to the medial epicondyle of the humerus (i.e. the funny bone). This produces numbness and tingling of the medial part of the palm and the fourth and fifth digits. Patients have difficulty making a fist because they cannot flex their fourth and fifth fingers at the distal interphalangeal joints. This gives the appearance of a "clawhand" then the patient attempts to straighten the fingers.

O   **Why are axillary rolls used in lateral decubitus positioning of the patient?**

To prevent compression of the dependent arm's axillary neurovascular bundle (arterial insufficiency, venous stasis and/or thrombosis, brachial plexus injury). The wedge may also prevent circumduction of the "down" shoulder which could result in stretching of the suprascapular nerve. Additional useful techniques that complement axillary rolls include: placing the pulse oximeter probe, insertion of arterial line or checking the radial pulse on the dependent arm to detect arterial insufficiency; placing the NIBP cuff on the upper arm, with frequent checks for cyanosis or mottling of the skin on the dependent arm; being cognizant of the fact that a surgical resident leaning on and swinging the arm board upwards could contribute to stretch injury of the brachial plexus.

O   **Are there any special considerations in positioning a patient with rib fractures in the lateral position?**

The injured side should not be placed dependent. The weight of the patient may displace the rib fracture causing trauma to the pleura or lung. If there is an associated underlying lung contusion, V/Q mismatch is minimized with the fractured rib in the non-dependent position as preferential perfusion to the dependent lung will move blood flow away from the contused and poorly ventilated alveoli.

O   **Why are chest rolls needed for positioning a patient prone?**

To reduce intra-abdominal and intra-thoracic pressure.
Abdominal compression will impair diaphragmatic excursion, resulting in an acute restrictive pattern of ventilation. Compression of the vena cava will cause venous congestion and increased bleeding during back

surgery from the epidural venous plexus and may preclude venous return to the heart. Direct pressure on the aorta may raise the blood pressure causing vascular insufficiency distally. A further pulmonary restriction occurs when thoracic compression prevents the rib cage from freely swinging open to accommodate inspirations. Elevated support for the pelvis and chest minimizes the number of pressure points, especially, to the breasts and genitalia. The head may be able to assume a more neutral position. The increase in intra-abdominal pressure may contribute to the development of vision deficits postoperatively. Note that the positioning devices may also injure the patient by direct pressure-induced ischemia, as well as stretch injury (brachial plexus or ulnar nerve).

⭕ What is mid-cervical tetraplegia?

This is unexplained postoperative paraplegia, which is rare, from stretching or compression of the cervical spinal cord causing ischemic injury in the midcervical segment (C_5) due to neck flexion with the patient in the sitting position. Patients considered at risk include those with significant degenerative disease of the cervical spine, cervical spinal stenosis and/or cerebral vascular disease. Cerebral perfusion pressure should be maintained at a minimum of 60 mm Hg, with the MAP transduced at the level of the head.

⭕ What are the potential complications associated with the sitting position?

* Hypotension, especially upon initial assumption of the position.
* Pneumocephalus, tension pneumocephalus.
* Flexed position of the neck causes mid-cervical quadraplegia, macroglossia, facial edema, venous bleeding.
* Brachial plexus injury.
* Stretch injury of the sciatic nerve.
* Venous air embolism.

⭕ Where should the mean arterial pressure be transduced in a sitting patient?

Mean arterial pressure should be measured with the transducer of the arterial line place at or corrected to the level of the head (Circle of Willis). The auditory meatus is an external landmark. This will give a meaningful measurement of cerebral perfusion pressure (CPP = MAP – cerebral venous pressure).

⭕ What happens to the distribution of V/Q ratios of the two lungs when an awake patient breathing spontaneously assumes the lateral decubitus position?

Not much. Preferential ventilation to the dependent lung (R>L) is matched by an increase in perfusion, so the V/Q ratio decreases from the non-dependent to the dependent lung, just as it does in upright and supine lungs.

⭕ What is the most common ophthalmologic diagnosis for postoperative visual loss associated with spine surgery?

Ischemic optic neuropathy.

⭕ How does ischemic optic neuropathy differ from central retinal artery occlusion as a cause for visual loss following surgery?

Ischemic optic neuropathy is associated with larger blood loss, hypotension, anemia, longer duration in the prone position and/or vaso-occlusive disease. The high percentage of patients with bilateral disease and reported cases occurring in patients whose heads are suspended in Mayfied tongs makes direct globe pressure an unlikely etiology. Recovery of vision is reported in 56% of cases.

The etiology of central retinal artery occlusion is thought to be direct pressure on the globe, emboli or low perfusion pressure in the retina. Supporting evidence includes: low estimated blood loss, lack of anemia, shorter duration of prone position, unilateral disease and no recovery of vision. Direct pressure on the globe may also cause unilateral periorbital bruising, proptosis, paresis of extraocular eye muscles and/or supraorbital paresthesias.

○   **What is the most frequent site of anesthesia-related peripheral nerve injury?**

Ulnar nerve.

○   **Which nerve injury associated with anesthesia is reported to have the highest median litigation-related payment?**

Spinal cord injury associated with delayed diagnosis of epidural hematoma.

○   **Explain the mechanism of femoral neuropathy following lithotomy positioning.**

Positional compression and stretch injury.

Flexion of the hip can compress the femoral nerve beneath the inguinal ligament and within the body of the psoas muscle, at the iliopsoas groove. Excessive hip abduction and external rotation causes additional stretch on the nerve. Direct trauma or retraction compression to the nerve and retroperitoneal hematoma during surgery or delivery should also be considered.

BLOOD THERAPY

What Lies Behind Us And What Lies Before Us Are Small Matters Compared To What Lies Within Us.
Ralph Waldo Emerson

○ **How does antithrombin III work?**

Antithrombin III is a circulatory serine protease inhibitor that irreversibly binds and inactivates thrombin and factor X. It also inhibits factors VIIa, IXa, Xa and XIa. Thrombin is necessary for clot formation and platelet activation.

○ **What is the main fibrinolytic enzyme?**

Plasmin.

○ **What are the major endogenous activators of plasminogen?**

Tissue plasminogen activator (TPA) released from endothelium and factor XIIa and kallikrein formed in the contact phase.

○ **What exogenous substances activate plasminogen?**

Streptokinase, urokinase and tissue plasminogen activator.

○ **When should heparin-induced thrombocytopenia be suspected?**

In association with thrombocytopenia (platelets < 100,000/μl), tachyphylaxis to heparin and thrombotic complications, appearing 7-10 days after the initiation of heparin therapy in those never exposed to heparin previously . Antibody-platelet interaction initiates activation and aggregation (complement-mediated, heparin-dependent IgG platelet antibody). In vitro platelet aggregation to heparin disappears in 4 to 8 weeks, but may persist up to 12 months. Administration of heparin to sensitized patients will decrease the platelet count dramatically and/or produce thromboemboli. Elective cardiac or vascular surgery should be delayed with resolution of platelet aggregation studies.
For urgent cardiac surgery, other strategies avoiding heparin exposure are necessary.

○ **What are the molecular events in heparin-associated thrombocytopenia?**

It is believed to be caused by a heparin-dependent IgG platelet antibody interaction with platelets which initiates platelet activation and aggregation.

○ **What is the nature of thrombosis in heparin-induced thrombocytopenia (HIT)?**

Arterial or venous and is a characteristic "white clot" (platelets and fibrin). Major thrombotic complications occur in 20% of HIT patients (coronary, cerebral, splanchnic and peripheral artery).

○ **When does the syndrome of heparin-associated thrombocytopenia usually occur in patients who were never previously exposed to heparin?**

Seven to 10 days after heparin administration.

○ **Is the heparin used in catheter flush solutions, or bonded to vascular catheters, sufficient to cause this syndrome?**

Yes.

O   **How does heparin work?**

Heparin binds to antithrombin III and increases its affinity for thrombin and the activated forms of X, IX, XI and XIII, effectively neutralizing each.

O   **How does a patient with antithrombin III deficiency usually present?**

Homozygotes usually die in infancy; 85% of heterozygotes have suffered a thrombotic event by age 50. The diagnosis should be suspected in a patient with thromboembolic disease or a resistance to anticoagulation with heparin administration.

O   **Can this antithrombin III disorder be acquired as well as congenital?**

Yes.

O   **What are some of the causes of acquired antithrombin III deficiency?**

Liver disease, malignancy, nephrotic syndrome, DIC, malnutrition or increased protein catabolism.

O   **What is the appropriate therapy for a patient with antithrombin III deficiency requiring anticoagulation?**

Fresh frozen plasma can be used as a source of ATIII when heparin is necessary. Antithrombin III concentrate is available. Alternate anticoagulant drug therapy should be considered.

O   **How does sodium warfarin (Coumadin) work as an anticoagulant?**

Inhibition of vitamin K epoxide reductase, limiting carboxylation of vitamin K-dependent coagulation factors (II, XII, IX, X and prothrombin).

O   **What other factors does coumadin inhibit?**

Proteins C, S and Z.

O   **What is the molecular abnormality in Hemophilia A?**

X-linked recessive disorder due to defective factor VIII:C molecules.

O   **What are the clinical manifestations of Hemophilia A?**

Bleeding into joints and muscles, epistaxis, hematuria and bleeding after minor trauma.

O   **What is the laboratory abnormality associated with Hemophilia A?**

Prolongation of aPTT.

O   **What is the minimum level of factor VIII required for hemostasis?**

30%.

O   **What is the molecular abnormality in Hemophilia B?**

X-linked hereditary deficiency of factor IX (Christmas factor).

○   **Is Hemophilia B clinically distinguishable from Hemophilia A?**

No.

○   **What is the molecular abnormality in Von Willebrand's disease?**

Defective vWF, or low levels of a normal vWF resulting in an inability of platelets to bind to collagen. vWF is a carrier for coagulation factor VIII, so bleeding time is prolonged and factor VIII activity is decreased.

○   **What is the most common complication of massive transfusion?**

The traditional answer: dilutional thrombocytopenia. In current practice, this may not be true when PRBCs are used for massive transfusion. It has been shown that coagulation factors (FFP) are necessary after 12 or more units and patients who receive 20 or more PRBCs require platelet therapy

○   **Which clotting factors are most likely to be decreased as a result of massive transfusion?**

Factors V and fibrinogen. With the use of **PRBCs,** fibrinogen levels decrease significantly in contrast to the use of whole blood, in which fibrinogen levels remain unchanged unless DIC is present. Factor VIII is probably stored in endothelial cells and released during surgical stress.

○   **What is a type and screen and how is it performed?**

Type and Screen is ABO-Rh typing and antibody screening. ABO typing is performed by testing RBCs for the A and B antigens and the serum for A and B antibodies. Recipient serum is mixed with commercially prepared type O red blood cells (RBCs) and incubated. If no agglutination is observed, the screen is negative. If the screen is positive, serum is tested using selected reagent RBCs to identify the antibodies present.

○   **What are the three phases of type and crossmatch of blood?**

Immediate phase, incubation phase and antiglobulin phase.
1. The first phase combines recipient serum and donor cells to test ABO group compatibility at room temperature. It also identifies MN, P and Lewis incompatibilities. This phase takes approximately five minutes.
2. The second phase incubates the products from the first in albumin at 37 degrees Celsius, enhancing incomplete antibodies. This phase primarily detects antibodies in the Rh system.
3. The last phase is the indirect antiglobulin test. Antiglobulin serum is added to the previously incubated test tubes. This phase aids in the detection of incomplete antibodies in Rh, Kell, Duffy and Kidd systems.

○   **What is the incompatibility risk of typed blood, screened blood and fully crossmatched blood?**

The risk of incompatibility of ABO/Rh-compatible blood is 0.1-0.2% (99.8% SAFE) if the patient has never been
transfused. The risk increases to 1.0% if the patient has had a previous transfusion. Adding a negative antibody screen decreases the risk to 0.06% (99.94% SAFE). Fully crossmatched blood should carry a risk less than 0.05% (99.5% SAFE).

○   **What is the most common blood group? What percentage of the population is Rh positive?**

The most common blood group is type O. 45% of Caucasians, 49% of American blacks, 79% of American Indians and 40% of Asians are blood type O. Approximately 85% of the population is Rh positive and

15% Rh negative.

O   **What is the formula to calculate oxygen delivery?**

Tissue oxygen delivery (DO2) is the product of blood flow and arterial oxygen content, and at the whole body level represented by the product of cardiac output and the arterial oxygen content. DO2=CO [(Hb x 1.39) SaO2+0.003 PaO2]. Where CO = cardiac output, Hb = hemoglobin, SaO2=arterial oxygen saturation and PaO2=partial pressure of oxygen in arterial blood.

O   **What is the effect of normovolemic-hemodilution on heart rate, blood pressure and cardiac output (CO) in elderly patients?**

In healthy elderly patients, with normovolemic-hemodilution, the hematocrit is reduced from 41% to 28%, stroke volume increases with heart rate and blood pressure remains unchanged. Cardiac output is increased secondary to decreased viscosity and systemic vascular resistance and increased contractility. There is a reduction in oxygen delivery as a result of the failure to fully compensate for the lowered oxygen carrying capacity by an increased cardiac output. Oxygen delivery is maximum in the hematocrit range of 35% to 45%.

O   **How can you estimate the volume of blood to be removed preoperatively when you are using the normovolemic-hemodilution/ autotransfusion technique to reduce the loss of red cells intraoperatively?**

The volume can be calculated according to the following formula:
V=EBV ({HCToriginal – Hctfinal}/Hctaverage), where V= volume to be removed and EBV= estimated blood volume (65 ml/kg multiplied by weight (kg)).

O   **What is "Critical Oxygen Delivery?"**

Oxygen consumption is usually independent of delivery due to compensatory increased extraction. Critical oxygen delivery is the point at which oxygen delivery is no longer capable of supporting cellular respiration and oxygen consumption becomes directly proportional to oxygen delivery. Progressive lactic acidosis results from cellular hypoxia.

O   **What is the relationship between oxygen extraction ratio (O2ER) and anemia?**

As the hematocrit decreases below normal, there is a decrease in systemic oxygen delivery, but the oxygen extraction ratio increases, which helps maintain a constant oxygen uptake in the tissues. The point at which the compensatory increase in oxygen extraction begins to fail corresponds to an oxygen ER of 0.5 (50%). Many institutions use this value as a transfusion trigger, when this information is available.

O   **According to the CDC-RBC panel, what are the indications for perioperative red blood cell transfusion?**

The Consensus Development Conference-RBC panel (September 1984) concluded that the sole indication for erythrocyte transfusion was to increase oxygen carrying capacity. In a healthy individual, a Hgb of 7 or greater was considered safe, and a Hgb of 10 appropriate for those with compromised critical organs.

O   **What does Prothrombin Time (PT) measure? How is it performed?**

The extrinsic and common pathways of the coagulation system are measured by the PT. The time to clot formation is measured after the addition of tissue thromboplastin to the patient's plasma.

O   **What does activated partial thromboplastin time (aPTT) measure? How is it performed?**

The intrinsic and common arms of the "tissue factor pathway of coagulation" are measured by the PTT. After the blood sample is exposed to celite for activation and a reagent is added (partial thromboplastin), time to clot formation is measured.

O   **What is the difference in volume and components between Fresh Frozen Plasma (FFP) and cryoprecipitate?**

The main difference is that cryo has much more fibrinogen. FFP (225 ml) contains 1 unit/ml of all procoagulants and 3-4 mg/ml of fibrinogen. A single donor unit of cryoprecipitate (10 ml) contains 80-145 units of factor VIII, 250 mg of fibrinogen, von Willebrand factor, factor XIII and fibronectin.

O   **How is FFP prepared?**

After the removal of red blood cells from whole blood, the remaining platelet-rich plasma is further centrifuged to separate the platelets from the plasma. The remaining plasma contains all the blood coagulation factors, fibrinogen and other plasma proteins. The plasma is frozen within six hours of donation to prevent inactivation of temperature sensitive coagulation factors V and VIII.

O   **How is FFP administered?**

Prior to the administration of FFP, it must be thawed in a water bath at 30-37 degrees Celsius with agitation, which takes approximately 30 minutes. After thawing, the units of FFP are stored at 1 to 6 degrees Celsius and must be transfused within 24 hours. FFP should be administered through a component administration set with a 170-micron filter.

O   **What are the indications for the administration of FFP?**

According to the ASA Task Force 2, there are six indications for the administration of FFP:
• Replacement of isolated factor deficiencies (as documented by laboratory evidence).
• Reversal of warfarin effect.
• Use in antithrombin III deficiency.
• Treatment of immunodeficiencies.
• Treatment of thrombotic thrombocytopenic purpura.
• Massive transfusion (rarely, and only when factors V and VIII are < 25% of normal).
Requirements for factor deficiencies in a massive transfusion would be a PT and PTT ≥1.5 times the normal value.

O   **How is cryoprecipitate prepared and administered?**

Cryoprecipitate is prepared from a unit of FFP. It is the cold-insoluble white precipitate that forms when a bag of FFP is thawed at 1-6 degrees Celsius. This cold-insoluble material is removed following centrifugation and immediately frozen at minus18 degrees Celsius and can be stored for up to one year. Cryoprecipitate must be transfused rapidly and within four to six hours of thawing if given to replace factor VIII levels. Units are usually pooled and should be given through a 170-micron component filter.

O   **What are the indications for cryoprecipitate administration?**

Cryoprecipitate is used for the treatment of congenital or acquired fibrinogen and factor VII and XIII deficiencies. Cryoprecipitate can also be administered prophylactically for nonbleeding perioperative or peripartum patients with congenital fibrinogen deficiencies or von Willebrand's disease unresponsive to desmopressin (DDAVP).

O   **What is the difference between high purity and intermediate purity factor VIII concentrates? What are the indications for transfusing them?**

The intermediate purity concentrate contains significant therapeutic quantities of the von Willebrand's component of factor VIII, whereas the high purity preparations contain principally the Hemophilia A component of factor VIII (VIII-C). Intermediate purity factor VIII concentrates are preferred for von

Willebrand's disease and recombinant or highly purified factor VIII concentrate for Hemophilia A.

○   **How is platelet concentrate prepared and how many platelets are in a platelet transfusion?**

Platelet concentrate is prepared from whole blood within eight hours of collection. After the collection of approximately 500 ml of whole blood into collection bags containing citrate-based anticoagulant preservative solution, the blood is centrifuged. Following centrifugation, the platelet rich plasma (PRP) is separated into an attached empty satellite bag. This PRP is centrifuged again and separated into one unit platelet concentrate and one unit of plasma. Each unit of platelets contains approximately 5.5×10^{10} platelets in 50-70 ml of plasma. An adult dose pack of platelets contains 6-7 units of platelet concentrate.

○   **How are platelets-pheresis units ("single donor") prepared?**

Platelets-pheresis units are obtained by performing apheresis on volunteer donors. During this procedure, large volumes of donor blood are processed into extracorporeal circuit and centrifuged to separate their components. The red cells and plasma are returned to the donor. From a single donor, the equivalent of 5-8 units are obtained and suspended in a volume 200-400 ml of plasma.

○   **How are platelets administered?**

Both platelets and platelets-pheresis may be stored at room temperature (20-24 degrees C) for up to five days with continuous gentle agitation to prevent platelet aggregation. Platelets can be infused through a platelet or standard component administration set with a 170-micron filter. Microaggregate filters (20-24 microns) should not be used because they will remove most of the platelets.

○   **Is it necessary to administer ABO-specific platelets?**

The administration of ABO-specific platelets is not required because platelet concentrates contain few red blood cells (where ABO antigens are expressed). However, the administration of pooled platelet components of various ABO types can transfuse plasma containing anti-A and/or anti-B, resulting in HLA (Human leukocyte antigen) antibody formation.

○   **What are the indications for platelet transfusion?**

Correction of a deficiency in either platelet number (thrombocytopenia) or platelet function in patients at risk for bleeding or with evidence of clinically significant bleeding.
Perioperative factors to consider for the transfusion of platelets for a borderline platelet count of 50-100,000/dL include: the type of surgery, anticipated and actual blood loss, extent of microvascular bleeding, presence of medications (aspirin) and disorders known to affect platelet function or coagulation (uremia). The prophylactic administration of platelets is not recommended in patients with chronic thrombocytopenia caused by increased platelet destruction (idiopathic thrombocytopenic purpura). Prophylactic platelet transfusion is rarely indicated when the count is > 100,000/dL and is usually indicated perioperatively when the count is below 50,000/dL. Spontaneous bleeding occurs with counts < 20,000/dL.

○   **How much does the transfusion of one unit of platelets increase the platelet count?**

In the adult, one unit of platelet concentrate generally increases the platelet count by approximately 5,000-8,000/mm3.

○   **Should packed red blood cells (PRBC) be diluted before administration to ensure rapid infusion?**

When additive solutions such as Adsol® are used, no dilution is necessary. For PRBC stored in preservatives in which the hematocrit may be as high as 70-80%, 60-100 ml of 0.9% saline can be added to facilitate rapid infusion and minimize hemolysis. Although the infusion flow rate of the diluted unit and total volume infused will be increased compared with the undiluted state, the time required for transfusion of 90% of the red cell mass is unchanged.

○ **Which solutions are considered "incompatible" with PRBC?**

Lactate Ringers (theoretical clot formation due to calcium) and 5% dextrose in water or 0.2% saline and plasmanate (hemolysis).

○ **What is the potassium load with transfusion?**

The extracellular concentration of potassium in stored blood steadily increases with time. The amount of potassium transfused is typically < 4 mEq per unit. Transfusion rates exceeding 100 ml/min may predispose to hyperkalemia (and hypocalcemia).

○ **Does a massive transfusion produce hyperkalemia?**

Except with patients in whom blood replacement fails to restore perfusion and reverse the acidosis, hyperkalemia rarely occurs in a massive transfusion. There is a progressive fall in the serum potassium levels in a massive transfusion, and this fall is related to the volume transfused. Hypokalemia is commonly encountered perioperatively due to citrate metabolism to bicarbonate producing a metabolic alkalosis and intracellular shifts of potassium.

○ **What is the incidence of hepatitis transmission with transfusion?**

Posttransfusion hepatitis may be evident clinically, but the majority of cases are subclinical. The incidence of hepatitis C (HCV) transmission is approximately 1 in 103,000. The incidence of hepatitis B (HBV) transmission is estimated to be 1 in 63,000. Hepatitis A, for which there is not a carrier state, is rarely seen in association with transfusion. (Schreiber et al. NEJM 334: 1685, 1996. Corresponding viral windows are HCV: 82 days and HBV: 59 days).
HIV I and II combined risk 1:493,000, Hepatitis A 1:1x106 , Hepatitis B 1:63,000, Hepatitis C 1:103,000 (American Association of Bloodbankers (AABB) technical manual ed 13).

○ **What is the incidence of HIV-1 transmission with transfusion?**

The most recent estimates of the risk of acquiring HIV from transfusion are 1 in 450,000 to 1 in 600,000. With the use of nucleic acid technology (NAT) the window of infectivity, which is the time from being infected to a positive test result, has decreased to 11 days. Prior to the implementation of testing for HIV-I p24 antigen in 1996, it was
estimated that there were 25 units of HIV contaminated blood, not detected by testing, made available for transfusion yearly of the 12 million units collected. Antigen testing would reduce that number by 25%.

○ **What is the cause and incidence of febrile reactions to blood?**

The febrile reaction is the most common mild transfusion reaction and occurs in 1-3% of transfusions. It is caused by alloantibodies (leukoagglutinins) to white blood cells, platelets or other donor plasma antigens. Fever is presumably caused by pyrogens liberated from lysed cells. It occurs more commonly in previously transfused patients. Bacterial contamination of platelets or gram-negative sepsis may produce similar findings.

○ **What is transfusion-related acute lung injury (TRALI)?**

TRALI is a form of noncardiac pulmonary edema most commonly occurring within hours of transfusion of whole blood, PRBCs and FFP. Antibodies to leukocytes, usually of donor origin, are identified in the majority of cases. This reaction should be suspected in any patient who develops dyspnea, hypotension and fever with bilateral pulmonary edema after a transfusion in which volume overload or cardiac dysfunction is unlikely. Symptoms usually resolve within 96 hours in response to oxygen, mechanical ventilation, and fluid support to maintain blood pressure and cardiac output. The syndrome is fatal in 5% of cases.

○ **An immunosuppressed patient requires a blood transfusion. You noticed "irradiation" on the blood product sent from the blood bank. Why?**

Graft-versus-host disease has been recognized after blood transfusion in immune-compromised patients. Viable lymphocytes in the transfused blood can damage tissues in the immunodeficient recipient if a response develops against the patient's HLA antigens. Irradiation of red cell, granulocyte and platelet transfusions inactivates lymphocytes. Cytomegalovirus transmission is also minimized.

○ **A patient being seen for her preoperative evaluation prior to knee surgery would like to donate her own blood. Her surgery is in two days. Recommendations?**

The most practical schedule for obtaining more than one unit of autologous blood is to draw units at weekly intervals for three weeks, preferably having the last unit withdrawn one week and no fewer than 72 hours prior to surgery. Donation two days prior to surgery is extremely unlikely to affect homologous blood transfusion requirements.

○ **Should FFP be used to neutralize heparin?**

FFP is contraindicated to neutralize heparin. FFP is a source of antithrombin III and transfusion could instead potentiate the action of heparin. Heparin resistance may result from low antithrombin III, which is remedied with FFP transfusion.

○ **What is the cardiovascular effect of acute anemia in an otherwise healthy patient?**

Basic cardiac output can rise fivefold to maintain oxygen delivery. As plasma volume increases, the hematocrit decreases (euvolemia is achieved without red blood cell transfusion), resulting in reduction in blood viscosity and peripheral vascular resistance. Heart rate does not increase in the absence of hypovolemia. Redistribution of blood flow to the heart and brain occurs with increased tissue oxygen extraction. Oxygen delivery is shown to be maximum in the hematocrit range of 35% to 45%.

○ **At what hemoglobin level does the oxyhemoglobin dissociation curve begin shifting to the right?**

The shift begins at hemoglobin levels of approximately 9-10 g/dl and is prominent at 6.5 g/dl. This change results from increased levels of 2,3-DPG and requires 12 to 36 hours to develop.

○ **If there is a greater than 40% probability of transfusing a patient during surgery, what would be the appropriate preoperative order to Transfusion Services?**

Type and crossmatch. ABO group and Rh type of the patient is determined, an antibody screening test is performed and compatible units of blood are made available before surgery.

○ **When would it be appropriate to require preoperative type and screen blood orders?**

If there is only a modest possibility of transfusion (<10%), and in cases with possible blood loss where the patient is multiparous or has had a prior transfusion (indicating possible difficulty cross-matching in an emergency). ABO group and Rh type of a patient are determined and a screening test is performed on a patient's serum for "unexpected" red cell alloantibodies. The screening test takes 30 to 120 minutes to complete and remains valid for 72 hours. If the antibody screen is negative, fully crossmatched blood can be available within 15 to 30 minutes.

○ **What is the difference between the whole blood lost by the patient and stored whole blood for transfusion?**

In stored whole blood, platelet function is 5% of normal after 48 hours of storage at 4 degrees C. There is also progressive loss of factors V and VIII to 15% and 50% of normal, respectively, after 21 days of storage.

○ **One of the complications of massive transfusion is citrate toxicity. How is citrate metabolized?**

Citrate is metabolized by the liver. Adults with hepatic dysfunction, hypothermia or those with a transfusion rate greater than 1 unit of blood every 5 minutes are at risk. The signs of citrate intoxication are those of acute hypocalcemia, as citrate binds calcium.

○ **A patient with hemophilia A is to have surgery. What is the half-life of factor VIII and how do you decide the dose of factor VIII needed preoperatively?**

Factor VIII has a half-life of 6-10 hours. The dose of factor VIII needed can be calculated on the assumption that each unit of factor VIII infused per kilogram of body weight raises plasma VIII levels by 2%. The minimal factor VIII concentrations necessary for hemostasis during major surgery is 30 to 40% of normal, but many recommend increasing factor VIII levels to more than 50% prior to surgery. FFP contains 1 unit factor VIII activity per ml, cryoprecipitate 5-10 units/ml and factor VIII concentrates 40 units/ml. Twice-a-Day transfusions are recommended following surgery. DDAVP may be a good adjuvant. In the patient with no factor VIII activity, 20 units/kg should be the initial dose, followed by 1.5 units/kg/hr. Additional factor VIII is given on the basis of factor levels for 6 to 10 days postoperatively.

○ **A Jehovah's Witness is to undergo D&C. The surgeon discussed the possibility of hemorrhage with the patient, but the patient refused transfusion based on her religious belief. During the procedure, the bleeding becomes life-threatening and the patient subsequently expires. Is the surgeon liable for the patient's death?**

If the bleeding occurred within the standards of care, the surgeon would not be liable. The patient's refusal to accept transfusion does not protect the surgeon from liability for any negligent action that may have necessitated transfusion.

○ **Is hepatitis a risk factor when albumin is given?**

No. Albumin is a blood-derived colloid and is freed of hepatitis and other viruses by heating after chemical stabilization of the protein.

○ **Blood is routinely screened for which infectious agents?**

• Hepatitis C antibody
• Antibody to hepatitis B core antigen
• HIV-1
• HIV-2
• HIV Ag (p24 antigen)
• HTLV I/II
• Serologic test for syphilis

○ **A patient with Type I von Willebrand's disease is to have a breast reduction. What should be the first line of therapy?**

DDAVP 0.3 μg/kg, 30 minutes before surgery, to increase vWF levels. Cryoprecipitate or factor VIII concentrates are administered to non-responders.

○ **What is citrate toxicity?**

Citrate is an anticoagulant used in stored blood products. Citrate binds ionized calcium, causing acute ionized hypocalcemid ie: muscle tremors, hypotension, decreased cardiac output, myocardial irritability and ventricular fibrillation. Treatment is the administration of exogenous calcium. Citrate also binds ionized magnesium; consider hypomagnesemia, especially for dysrhythmia (Torsades de pointes).

O   **Compare the terms: "type and hold," "type and screen" and "type and cross."**

Type and hold: ABO and Rh types are determined. Type and screen: ABO and Rh types are determined. Additionally, the patient's serum is screened against group O donor RBCs with known antigens that will react with antibodies that are commonly implicated in hemolytic transfusion reactions. Type and cross: a type and screen plus a crossmatch. Crossmatching involves adding the patient's serum to actual donor RBCs to detect antigen/antibody reactions.

O   **What are the hemostatic uses for DDAVP?**

DDAVP (desmopressin acetate) is an analogue of vasopressin without vasopressor activity. Infusion of DDAVP increases the release of von Willebrand's factor and factor VIII from the endothelium; intravenous peak effect in 15 to 30 minutes, with an increase in vWF seen over 3 hours and an increase in factor VIII over 4 to 24 hours. It is useful in treating the coagulopathy associated with von Willebrand's disease and hemophilia A. DDAVP has also shown utility in treating uremia-induced platelet dysfunction.

O   **Is stored blood acidic or basic? What happens with transfusion?**

Stored CPDA-1 blood is acidic with a pH between 6.6 and 6.9. Citrate in the anticoagulant and erythrocyte metabolism producing lactate and CO_2 contribute to the acidity. With adequate tissue perfusion, citrate and lactate are metabolized to bicarbonate.

O   **What is the most common transfusion transmitted infection?**

Ninety percent of post-transfusion hepatitis is caused by the hepatitis C virus; less than one third of these patients develop jaundice.

O   **How does epsilon-aminocaproic acid (EACA) work?**

Epsilon-aminocaproic acid (Amicar) is a synthetic monoamine carboxylic acid that interferes with the conversion of plasminogen to plasmin, thus attenuating primary fibrinolysis.

O   **What is aprotinin and how does it work?**

Aprotinin is a serine protease inhibitor with has been used to diminish perioperative blood loss and transfusion requirements. The exact mechanism is unclear but may be due to inhibition of plasmin-mediated fibrinolysis. There is also evidence that aprotinin maintains platelet adhesiveness by preventing plasmin-mediated degradation of platelet glycoproteins.

O   **Is there any role for prophylactic FFP and platelets with RBC transfusion?**

More data suggests there is no role for prophylaxis (e.g., two units FFP for every 10 units RBC transfused). Transfusion of blood components should ideally be guided by laboratory evidence of coagulopathy or clinical evidence of bleeding. After two blood volumes of blood loss, FFP is usually required.

O   **Which blood products should be filtered?**

All blood products should be filtered through a 170 micron filter to remove small clots and debris. Smaller pore filters can be used to filter microaggregates in patients with a history of febrile transfusion reaction. Leukocyte-depleting filters should be used to prevent alloimmunization in susceptible patients.

O   **How can you calculate maximum allowable blood loss?**

An estimate of allowable blood loss can be calculated by using estimated blood volume (EBV), initial hematocrit and desired ending hematocrit.

Blood loss = EBV x Hct(initial)-Hct(final) }/ Hct(average) . The calculation assumes euvolemia is maintained.

○ **What is the activated clotting time?**

Activated clotting time (ACT) is a modified, accelerated whole blood coagulation time. An activator (celite or kaolin) is added to a blood sample, causing contact activation of the intrinsic pathway, and the time to clot formation is measured. Normal automated Hemochron ACT is between 90 and 130 seconds.

○ **What is hydroxyethyl starch?**

Hydroxyethyl starch (hetastarch) is a synthetic colloid solution available as a 6% solution in 0.9% sodium chloride or lactated Ringers for volume expansion. It has been reported to affect coagulation by decreasing factor VIII:C levels and interfering with clot formation by direct movement of hetastarch molecules into the fibrin clot. It is recommended that dosage be less than 20 ml/kg to minimize difficulties with crossmatching and bleeding. Either 1:1 or 1:2 replacement is suggested for blood loss to maintain euvolemia.

○ **A patient undergoing a vascular procedure receives high-dose heparin. Shortly thereafter, the surgeon reports clot formation. Laboratory work shows normal PTT. What is the likely diagnosis and how is it treated?**

Antithrombin III deficiency. The treatment is with FFP transfusion or a AT III concentrate to increase antithrombin III levels.

○ **How can you reverse warfarin anticoagulation?**

Warfarin is a vitamin K antagonist which inhibits hepatic production of factors II, VII, IX and X and proteins C, S and Z. The half-life is approximately 36-42 hours. Reversal of warfarin anticoagulation is achieved by administering either vitamin K or FFP 5 to 8 ml/kg.

○ **What is the significance of pulmonary edema in the transfused patient?**

The most common cause of pulmonary edema after transfusion is cardiogenic, due to fluid overload, with or without left ventricular dysfunction. Rarely transfusion can provoke a non-cardiogenic pulmonary edema due to transfusion related lung injury, massive transfusion or gram-negative sepsis.

○ **How do you correct hemophilia B?**

Factor IX deficiency is corrected with FFP to at least 30% of normal or with the administration of recombinant or monoclonal purified factor IX.

○ **How does von Willebrand's disease manifest itself?**

Most patients have a history of bleeding excessively with surgery, tooth extractions, trauma or following ingestion of aspirin or NSAIDs. Nosebleeds or menorrhagia are the most frequent clinical problems. Typical laboratory findings: prolonged PTT and bleeding time, with qualitative platelet dysfunction.

○ **How is von Willebrand's disease treated?**

DDAVP, cryoprecipitate or FFP. Desmopressin will increase plasma von Willebrand factor and factor VIII concentrations two- to fivefold.

○ **A patient develops postoperative bleeding. What common causes should you consider?**

Surgically correctable bleeding, clotting factor problem, platelet deficiency, DIC, hypothermia or residual heparin effect.

O   **If a patient is receiving blood and has a potential hemolytic transfusion reaction, what should you do if they still need blood?**

Use type O Rh-negative packed red blood cells. Stop the blood transfusion. Confirm the diagnosis of major transfusion reaction, repeat donor and recipient blood types, avoid further transfusions unless absolutely necessary. If you must continue to transfuse, consider universal donor blood as an error might have occurred in the typing.

O   **What are potential problems with massive blood transfusion?**

Hypothermia, thrombocytopenia, hypokalemia, hyperkalemia, dilution of clotting factors, acidosis, ARDS, pulmonary edema, hypocalcemia and hypomagnesemia due to citrate intoxication, hepatitis or other infectious diseases.

O   **What is the fastest way to reverse coumadin?**

FFP administration.

O   **What are the manifestations of beta thalassemia major?**

This is the most severe form of beta thalassemia and has manifestations which include: frontal bossing, overgrowth of the maxilla, splenomelagy, congestive heart failure, possible pericarditis and SVT. Multiple transfusions may cause iron-overload, diabetes, hypothyroidism, adrenal insufficiency, liver failure and/or myocardial damage.

O   **What is the main treatment for beta thalassemia major?**

Chronic transfusion therapy, to keep the Hgb over 9 g/dL.

O   **What is the treatment for febrile non-hemolytic reaction?**

Acetaminophen, NSAIDs, antihistamines and leuko-depleted blood products.

O   **What is the normal blood volume in adults, children, infants and neonates?**

Adults 70 (men 75 and women 65); children 75; infants 80; full-term neonates 85 (ml/kg).

O   **How do you maintain urine output in the patient with a hemolytic transfusion reaction?**

Intravenous fluids, mannitol, furosemide, and alkalinize the urine with sodium bicarbonate.

O   **What are the key laboratory values suggestive of acute DIC?**

There is no one pathognomonic test for DIC; prolonged PT and PTT in 75% and 50 to 60% of patients, respectively, reduced platelet count and fibrinogen with elevation of fibrin degradation products.

O   **What are the major causes of DIC?**

Septicemia, amniotic fluid embolism, trauma, hemolytic transfusion reactions, massive transfusion, liver disease, viremias, burns and leukemia.

O   **What is the drug antagonist for heparin?**

Protamine (1 mg protamine for each 100 units of heparin given, repeating the ACT measurement 3-5 minutes after reversal). The protamine dose may be calculated based on the heparin-dose response curve.

○ **What happens to clotting if too much protamine is given to antagonize heparin?**

Excess protamine has anticoagulant activity (1/100 that of heparin).

○ **List 3 ways of collecting autologous blood for transfusion.**

Pre-donation of the patient's blood days or weeks prior to surgery, *intraoperative isovolemic hemodilution* using blood withdrawal and simultaneous volume replacement with cell-free substitutes or *perioperative blood salvage* during and immediately after surgery.

○ **What are the relative contraindications to autologous blood donation?**

Severe aortic stenosis, severe left main coronary artery disease, anemia, recent myocardial infarction or unstable angina, hypertrophic cardiomyopathy, active bacterial infection or low blood volume (weight < 100 pounds).

○ **What is acute normovolemic hemodilution (ANH)?**

A point-of-care method of autologous blood procurement. Whole blood is removed at the start of the operative procedure (1 to 1.5 liters, to a hematocrit of 27 to 33%) with reconstitution of the patient's circulating blood volume with crystalloid or colloids solutions to maintain normovolemia. Blood is stored in the operating room at room temperature and is re-infused during or immediately following surgery.

○ **What is the rationale for acute hemodilution?**

During surgery, the patient will lose blood at a lower hematocrit and the fresh whole blood withdrawn immediately prior to surgery will be available for reinfusion. This procedure may reduce total red cell volume loss, enhance the maximum allowable blood loss before blood transfusion, as well as, reduce the need for transfusion of allogeneic blood.

○ **Describe the process of intraoperative autotransfusion.**

Intraoperative autotransfusion is defined as the reinfusion of patient blood salvaged during the operation. Red "cell savers" collect and anticoagulate the salvaged blood with citrate or heparin as it leaves the surgical field, filter to remove debris and clots, wash with saline and concentrate red blood cells (RBC) by centrifugation, and the concentrate is then reinfused to the patient suspended in saline in aliquots of 125-225 ml with an Hct of 45-65%.

○ **What are the potential complications of IBS (intraoperative blood salvage)?**

Cost, contamination, removal of essential blood components (clotting factors and platelets) and air embolism.
   a) Reinfusion of materials that might remain after the washing process such as fat, microaggregates, air, red cell stroma, free hemoglobin, heparin, bacteria, tumor and debris from a contaminated surgical field.
   b) Massive air embolism has been reported. Direct return of blood to the patient from the cell saver device and the use of pressure infusor devices applied to the collected blood bags is not recommended.
   c) Dilutional coagulopathy is associated with large-volume IBS because washing removes clotting factors and most of the platelets. DIC-like coagulopathy has also been reported especially with the older cell saver devices.

○ **What is isovolemic hemodilution?**

During surgery, acute blood loss is replaced with an equal volume of an isoosmotic solution, resulting in acute isovolemic hemodilution.

○   **In isovolemic hemodilution, what mechanisms serve to maintain oxygen delivery?**

Increase in cardiac output, redistribution of blood flow to organs with greater oxygen requirements, increased oxygen extraction and decreased hemoglobin oxygen affinity.

○   **What is the primary reason for increase in cardiac output with isovolemic hemodilution?**

Anemia must be fairly severe (hemoglobin < 7 g/dL) before cardiac output increases. The rise in cardiac output is related mainly to a decrease in blood viscosity and enhanced sympathetic stimulation. As hematocrit decreases, a reduction in blood viscosity causes a decrease in peripheral vascular resistance and increase in stroke volume (increased venomotor tone and venous return), so that cardiac output rises without an increase in blood pressure.

○   **What happens to the oxygen transport during hemodilution?**

Over a wide range of hematocrits (usually between 30 and 45%), isovolemic hemodilution is self-correcting. The decrease in the oxygen carrying capacity of the blood due to decreased red blood cells is matched by improvement in oxygen transport due to improved blood flow to the tissues. Decreasing hematocrit from 40% to 20% decreases the viscosity by 50%.

○   **How does healthy heart compensate for anemia during hemodilution?**

Redistribution of blood flow to the coronary circulation, as under basal conditions the heart already has a high extraction ratio (between 50-70% vs. 30% in most tissues).

○   **What is extraction ratio?**

The extraction ratio (ER) defines what fraction of the total oxygen delivered is consumed or extracted by the tissues; ER = oxygen consumption/oxygen delivery. In healthy resting adults the overall extraction ratio of oxygen from capillary blood is about 25%, but may increase to 70-80% during maximal exercise in well trained athletes.

○   **What is the reason for decreased hemoglobin oxygen affinity in anemia?**

Increased 2,3-diphosphoglycerate. In chronic anemia, increased oxygen extraction by tissues produces increased concentration of deoxyhemoglobin in the RBC, which stimulates the production of 2,3-DPG and lowers the affinity of hemoglobin A for oxygen.

○   **Which data may be useful in determining a red blood cell transfusion threshold?**

Cardiac output, arterial and mixed venous oxygen, and the whole body extraction ration.

○   **What happens once the critical threshold for hemoglobin is reached during hemodilution?**

According to the studies, at Hct of 10% and a whole body ER of approximately 50%, no further increase in oxygen consumption (VO_2) occurs; the tissue converts to anaerobic metabolism, which leads to metabolic acidosis and hemodynamic instability. Death occurs due to high output failure with severe tissue hypoxia.

○   **What type of transfusion reactions may occur?**

Hemolytic transfusion reactions (anti A or anti B antibodies during a ABO incompatible transfusion), allergic reactions and febrile nonhemolytic transfusion reactions. Most of the serious transfusion reactions are immunologically mediated and febrile non-hemolytic is the most common..

○   **What causes immediate hemolytic transfusion reactions?**

This is usually due to ABO incompatibility but may also be due to Kell, Kidd, Lewis and Duffy antigens. When incompatible blood is administered, antibodies and compliment in the recipient's plasma attack the corresponding antigens on donor RBCs. The resulting hemolysis may take place in the intravascular space (most catastrophic) and/or in the extravascular space.

O   **What are the signs and symptoms of a hemolytic transfusion reaction?**

During general anesthesia; hypotension, hemoglobinuria and diffuse bleeding. Oliguria may develop due to renal failure. Clinical manifestations in the awake patient may include fever, chills, nausea, and vomiting, diarrhea, and rigors. The patient become hypotensive and tachycardic, restless, flushed and dyspneic (histamine). Chest, flank and back pain result from diffuse intravascular occlusion by agglutinated RBCs.

O   **How do you manage a hemolytic transfusion reaction?**

If a reaction is suspected, the transfusion should be stopped immediately. Notify transfusion services and send blood samples for compatibility testing. Management has four main objectives 1) maintenance of systemic blood pressure (volume, pressors, inotropes, detect hyperkalemia), 2) preservation of renal function (fluid, mannitol, diuretics to promote urine output), 3) prevention of DIC (prevent stasis and hypoperfusion by avoiding hypotension and supporting cardiac output) and 4) treat bronchospasm.

O   **What tests are indicated to establish the diagnosis of hemolytic transfusion reaction?**

1) Direct antiglobulin (Coombs) test – examines recipients' RBCs for the presence of surface immunoglobulins and complement.
2) Serum haptoglobin level, plasma and urine hemoglobin, and bilirubin indicate hemolysis
3) Repeat crossmatch with recipient and donor blood

O   **If a patient experiences a fever with or without chills during blood transfusion, what is the differential diagnosis?**

Fever occurs in 0.1 to 1% of transfusions and must be considered an ominous sign.

*   Febrile nonhemolytic reactions due to leukocyte antibodies can be treated with acetaminophen. Typically a temperature increase of more than 1° C occurs within 4 hours of a blood transfusion and for most patients is unpleasant but temporary
*   Bacterial contamination of blood products (especially platelets)
*   Acute hemolytic transfusion reaction
*   Administration of thrombocytes as a result of antibodies against thrombocytes or cytokines in the product

O   **What causes hypocalcemia after blood transfusion?**

Citrate in stored blood binding calcium resulting in acute ionized hypocalcemia.

O   **Should you routinely administer calcium salts IV to prevent hypocalcemia during blood transfusions?**

No, calcium administration is rarely necessary. Citrate is metabolized efficiently by the liver, and decreased ionized calcium levels should not occur unless the rate of transfusion exceeds 1ml/kg/min or about 1 unit of blood per 5 minutes in an adult. Risk factors include impaired liver function, hypoperfusion and hypothermia. Low ionized calcium levels do not correct readily giving IV calcium salts in doses generally recommended (1 g), but return towards normal when hemodynamic status improves. Therefore, even in patients with low-output states, the emphasis should be placed on correcting the underlying disorder.

O   **Describe the storage defect in blood.**

↓ pH due to RBC conversion of glucose to lactate
↓ 2,3-DPG
↓ ATP
↓ Glucose
↑ Plasma potassium, ammonia and hemoglobin
↑ Ionized phosphate with ↓ 2,3-DPG
WBC and platelet function lost after 24/48 hours
↓ Labile clotting factors (V, VIII)

○   **What is a massive transfusion?**

Any patient who receives a transfusion of one or more blood volumes in less than 24 hours, which is equivalent to 10 or more units of packed RBC transfused in an adult.

○   **What causes coagulopathy in massively transfused patients?**

Multifactorial etiology: dilutional thrombocytopenia, depletion of coagulation factors (V, VIII, and fibrinogen) and DIC. Risk factors include the volume of blood given and the duration of hypotension and hypoperfusion. Hemolytic transfusion reaction also causes coagulopathy and should be considered.

○   **How should dilutional coagulopathy from massive packed cell transfusion be treated?**

During massive transfusions of packed RBCs, patients receive only a small residual plasma volume (50 mls) which contains clotting factors. Investigations of patients receiving large-volume isovolemic transfusions suggest that clinically significant dilution of fibrinogen; factors II,V,VIII; and platelets will occur after volume exchange of approx. 140%, 200-230%, and 230% (1.4, 2, 2.3 blood volumes), respectively. Resuscitation from hypovolemia will result in reaching these thresholds at smaller percentage volume exchanges. Treatments includes: cryoprecipitate (fibrinogen), FFP (clotting factors) and platelet transfusions.

○   **What is the purpose of compatibility testing prior to blood transfusion?**

These tests are designed to prevent lethal antigen-antibody interactions between donor and recipient blood.

○   **An patient is brought into the emergency room exsanguinating from blood loss. There is not enough time for complete compatibility testing. What is the first choice for blood products?**

The first choice is to transfuse type-specific, partially cross-matched blood. This incomplete crossmatch takes 1-5 minutes and is accomplished by adding the patient's serum to donor RBCs at room temperature, centrifuging it and then looking for macroscopic agglutination (confirms no clerical or laboratory errors). ABO-Rh typing alone results in a 99.8% chance of a compatible transfusion. The addition of an antibody screen increases the safety to 99.94%, and a complete crossmatch increases this to 99.95%.

○   **What is the second preference?**

Type-specfic uncrossmatched blood.

○   **What is the last option?**

O negative packed RBCs.

○   **What are the indications for administration of cryoprecipitate?**

1.   Hemophilia A (F VIII deficiency) – should try DDAVP first
2.   Von Willebrand Disease (bleeding unresponsive to DDAVP)
3.   Hypofibrinogenemia (fibrinogen <80 mg/dl) - cryoprecipitate is preferable to commercially prepare fibrinogen, which has a high risk of hepatitis.

4.   Sometimes used if platelet dysfunction with renal failure does not respond to DDAVP or dialysis.

○   **How does perfluorochemicals (PFCs) transport oxygen?**

PFCs are chemically inert liquids in which the solubility for oxygen is nearly 20 times that of water. Since PFCs transport oxygen by simple solubility, the oxygen carrying capacity is directly proportional to the percentage of PFCs in the blood stream and to the partial pressure of oxygen inspired. Direct diffusion of oxygen is off-loaded to peripheral tissues.

○   **What are the limitations of PFCs?**

a) Short plasma half-life of 12 hours, b) requires a high inspired oxygen ie: 400 mm Hg or greater of partial pressure, c) completely immiscible with water and must be prepared as an emulsion, d) costly, e) rapidly removed from the circulation and retained in the reticuloendothelial system for about one week, and f) can be used only in a single, low dosage in humans.

HEMOSTASIS

It's Not The Size Of The Dog In The Fight - It's The Size Of The Fight In The Dog.
Mark Twain

○ **List the vitamin K-dependent coagulation factors.**

Factors II, VII, IX, and X. Vitamin K activates each factor with the addition of a carboxyl group, which then enables them to bind via calcium to the phospholipid surface.

○ **Which of the vitamin K-dependent coagulation factors has the shortest half-life?**

Factor VII, with a half-life of 6 hours.

○ **How does coumadin work as an anticoagulant?**

Coumadin is a vitamin K antagonist that block the carboxylation of the vitamin K-dependent factors by competing with vitamin K for binding sites on the hepatocyte where the carboxylation occurs.

○ **Where are the coagulation factors produced?**

All are manufactured in the liver except factor VIII which is synthesized by vascular endothelium.

○ **Describe how heparin functions as an anticoagulant.**

Heparin alone has no intrinsic anticoagulant activity. Heparin acts as a catalyst to accelerate the interaction between antithrombin III and the activated forms of factors XIII, XII, XI, X and II. Heparin-induced thrombocytopenia is caused by heparin-dependent antibodies which agglutinate platelets.

○ **What is the treatment for antithrombin III (antithrombin III) deficiency?**

Depends on the patient's risk of recurrent thromboembolic disease. Patients with a history of arterial or venous clot may require anticoagulation (warfarin, heparin, or low molecular weight heparin). AT-III concentrates (or FFP) have been used in the perioperative period for surgical prophylaxis in patients with known deficiency.

○ **Describe the most commonly used tests used to evaluate primary hemostasis.**

Platelet count and bleeding time.

Normal platelet count is between 150,000 and 450,000/mm^3. Patients with platelet counts greater than 100,000/mm^3 and normal function have normal primary hemostasis. Ivy bleeding time performed in a standardized fashion is 4 to 9 minutes and is abnormal if greater than 15 minutes. Unfortunately, there is lack of correlation between bleeding time and intraoperative bleeding.

○ **How does one reverse the effects of coumadin?**

Wait 4 to 5 days until the PT normalizes, or give Vitamin K IM and 2 units of fresh frozen plasma IV.

○ **What drug is used to reverse the anticoagulant effects of heparin?**

Protamine. Protamine (positively charged protein) binds and neutralizes heparin (negatively charged polysaccharide), with the complex then cleared by the reticuloendothelial system.

O   **What are the potential side effects of protamine?**

Hypotension secondary to systemic vasodilation, marked pulmonary hypertension or anaphylaxis. These are immune-mediated and idiosyncratic reactions. Patients at risk include: those with an allergy to salmon, vasectomized males, prior exposure with sensitization and diabetic patients taking NPH insulin.

O   **What is the treatment for adverse events after IV protamine administration following cardiopulmonary bypass?**

IV protamine sulphate has been reported to cause hypotension and bradycardia. Severe adverse reactions include: anaphylaxis (bronchospasm, vasodilatation and capillary leak) and anaphylactoid reactions (circulatory collapse, capillary leak, noncardiogenic pulmonary edema and acute pulmonary hypertension). Irreversible circulatory collapse associated with coronary spasm and reduced cardiac output can also occur. Standard emergency resuscitation and treatment of shock is indicated: discontinue the drug, 100% oxygen, epinephrine, IV fluids, bronchodilators, antihistamines (H_1 antagonists) and corticosteroids with invasive hemodynamic monitoring and inotropic support as needed.

O   **How is the effectiveness of coumadin therapy evaluated?**

Monitoring International Normalized Ratio (INR) or prothrombin time (PT). The recommended therapeutic range for standard oral anticoagulant therapy is an INR = 2 to 3, and with high-dose therapy an INR = 2.5 to 3.5.

O   **What is INR?**

INR is a means of converting the PT ratio to a value obtained using a standardized PT method. The INR is calculated as $(PT_{patient}/PT_{normal})^{ISI}$ where ISI is the international sensitivity index assigned to the test system. This testing system was devised to improve the consistency of dosing coumadin.

O   **What does PTT measure and what are the normal values?**

aPTT is the activated partial thromboplastin time. Maximal activation of the contact factors XII and XI is achieved with the addition of diatomaceous earth, kaolin or crushed glass to the test tube before the addition of partial thromboplastin. Normal aPTT is 25 to 35 seconds.

PTT is the partial thromboplastin time and is used to assess all the coagulation factors in the intrinsic and common pathways, except factor XIII. Normal values are 40 to 100 seconds, with > 120 seconds abnormal.

O   **What does PT measure and what are the normal values?**

PT is prothrombin time. It is a measure of the coagulation reactions of the extrinsic and common pathways, and the patient's response to oral anticoagulant therapy. Normal values are 10-12 seconds.

O   **What is the ACT and when is it used?**

ACT is activated clotting time, which is used primarily to monitor heparin therapy during cardiopulmonary bypass. Baseline values are usually 100-120 seconds and an ACT of 480 seconds or longer is considered acceptable anticoagulant activity of heparin for instituting cardiopulmonary bypass.

O   **What are the uses and limitations of measuring activated clotting time (ACT)?**

ACT is used to monitor heparin effect during cardiopulmonary bypass (CPB), interventional cardiology and hemodialysis. Limitations include:

- new technology (instruments and reagents) gives varying results for IV heparin dosing when trying to achieve a standard target ACT for CPB (480 seconds using Hemochron 801)
- choice of activator (celite or kaolin); if aprotinin is administered concomitantly, the celite ACT becomes significantly higher than the kaolin ACT due to decreased thrombin generation; insufficient anticoagulation using C-ACT may result
- ACT may lack correlation with heparin levels because of its lack of specificity for heparin and variability during hypothermia and hemodilution on CPB. Changes in the ACT can reflect changes in [heparin-ATIII], changes in [thrombin] or both.

⃝ Describe when a thromboelastogram (TEG) may be helpful.

TEG is a viscoelastic measure of coagulation function. TEG assesses coagulation by measuring viscosity and elasticity of the clot as it forms. TEG provides a rapid interpretation of coagulation function (which would otherwise require analysis of a combined number of tests) particularly useful in patients receiving massive transfusions or at risk of bleeding from multiple causes (platelet dysfunction, factor deficiencies, fibrinolysis) i.e.: liver transplantation or cardiac surgical patients. The accuracy of TEG may be greater than that of routine coagulation tests in predicting clinical bleeding.

⃝ What is the most common inherited bleeding disorder?

Von Willebrand disease, which is a qualitative platelet disorder, in which there is a deficiency of factor VIII antigen and factor VIII:vWF (von Willebrand factor).

⃝ What are the two key functions of von Willebrand factor (factor VIII:vWF)?

Von Willebrand factor is necessary for platelet adhesion to collagen in the subendothelial layer of injured blood vessels and formation of the hemostatic plug through regulation and release of factor VIII antigen.

⃝ What is the treatment for Von Willebrand's disease?

Depends on the type (1,2 or 3), severity of the disorder and type of surgery. The aim of treatment is to correct the dual defect of hemostasis: the abnormal intrinsic coagulation pathway caused by low factor VIII levels and the prolonged bleeding time resulting from abnormal platelet adhesion. Desmopressin (DDAVP) is the treatment of choice for type 1 VWD because it corrects the FVIII/VWF levels and the prolonged bleeding time in the majority of cases. In type 3 and in severe forms of type 1 and 2 VWD, DDAVP is not effective and plasma virally-inactivated concentrates containing FVIII and VWF (von Willebrand factor) are the mainstay of treatment.

⃝ What are the laboratory findings in patients with von Willebrand's disease?

A prolonged bleeding time, normal platelet count, decreased factor VIII activity, and decreased plasma factor VIII:vWF. A history of easy bruising or excessive bleeding during surgery or following ingestion of aspirin or nonsteroidal antiinflammatory drugs may be the only clue to this disease.

⃝ Does Ketorolac have a significant effect on platelet function?

Yes. Ketorolac is a cyclo-oxygenase inhibitor which decreases prostaglandin synthesis (thromboxane B_2) resulting in a reversible impairment in platelet aggregation. Bleeding time is prolonged. Platelet dysfunction following ketorolac 0.4 mg/kg IV may persist beyond 24 hours.

⃝ How do you reverse fibrinolytic agents?

Fibrinolytics (streptokinase, urokinase, alteplase, reteplase and tenecteplase) are used for the acute treatment of DVT and myocardial infarction to break up thrombi by activating the conversion of plasminogen to plasmin, which degrades fibrin.

Management of toxicity:
- Discontinue the drug
- Consider treating hemorrhage with fresh blood, packed pRBC, cryoprecipitate, fresh-frozen plasma, platelets, desmopressin and tranexamic acid or aminocaproic acid if hemorrhage is unresponsive to conventional therapy
- Avoid dextrans for volume expansion due to platelet inhibiting effect

○   **Which commonly used herbs may increase bleeding.**

Feverfew, garlic, ginger, ginkgo biloba, ginseng and vitamin E.

HYPOTHERMIA

The Most Effective Means Of Cooling A Man Is To Give Him An Anesthetic.
Pickering, 1958

○ **Why is the maintenance of body temperature of biological importance?**

Homeothermic organisms have a relatively constant body temperature ensuring optimum enzymatic function. These protein catalysts integrate the body's complex biochemical reactions. Their action is temperature dependent.

○ **What is core temperature?**

Central compartment (core) blood temperature corresponding to the vessel-rich group organs. The body is divided into three temperature compartments: central, peripheral and the skin.

○ **What is 'normal' body temperature?**

37°C +/- 0.2°C, in humans.

○ **Are certain groups of patients more susceptible to becoming hypothermic?**

Heat loss during anesthesia (the heat of vaporization is possibly the largest source) is greatest at extremes of age. Geriatric patients have reduced autonomic vascular control and neonates have a large surface area-to-mass ratio.

The high risk surgical procedures are those involving exposure of large skin, serosal and mucosal surfaces during lengthy procedures under general anesthesia (with no humidification of gases) in a "cold" operating room, with the patient receiving cold IV solutions. Disruption of the hypothalamic thermoregulatory center will cause the patient to become poikilothermic.

○ **What factors make newborns more susceptible to hypothermia?**

- increased heat loss due to increased surface area-to-mass ratio
- high respiratory water loss and thin subcutaneous tissues causing increased thermal conductance
- diminished thermoregulatory response
- diminished ability to produce endogenous heat (reduced shivering thermogenesis)

Sedative drugs, hypoglycemia and cerebral damage further increase heat loss.

○ **What are the consequences of hypothermia in neonates?**

Hypothermia can result in acidosis, hypoxemia, apnea, hypoventilation, and cardiac arrest. Pulmonary vasoconstriction may cause an increase in pulmonary artery pressure, right-to-left intracardiac shunting and cardiopulmonary decompensation.

○ **How do full term infants compensate for this heat loss?**

Physiologic cold responses include non-shivering thermogenesis > vasoconstriction and shivering behavior.

Heat production is achieved primarily by non-shivering thermogenesis (metabolism of brown fat stores). Voluntary muscle activity is restricted during the perioperative period and shivering thermogenesis is not significant until the infant reaches at least one year of age. Vasoconstriction can occur in both full-term and premature infants, decreasing cutaneous blood flow and conductive heat loss.

○   **Are the elderly more prone to hypothermia?**

Yes, primarily due to impaired temperature regulation.

Factors that increase their susceptibility include; less insulation due to smaller amounts of subcutaneous tissue, decreased reflex cutaneous vasoconstriction, and decreased heat production (decline in basal metabolic rate by 1% per year after age 30 years).

○   **What mechanisms are used to reduce hyperthermia?**

Vasodilation and sweating.

○   **Where is the best non-invasive site for measuring core temperature?**

External auditory meatus. The thermoregulatory center is in the hypothalamus. The closer a temperature monitoring site is to this area the more reflective measurements will be of the 'core' temperature. Since the tympanic membrane is in close proximity to the internal carotid artery and brain stem it is considered the "Gold Standard." It has also been suggested that a nasopharyngeal probe placed close to the ethmoid plate similarly reflects brain temperature.

○   **What are the most common sites for measuring core temperature?**

Sites for accurate monitoring of core temperature includes probe in the lower one-third of the esophagus, tympanic membrane, and pulmonary artery catheter. Repeated measurements of tympanic membrane temperature is not practical for a variety of reasons, such as danger of eardrum perforation. Central core temperature is higher than skin temperature by 3 to 4°C. Transitional zones (peripheral compartment) includes: axillary temperature (1 °C less), bladder, and mouth. Rectal temperatures are unreliable. Skin temperature (outer shell) is influenced by changes in the external environment.

○   **Is forehead temperature a good reflection of core temperature?**

No.

○   **Define hypothermia**

A core temperature of less than 36°C.

○   **What is the typical pattern of unintentional hypothermia during general anesthesia?**

Typically: a precipitous drop in core temperature during the first hour (phase I redistribution), followed by a gradual decline during the next 3 to 4 hours (phase II heat loss), eventually reaching a steady state (phase III equilibrium).

○   **Can hypothermia be beneficial?**

Yes. Mild hypothermia reduces metabolic oxygen requirements (9% for every degree in temperature drop) which may limit warm ischemia, cerebral and myocardial injury. Preservation of vital organs for transplantation is inherent upon rendering the organ metabolically inert by reducing the core temperature to 4 °C through cold preservation techniques. For organ specific protection, lowering the body temperature to 33 °C for 12 or 24 hours in comatose survivors of cardiac arrest has been shown to improve neurologic outcome.

○   **When does hypothermia become detrimental?**

It really depends on who you ask.   The ideal is maintenance of normal body temperature. For whole body hypothermia, the surgeon may respond 34°C (platelet dysfunction, fibrinolysis and bleeding begin to increase in a linear fashion), the anesthetist may respond 37°C (delayed reversal of muscle relaxation or increased risk of myocardial ischemia) or 32°C (arrhythmia, cold diuresis, delayed awakening). There may be an increased risk of infection in hypothermic patients as well. The detrimental physiological effects of mild hypothermia (32 to 35°C) include depression of mental status, tachycardia, shivering and muscle weakness.

O   **What is the effect of general anesthesia on basal metabolic rate?**

A reduction of approximately 15%. Greater if muscle relaxants are used (up to 50%) and some degree of hypothermia occurs.

O   **What are the effects of hypothermia on the central nervous system?**

Mild hypothermia (32-35°C)
- Decrease in cerebral blood flow, increase in cerebral vascular resistance, normal arteriovenous oxygen difference.
- Decrease in cerebral metabolic oxygen and glucose consumption 7 to 10% per °C decrease in temperature.
- MAC of volatile agents is reduced by approximately 5 to 7% per °C decrease in temperature.
- Delayed emergence, sedation, confusion < 33°C.
- Narcosis at < 30°C.
- Increase in latency in motor and SSEP.
- Slowing of the EEG, isoelectric at 20°C.

O   **What changes does hypothermia produce in the cardiovascular system?**

- Preload: increase in CVP.
- Afterload: increase in systemic vascular resistance due to vasoconstriction, with vasodilation below 20° degrees.
- Heart rate and rhythm: bradycardia and arrhythmias (nodal, PVC, AV-block and ventricular fibrillation or asystole).
- Contractility: decreases, reduced cardiac output.
- Effect on coronary blood flow is variable, coronary artery resistance decreases.
- Pulmonary vascular resistance is increased.
- Increased myocardial oxygen demand with shivering (300%).
- EKG: sinus bradycardia, prolonged PR and QT intervals, widened QRS complexes.

If the sympathetic adrenergic response is functional, the initial response is sympathetic stimulation with an increase in heart rate, blood pressure and cardiac output.

O   **Is respiratory function compromised by hypothermia?**

Yes. Hypothermia has been cited as one of the primary reasons for reintubation in the recovery room following general anesthesia.

Pulmonary Effects of Hypothermia
- Increase in pulmonary vascular resistance.
- Decrease in hypoxic pulmonary vasoconstriction.
- Increased V/Q mismatch and hypoxemia.
- Depression of the hypoxic ventilatory drive, no change in the CO_2 ventilatory response.
- Bronchodilation (increase in anatomic dead-space).
- Increase in carbon dioxide and oxygen solubility, a rule of thumb is that the body temperature (°C) should equal the $PaCO_2$ in mm Hg.
- The pH rises 0.015 units per centigrade decrease in temperature.

○   **How does hypothermia effect the metabolism of anesthetic drugs?**

Hypothermia impairs both hepatic metabolism and renal clearance of drugs due to a reduction in blood flow. Half-life is prolonged for vecuronium (liver) and pancuronium (kidney). Metabolism of drugs dependent on Hoffman elimination or esterases is delayed (cis-atracurium and atracurium). Protein binding increases as body temperature decreases.

○   **T/F: Inhalational induction of anesthesia is facilitated by the decrease in MAC seen in hypothermic patients?**

False. The MAC of inhalational agents is decreased 5 to 7% per °C decrease in core temperature, but decreased cardiac output and increased blood solubility offset this effect resulting in no change in the speed of inhalational induction.

○   **What are the hematologic consequences of hypothermia?**

•   Thrombocytopenia secondary to platelet aggregation and sequestration in the portal circulation.
•   Increased fibrinolysis and DIC with tissue damage.
•   Reduced clotting factor activity.
•   Sequestration of leukocytes.
•   Increase in blood viscosity due to increase in hematocrit and plasma protein (2 to 3% with each centigrade decrease in temperature).
•   Increase in hematocrit and rouleaux formation.
•   Shift of the oxygen-hemoglobin dissociation curve to the left.
•   Decrease in plasma volume (cold diuresis and impaired sodium resorption).

○   **How is renal function affected by hypothermia?**

Renal blood flow and GFR are decreased. Cold-induced diuresis and impaired tubular transport sodium, chloride and water may lead to hypovolemia. Reabsorption of potassium is decreased. The ability to concentrate or dilute urine is impaired.

○   **What are the consequences of shivering?**

A significant increase in oxygen consumption and CO_2 production. This may result in myocardial ischemia or hypoxemia and respiratory acidosis, respectively.

○   **Which modalities are available in order to treat shivering?**

Ideally, passive or active rewarming will prevent perioperative hypothermia. The most effective drug therapy is IV meperidine 12.5 to 25 mg.

○   **How do you respond to the surgeon who demands that the operating room temperature be reduced because of the increased risk of wound infection?**

Recent evidence shows that the risk of wound infection is increased in hypothermic patients, possibly due to impaired neutrophil function and vasoconstriction with hypoperfusion of peripheral tissues and tissue hypoxia. The ideal temperature for vascular surgery is 70°F.

○   **Can warming fluids aid in the prevention of hypothermia?**

Yes. One unit of refrigerated blood or one liter of room-temperature crystalloid decreases the body temperature about 0.25°C. If a massive transfusion is anticipated then a rapid infusion system that can deliver blood at 37°C at rates of 250-500ml/min can be used.

○   **What are the consequences of postoperative rewarming?**

If a patient is hypothermic in the immediate postoperative period, and then rewarmed, the physiologic consequences include vasodilation, shivering, and increased basal metabolic rate (increased O_2 consumption and CO_2 production). Vasodilation may unmask underlying hypovolemia resulting in hypotension and tachycardia.

○   **Why is shivering undesirable in the postoperative period?**

Shivering will increase oxygen consumption (up to 400%). In addition, peripheral vascular resistance and CVP are increased, all of which may be especially detrimental in patients with compromised cardiac function and microsurgery for replantation and rotational flaps. In an awake patient, shivering may cause significant discomfort.

○   **What postoperative complications are associated with mild hypothermia?**

Hypothermia to core temperatures near 34°C may be associated with myocardial ischemia, impaired resistance to surgical wound infections, coagulopathies and postoperative shivering.

○   **What are the causes of intraoperative hypothermia?**

•   Altered normal thermoregulatory mechanisms
•   Peripheral vasodilation with increased heat loss
•   Reduced heat production from muscle
•   Reduced basal metabolic rate
•   No shivering
•   Decrease in the threshold for peripheral vasoconstriction
•   Altered sympathetic response to hypothermia
•   Cold environment (room temp, skin preparation solutions, irrigation, cold IV fluids)
•   Exposure of pleural, pericardial and peritoneal surfaces
•   Prolonged surgery (rate of heat loss in greatest in the first hour, with as much as 1°C reduction in core temperature within the first 15 minutes of induction)

○   **Mechanisms of intraoperative heat loss?**

•   Heat of vaporization (respiratory tract moisture and heat loss)
•   Conduction (heat loss from warm body surfaces in contact with colder surfaces)
•   Convection (cold air mass moving across exposed areas of a patient)
•   Radiation (heat from the patient into the atmosphere)

○   **What are the causes of intraoperative hyperthermia?**

•   Prevention of convective heat loss by covering the patient
•   Prolonged closed or semi-closed systems that increase heat and moisture from the carbon dioxide-soda lime reaction
•   Malfunction or overuse of a humidifier, heat-moisture exchanger or fluid warmer
•   High ambient temperature
•   Sepsis
•   Malignant hyperthermia, thyroid storm
•   Thermal instability (osteogenesis imperfecta)
•   Drugs

○   **Describe methods of intraoperative rewarming.**

Warming the blood (cardiopulmonary bypass, counter-current heat exchanger using an endovascular heat-exchange catheter, fluid warmers); surface skin rewarming methods (circulating-water warming garment, forced air warming, heating blanket, myler foil wrapping); lavage body cavities; airways (humidifier and heat-moisture exchanger).

○   **Discuss the physiology of deliberate hypothermia.**

Deliberate hypothermia is used as a neuroprotective strategy to decrease cerebral metabolic requirements in patients at risk for cerebral hypoperfusion and postoperative neurocognitive dysfunction. The temperature required to achieve electrocortical silence ranges from 12.5°C to 27.2°C (median 18°C).

○   **Where is the thermoregulatory center found in poikilothermic animals?**

The hypothalamus and thalamus. Hypothalamic and thalamic pathways can result in cortical excitation which is involved in behavioural changes. Efferent vasomotor, piloerector, sweating and shivering efferents are generated in the hypothalamus. *CNS thermosensors* are found in the pre-optic nucleus and anterior hypothalamus. The posterior hypothalamus is the location of the *set point for thermoregulation*.

AUTONOMIC PHARMACOLOGY AND PHYSIOLOGY

If winning isn't everything, why do they keep score?
Vince Lombardi

○ **A patient using echothiophate drops for treatment of glaucoma is scheduled for an emergency appendectomy. She was slow to recover muscle strength following succinylcholine. Diagnosis?**

Echothiophate inactivates plasma cholinesterase, thus prolonging the duration of action of succinylcholine.

○ **A patient develops a fever during hernia repair under general anesthesia. He was exposed to succinylcholine, atropine, fentanyl, midazolam, propofol, isoflurane, nitrous oxide and oxygen. What is the most likely diagnosis?**

Malignant hyperthermia until proven otherwise. An increase in end-tidal CO_2 and unexplained tachycardia is usually the first sign. In children, in the face of normocarbia, a rise in temperature is most likely due to the anticholinergenic effect of atropine on sweat glands or overbundling.

○ **What is the advantage of using glycopyrrolate as an anticholinergic medication versus atropine?**

Glycopyrrolate does not cross the blood-brain barrier (no central anti-cholinergic syndrome possible) and it has a longer duration of action than atropine (6-8 hours, with 2 hours of vagolytic activity). Onset of action is better matched with neostigmine compared to atropine, avoiding the initial tachycardia and arrhythmia seen with neostigmine-atropine.

○ **A patient appears to be disoriented after receiving atropine for treatment of bradycardia. What is the diagnosis and treatment?**

Immediately rule out causes secondary to neurologic or metabolic disorders (hypotension, hypoxemia, hypercarbia, acidosis, hypoglycemia and electrolyte disorders). Atropine can cross the blood-brain barrier and cause CNS symptoms in relatively large doses (1-2 mg). Physostigmine is an anticholinesterase that penetrates the blood-brain barrier and may reverse the CNS effect of atropine.

○ **What is a commonly used α_2-agonist for treating hypertension and its mechanism?**

Clonidine. α_2-agonists act at the pre-synaptic membrane to inhibit further release of catecholamines. This is a classic feedback mechanism. The sympatholytic effect results in a decrease in sympathetic outflow from the CNS medullary pressor centers, reducing activity in peripheral sympathetic neurons without affecting baroreceptor reflexes.

○ **A patient on isoproterenol 3 µg/kg/min is hypotensive. Why?**

Isoproterenol is a pure beta-adrenergic agonist. The β_2-vasodilating effect reduces systemic vascular resistance and diastolic blood pressure. Recommended infusion rate is 2-10 ug/min to clinical response. A dose of 3 µg/kg/min is too high.

○   **A parkinsonian patient requires urgent coronary artery bypass graft surgery while he is taking selegiline (selective inhibitor of monoamine oxidase type B). Should the patient stop taking MAO inhibitors prior to surgery?**

Although controversial, MAO inhibitors may be continued perioperatively. Decreased presynaptic metabolism of catecholamines and serotonin by MAOIs may be responsible for hemodynamic instability, hyperpyrexia and death when these patients are exposed to stress and anesthesia. Avoid meperidine (hyperpyrexic coma) and indirect acting sympathomimetic drugs (hypertensive crisis). Anticipate hemodynamic instability. If an adverse drug reaction occurs convert from a narcotic-based anesthetic to a volatile anesthetic technique with postoperative sedative infusion. All patients are considered to be at some level of risk.

○   **A patient with a history of CAD and bronchospasm presents with supraventricular tachycardia (SVT). What would be a reasonable medication to give?**

Verapamil, digoxin or beta-blockers. Adenosine is the drug of choice for terminating SVT but contraindicated in patients with asthma and those taking dipyridamole.

○   **How are acetylcholine and esmolol metabolized?**

Acetylcholine is hydrolyzed by acetylcholinesterase (tissue esterase or true esterase). Esmolol is metabolized by red blood cell esterases. These two enzymes are distinct from plasma esterase or pseudocholinesterase, whose function is not known but which is known to break down succinylcholine.

○   **What is the presumed mechanism of adrenergic denervation hypersensitivity?**

No signal is sensed after denervation, so cells respond by putting out more receptors to "catch" a signal. In the transplanted heart, surgical denervation of the postganglionic sympathetic nerves results in up-regulation of beta-adrenergic receptors and down-regulation of muscarinic receptors. Increased beta-adrenergic receptor density and adenylate cyclase stimulation account for the augmented chronotropic response to catecholamine stimulation.

○   **How is norepinephrine and epinephrine release by the adrenal medulla regulated differently from that of the neurotransmitter?**

The adrenal medulla is homologous to sympathetic ganglia. Cholinergic preganglionic fibers of the sympathetic nervous system (SNS) release acetylcholine and stimulate the adrenal medulla to release catecholamines. Stimuli include hypotension, hypothermia, hypoglycemia, hypercapnia, hypoxemia, fear and pain. Norepinephrine is the adrenergic neurotransmitter of the SNS that is released by postganglionic fibers at end-organ tissues (heart, smooth muscle and glands).

○   **Metoprolol is a selective β_1 antagonist. Why is it that in large doses metoprolol increases airway resistance?**

Selectivity is relative and dose-related. At large doses, β_2 receptors are also blocked causing bronchoconstriction.

○   **A newborn of a mother treated with propranolol for hyperthyroidism during pregnancy is diagnosed with bradycardia and hypoglycemia. What is the most likely explanation?**

Beta antagonists can cross the placenta and cause these symptoms in the fetus, especially towards the end of the third trimester. Non-selective beta-blockers decrease glycogenolysis that ordinarily occurs in response to the release of epinephrine during hypoglycemia.

○   **A patient on MAO inhibitors becomes hypotensive intraoperatively. Which drug would be a better choice: phenylephrine or ephedrine?**

Phenylephrine. MAOI cause intraneuronal accumulation of amines within the presynaptic nerve terminals. The effects of indirect-acting sympathomimetic amines such as ephedrine are enhanced, while direct-acting sympathomimetics such as phenylephrine activate adrenergic receptors directly and actions are close to expected. It would be prudent to use a direct acting sympathomimetic to avoid an exaggerated hypertensive response.

○ **Do beta-adrenergic blockers affect plasma potassium concentration?**

Beta-adrenergic blockers inhibit the uptake of potassium into skeletal muscle; therefore the plasma concentration of potassium is increased.

○ **A patient was brought to the OR with dopamine running into a peripheral IV. The patient is complaining of intense pain at the IV site. Diagnosis and initial management?**

Infiltration of the IV and extravasation of dopamine into skin or subcutaneous tissues, like norepinephrine, produces intense local vasoconstriction which should be treated by local infiltration of phentolamine.

○ **During an epidural C-section, the patient complains of severe nausea. Diagnosis?**

The nausea may be due to hypotension from sympathetic blockade, anxiety, exteriorization of the uterus or mesenteric traction and pain from insufficient sensory block height.

○ **What is the mechanism of sedation with scopolamine?**

Scopolamine crosses the blood brain barrier and depresses the reticular activating system, producing sedation. Paradoxical restlessness and delirium are possible. Other properties include; antisialagogue, amnestic, prevention of motion sickness and minimal effect on heart rate.

○ **Following a reversal of neuromuscular blockade with atropine-neostigmine, a patient becomes restless and combative. Diagnosis?**

Hypoxia and/or hypercarbia. Then consider the possibility that atropine can enter the CNS and produce a central anticholinergic syndrome ("mad as a hatter"). Physostigmine, a tertiary amino anticholinesterase, can be used to treat this syndrome.

○ **What are the main divisions of the autonomic nervous system and where are they located?**

Sympathetic and parasympathetic divisions. The sympathetic nervous system originates from the thoracolumbar region of the spinal cord (T_1 to $L_{2,3}$) with preganglionic fibers synapsing in ganglia that are distant from effector organs. The parasympathetic, or craniosacral nervous system, has cranial outflows from cranial nerves III, VII, IX and X and sacral branches that converge to form the pelvic nerves. The ganglia are proximal to or within the innervated organ.

○ **How does the sympathetic nervous system innervate its end organs?**

Efferents exit the cord in the anterior nerve roots and travel a short distance into the ventral white rami, where they synapse in the paired paravertebral ganglia. Long postganglionic unmyelinated nerves leave via the gray rami, re-enter the spinal nerve and innervate the target organs.

○ **How does the parasympathetic nervous system innervate its end organs?**

The craniosacral outflow tracts extend out as long preganglionic fibers that synapse at ganglia that are near the effector organs. Short postganglionic fibers make the terminal connections to elicit the end organ response.

○   **What are the neurotransmitters of the sympathetic and parasympathetic nervous systems?**

Acetylcholine is used as the preganglionic neurotransmitter at the level of the ganglia in both the sympathetic and parasympathetic nervous systems. It is also the postganglionic neurotransmitter of the parasympathetic nervous system. Norepinephrine is used in the postganglionic fibers of the sympathetic nervous system, except for those fibers which innervate sweat glands, which use acetylcholine.

○   **What are the subtypes of cholinergic receptors and where are they found?**

There are two main types of receptors that bind acetylcholine: nicotinic and muscarinic. Nicotinic receptors have two major subtypes; those found in the ganglia of the autonomic nervous system and those located at the neuromuscular junctions. Muscarinic receptors are also divided into the M_1 type, which are primarily in the ganglia and central nervous system, and the M_2 type located mainly on peripheral visceral organs.

○   **What happens to acetylcholine after it binds to its various types of receptors?**

Acetylcholine is hydrolyzed by acetylcholinesterase at cholinergic synapses and to a lesser extent pseudocholinesterase to acetate and choline. Choline is taken back up by the neuron and reused while acetate diffuses away and is eliminated.

○   **Where is acetylcholinesterase or "true cholinesterase" synthesized?**

It is a membrane-bound enzyme that is synthesized in the Golgi apparatus of neuronal cell bodies and red blood cells.

○   **Where is plasma cholinesterase or pseudocholinesterase synthesized?**

This is a soluble enzyme that is synthesized in the liver and circulates in the blood.

○   **What type of receptors does norepinephrine bind?**

Norepinephrine binds both types of adrenergic receptors: α_1 and $\beta_1 >> \beta_2$.

○   **What happens to norepinephrine after it binds to alpha-1 and beta-adrenergic receptors?**

There are several mechanisms for terminating the action of norepinephrine. The majority is taken up into the nerve ending and re-stored in synaptic vesicles to be re-released or deaminated by monoamine oxidase (MAO). Uptake by non-neuronal tissues or metabolism by MAO and/or COMT in the blood, liver and kidney also occurs, to a limited extent.

○   **What is the interaction between sympathetic and parasympathetic nervous systems?**

Most organs are innervated by both divisions of the autonomic nervous system. In general, each gets to antagonize the other in creating an end-organ response. This allows for tighter regulation of organ function and homeostasis.

○   **What is dysautonomia?**

Autonomic dysfunction due to generalized, segmental or focal disorders of the central or peripheral nervous system. The most serious anesthetic risk is orthostatic hypotension. Dysautonomic crises triggered by stress are characterized by hypertension, tachycardia, abdominal pain, diaphoresis and vomiting.

○   **What causes dysautonomia?**

Congenital, familial or acquired (infectious states, drugs or trauma). Each may lead to different signs or symptoms, depending on the location and degree of autonomic dysfunction. It can be seen in patients with diabetes millitus, Parkinson's disease, cystic fibrosis, Riley-Day Syndrome, Shy-Drager, amyloidosis, Guillain-Barré and spinal cord injuries.

○   What is spinal shock?

Acute high spinal cord injury (commonly at C_{5-6}) with mechanical disruption of sympathetic nervous system outflow from T_1 to L_2 producing loss of sensation, flaccid paralysis and loss of spinal reflexes below the level of injury. Diminished sympathetic activity results in hypotension and bradycardia secondary to vasodilatation, decreased preload (after an initial massive increase) and unopposed vagal activity.

○   What is the duration of spinal shock?

Symptoms may resolve within 72 hours or persist for six to eight weeks, or longer.

○   Can succinylcholine be used in a patient with spinal shock?

It is safe within the first 24 hours of spinal trauma. After that, the possibility of developing life-threatening hyperkalemia increases secondary to the proliferation of extrajunctional acetylcholine receptors. If unsure of the time of injury, rocuronium may be a good alternative for securing the airway.

○   What is autonomic hyperreflexia?

Following the period of spinal shock, there is a gradual return of spinal reflexes. Lacking any descending central regulatory control, the sympathetic nervous system becomes overreactive to external stimuli, either cutaneous or visceral. This may begin as early as a few weeks, or as long as two years after the injury to the spinal cord and is common with transection at T_5 or above, and unusual with injuries below T_{10}.

○   What are the signs of autonomic hyperreflexia?

With spinal cord lesions at T_6 or higher, interruption of normal descending inhibitory impulses allows cutaneous or visceral stimulation below the transection to induce unopposed hyperactive sympathetic discharge (vasoconstriction and hypertension) with baroreceptor-mediated reflex bradycardia and vasodilatation above. Other symptoms include visceral and muscle spasm, sweating, piloerection and uncontrolled motor activity below the level of the lesion. Extreme elevations in blood pressure (due to the fact that more than half the sympathetic system is unmodulated below the lesion and activated) can lead to retinal or cerebral hemorrhage, convulsions, or coma.

○   What is the treatment for autonomic hyperreflexia?

Prevention of the stimulus or pharmacological intervention. First, eliminate the predisposing factor, if possible, which is usually surgical manipulation by incision or bladder distention. Treatment for hypertension includes esmolol, labetalol, nitroglycerin or nitroprusside in the form of boluses or infusions. Other agents that have been used are ganglionic blockers, such as trimethaphan or alpha-adrenergic antagonists, such as phentolamine or phenoxybenzamine.

○   What are the anesthetic options for patients with a history of autonomic hyperreflexia?

General and regional techniques can offer adequate levels of anesthesia to prevent sympathetic hyperreflexia. Regional anesthesia eliminates noxious signals from the lower sacral nerve roots, thereby preventing the reflex. Some suggest that a spinal approach is better than epidural, especially with bladder distention in urologic procedures, as there may be sparing of the sacral roots with epidural anesthesia. With general anesthesia, the depth of anesthesia is more important than the choice of agent. However, one must always be prepared to treat a hypertensive crisis.

○   **What are the signs of autonomic dysfunction in patients with diabetes mellitus?**

Diabetic autonomic neuropathy primarily involves the heart and GI tract. Clinical signs include; orthostatic hypotension, hypertension, painless myocardial ischemia, diminished baroreceptor and cardiac reflexes, resting tachycardia and gastroparesis.

○   **What are the anesthetic concerns regarding the autonomic nervous system in patients with Guillain-Barré Syndrome?**

Guillain-Barré Syndrome is an acute demyelinating polyneuropathy characterized by ascending motor paralysis areflexia and variable paresthesias. These patients tend to have exaggerated hypo- and hypertensive responses and cardiac dysrhythmias, (atrial tachycardia or fibrillation) which are often unresponsive to carotid massage suggestive of hypoactive vagal innervation. Observation of the EKG and invasive hemodynamic monitoring may be prudent during positioning and other surgical anesthetic stimuli. Pharyngeal muscle weakness is also a concern for airway protection and may necessitate postoperative ventilation.

○   **What is the precursor of norepinephrine synthesis?**

Tyrosine.

○   **What is the rate-controlling step in the synthesis of norepinephrine?**

Conversion of tyrosine to dopa, a step controlled by the enzyme tyrosine hydroxylase.

○   **Where is norepinephrine converted to epinephrine?**

In the adrenal medulla, and to a limited extent in the brain. Phenylethanolamine-N-methyltransferase (PNMT) methylates NE to epinephrine.

○   **Biosynthesis of NE in sympathetic nerve terminals involve what intermediaries?**

Tyrosine, dopa and dopamine.

○   **Once dopamine is formed in the cytoplasm of the sympathetic nerve terminal, what happens to it?**

Dopamine is taken up into the storage vesicles in the sympathetic nerve terminal where it is converted to norepinephrine by dopamine-β-hydroxylase.

○   **Name two drugs that block the reuptake of norepinephrine causing an enhanced response to catecholamines?**

Cocaine and tricyclic antidepressants.

○   **Should beta-blockers be continued throughout the perioperative period?**

Yes. Beta-adrenergic antagonists decrease myocardial oxygen demand by decreasing heart rate and cardiac contractility. Abrupt withdrawal of beta-blockers may result in rebound increases in heart rate and blood pressure in patients with coronary artery disease causing ischemia, infarction or ventricular arrhythmias. Outcomes may be improved in those at high risk of ischemia by adequate pre and postoperative beta-blockade.

○   **Why is the administration of beta-agonists relatively ineffective in the treatment of chronic congestive heart failure?**

Tolerance or down-regulation of cardiac beta-receptors.

○　**T/F:　Administration of epinephrine is contraindicated in patients taking β-1 adrenergic blocking drugs (cardioselective).**

False. Unopposed alpha responses with the administration of epinephrine is a potential problem in patients taking nonselective beta blockers, but it is not contraindicated.

CLINICAL PHARMACOLOGY

Imagination Was Given To Man To Compensate Him For What He Isn't;
And A Sense Of Humor To Console Him For What He Is.
Unknown

O **Describe the pharmacology of mannitol.**

Mannitol ($C_6H_{14}O_6$) is an alcohol and a sugar (polyol) available as a sterile, nonpyrogenic solution for intravenous injection only. It is a vasodilator and obligatory osmotic diuretic available in concentrations of 5 to 20%. The 5% concentration has 5 g/100ml, 274 mOsmol/liter and is pH adjusted to 6.3 (4.5 to 7). Dose 0.25-1.5 gm/kg IV slow over 10 min. $T_{1/2}$ elimination is about 30 to 60 minutes. It is used mainly to reduce intracranial pressure and to treat patients with oliguric renal failure. Non-osmotic actions include: decrease in blood viscosity, decrease in SVR, mild positive inotropic effect on the heart, and free radical scavenger. Side effects include variable effects on blood pressure, acute heart failure in patients with impaired renal function, rebound phenomena with unexpected rise in ICP, hypovolemia, electrolyte disturbances and plasma hyperosmolarity.

O **What are the pharmacodynamics of midazolam?**

Profound anterograde amnesia, anxiolysis, central respiratory depression, anticonvulsant, specific benzodiazepine receptors (GABAa) enhances GABA. Decreases $CMRO_2$ and cerebral blood flow, but unable to produce isoelectric EEG. Preserves vasomotor responsiveness to CO_2.

O **Describe complications of naloxone use.**

Naloxone is a central opioid antagonist. Naloxone-related adverse effects include medical complications (convulsions, ventricular arrhythmia, pulmonary edema, hemodynamic instability), symptoms of heroin withdrawal and aggressive/agitated behaviour. Moderate increases in RR, HR, and BP occur after naloxone administration to children, but development of more serious complications is rare.

O **What is the mechanism of vancomycin-induced hypotension and how can it be minimized?**

Red man syndrome: chills or fever, fainting, tachycardia, hives, hypotension, cardiac arrest, itching, nausea or vomiting, rash or redness of the face, base of neck, upper body, back and arms from histamine release due to rapid infusion. Parenteral vancomycin should be administered as an infusion over at least 60 minutes.

O **What are the relative contraindications of metoclopramide?**

Metoclopramide is relatively contraindicated in patients: not tolerating an increase in GI motility (GI hemorrhage, obstruction or perforation); pheochromocytoma (may cause hypertensive crisis due to release of catecholamines); sensitive to metoclopramide, procaine, procainamide; seizure disorders; at risk for extrapyramidal side effects (epilepsy, renal failure, Parkinson's disease) or bronchospasm.

O **What are the cardiovascular effects of protamine?**

Unpredictable. The most common effect is hypotension especially if given rapidly in patients with poor LV function for heparin reversal after cardiopulmonary bypass. Causes include: mediator release (histamine, thromboxane), hypocalcemia and anaphylaxis. Systemic vasodilation and pulmonary vasoconstriction (increase PAP and PVR) are variable. Protamine has no direct action on the human heart. Maximum effect is at 1 minute, worn off by 4 minutes. Other adverse effects: bleeding, hypertension and noncardiogenic pulmonary edema.

O   **Describe the therapeutic action and mechanism of magnesium sulphate.**

Second most common intracellular cation after potassium; normal plasma level: 0.7 - 1.1 mmol/l, anticonvulsant level 2-3.5 mmol/l; exists in 3 forms: ionised, protein bound & ion bound
- Magnesium supplement
- Antiarrhythmic and direct cardioprotectant: Ventricular tachycardia: monomorphic or torsade de pointes
- Anticonvulsant (obstetrics: preeclampsia)
- Cofactor in enzymatic reactions involving energy metabolism and nucleic acid synthesis
- Also: hormone receptor binding, gating of calcium channels, transmembrane ion flux and regulation of adenylate cyclase, neuronal activity, control of vasomotor tone (coronary and systemic vasodilation), decreases cardiac excitability, depression of neurotransmitter release and muscle contraction, physiological calcium antagonist, inhibition of platelet aggregation.
- Toxic effects: hypotension, cardiac conduction defects/cardiac arrest (antidote: calcium chloride), CNS depression

O   **Describe the treatment of a cholinergic crisis.**

Atropine 35-70 μg/kg IV every 3-10 minutes until the muscarinic symptoms improve.
Pralidoxime may be used to improve muscle weakness which results from an overdose of neostigmine and pyridostigmine used to treat myasthenia gravis. Dosing: 1-2 g IV, then 250 mg IV every 5 minutes.
Supportive therapy for respiratory insufficiency may be needed.

O   **What is the duration of action of flumazenil?**

Onset: 1-2 minutes after IV injection, peak effect: 6-10 minutes, elimination: brain 20 to 30 minutes and plasma 54 minutes. Reversal of benzodiazepines depends on dose and plasma concentration of both drugs. The duration of action for reversal of: sedation, 30 minutes; psychomotor deficits, 45 minutes; anterograde amnesia, 60 minutes. Flumazenil also improves respiratory function by increasing tidal volume.

O   **What are the side effects of beta agonist drugs?**

Beta$_1$ agonists: tachycardia, arrythmias, hypertension, hypotension at higher doses.
Beta$_2$ agonists: fine tremor of the hands, restlessness, nervousness and headache are common. They can also cause flushing and palpitations. Rarely: arrhythmia, hypokalemia, hyperglycemia, muscle cramps, nausea and vomiting and allergic reactions. Elderly are at increased risk.

O   **Describe the main therapeutic uses of adenosine.**

The heart: inhibitory effect on the AV node resulting in cardiac arrest which makes it the drug of choice for AV nodal reentrant tachycardia (SVT). Important in myocardial pre-conditioning and may be helpful in heart failure. Adenosine induces collateral circulation, reduces noradrenaline/endothelin release and renin/angiotensin/aldosterone axis activation and protects against reperfusion.
The brain: Parkinson's disease, neuropathic pain, drug addiction, schizophrenia and Alzheimer's disease.
The lungs: marker of airway inflammation with provocative inhalational testing
The immune system: immunosuppression in chronic illness, inhibits tumor growth
The blood: inhibits platelet aggregation

O   **What is the duration of action of adenosine?**

Less than 10 seconds. Metabolism is very rapid by circulating enzymes in erythrocytes and vascular endothelial cells. Adenosine is deaminated to inactive inosine (further degraded to hypoxanthine and uric acid) and by phosphorylation to adenosine monophosphate (AMP).

O   **Describe the major side effects of flumazenil.**

Flumazenil is a drug mainly used for benzodiazepine reversal, as it is an inhibitor of GABA receptors. The main side effects include: nausea and vomiting, flushing, seizure, anxiety and agitations and withdrawal reactions (depression, insomnia, irritability, sweating, diarrhea, emotional lability, hypertension, panic, tachycardia). The risk of precipitating a withdrawal syndrome is increased with flumazenil doses higher than 1 mg and/or rapid administration and the degree of dependence. Cardiac effects reported in less than 1% of patients include: arrhythmias (atrial, nodal, and ventricular extrasystoles, bradycardia, and tachycardia), hypertension, and chest pain.

O   **Compare the action of Albuterol with Ipratorium.**

Albuterol is a selective Beta 2 agonist causing smooth muscle relaxation by increasing cyclic AMP intracellularly in the smooth muscle of the respiratory tract.
Ipratorium acts by blocking the muscarinic receptors in the bronchial smooth muscle and cause bronchodilation.
The combination of both agents causes better bronchodilation as compared to any of them used alone.
The side effects also differ based on the mechanism of action.

Beta-adrenergic bronchodilators may decrease serum potassium concentrations, especially when the recommended dose is exceeded and can cause EKG changes like flattened T waves, prolongation of the QT_c interval, and ST segment depression.

Ipratorium can cause an acute attack of Glaucoma or condition may be exacerbated if ipratropium-containing inhalation aerosol is sprayed directly into the eyes. In addition may lead to urinary retention.

O   **Discuss the extrapyramidal effects of anti emetics used in anesthesia practice.**

The anti emetics associated with the extrapyramidal side effects are Phenothiazines like, Chlorpromazine. Promotility agent Metoclopramide is also known to cause the same.
The mechanism of action for antiemesis of both group of drugs is by Dopamine antagonism in the Dopaminergic receptors in the CNS especially the chemoreceptor trigger zone(CTZ). This is also the reason for the side effects.
The extrapyramidal side effects include Tardive dyskinesia (abnormal involuntary that may affect the tongue, facial and neck muscles, extremities and sometimes muscles involved in breathing and swallowing) caused by chronic Phenothiazine administration. The other effects are Acute dystonias, ophisthotonus, occulogyric crisis,and muscle cramping and rigidity.Very rarely laryngospasm has been seen causing sudden respiratory distress. Akathisia , a feeling of unease and restlessness in the lower extremities is also seen.

O   **Describe the anesthetic implications of Clonidine as a pre medication.**

Clonidine is a centrally acting, selective, partial Alpha 2 agonist (220:1 A2 : A1). Its use as a premedication orally (5ug/kg) has following effects:
1. Blunting of reflex tachycardia due to direct laryngoscopy.
2. Decrease in intra operative cardiovascular lability.
3. Decrease in plasma catecholamine concentrations.
4. Decrease in the MAC of inhaled agents.
5. Decrease in perioperative myocardial ischemic episodes in pts with CAD.
6. Augmentation of pressor responses to ephedrine.

O   **Describe sedative effects of Midazolam and apneic potential of the drug.**

Midazolam enhances the inhibitory tone of GABA receptors in the CNS producing sedation. Can be given IV, PO, and the only benzodiazepine with reliable IM absorption. Produces dose dependent decrease in respiratory rate and tidal volume. Big dose and injected rapidly can cause transient apnea (>0.15 mg/kg IV) the effect is more pronounced in the presence of opioids.

O   **What are the effects of Muscarinic receptor antagonism?**

Cardiac: Tachycardia
Bronchial: Bronchodilation, drying of secretions.
GI tract: Smooth muscle relaxation and slowing of peristalsis.
GU tract: Lowering of bladder tone and increase of sphincter tone.
Eye: Mydriasis.
Secretory glands: Inhibition of salivary, tracheobronchial, lacrimal, digestive and exocrine sweat gland secretions.

○ Describe the side effects of Amiodarone.

The side effects are common particularly at daily doses higher than 400mg. They include:
Pulmonary alveolitis.
Prolongation of QT interval which may lead to torsade.
Corneal microdeposits, photosensitivity, cyanotic discoloration.
Displacement of Digoxin from protein binding sites and increase in its plasma concentration.
It may cause hypo or hyperthyroidism.

○ Describe Sodium Nitroprusside (SNP) metabolism.

A direct acting non selective peripheral vasodilator acting on both arterial and venous smooth muscle. Immediate short lived action caused by release of NO (nitric oxide). Metabolism begins with: transfer of an electron from Iron of oxyhemoglobin to SNP→Methemoglobin and unstable SNP→unstable SNP breaks down to release 5 Cyanide ions→ One cyanide ion combines with methemoglobin→Cyanomethemoglobin. Remaining cyanide ions are converted by Rhodanase enzyme from liver and kidneys to Thiocyanate, which is excreted. Cyanide ions also bind cytochrome oxidase which interferes with oxygen use resulting in toxicity. The thiosulfate ions are used as sulfur donors for this reaction.

○ Where is the site of action of Bronchodilators?

There are 2 types of Bronchodilators.
Anti cholinergic drugs : They act via acetyl choline antagonism at the muscarinic receptors.
B2 receptor agonists: These drugs act on the B2 receptor , increasing intracellular c-AMP concentration in the bronchial smooth muscle which leads to decreased Ca influx and consequent relaxation.

○ Describe the toxicity of Sodium Nitroprusside.

The SNP toxicity may occur due to cyanide accumulation (>40uM), if infusion rates are >2ug/kg/min or when sulfur donors and methemoglobin are exhausted.
Signs of toxicity are:
Tachyphylaxis to the infusion.
Increase in the mixed venous O_2.
Metabolic acidosis with lactate concentration >10 mM.
Increased cerebral venous oxygen content.
Awake pts may have mental status changes or seizures.

○ Describe Bleomycin toxicity.

Most serious toxic effect is dose related Pulmonary interstitial fibrosis which is estimated to involve 4% of all pts treated.
The other side effects are mucocutaneous reactions, alopecia and hyperpigmentation.
Some patients with lymphoma may develop acute reaction characterized by hyperthermia, hypotension and hypoventilation.

○ What are the side effects of Ketorolac ?

These include reversible inhibition of platelet aggregation by inhibition of thromboxane production.

Life threatening bronchospasm may occur in patients with nasal polyposis, asthma and aspirin sensitivity. Other side effects include modest increase in liver transaminase plasma levels, nausea, GI irritation and peripheral edema.

○ **Compare the anticholinergic drugs Glycopyrrolate and Atropine**.

	Atropine	Glycopyrrolate
Sedation	+	0
Antisialagogue	+	+ +
Tachycardia	+ + +	+ +
Smooth Muscle Relaxation	+ +	+ +
Mydriasis	+	0
Prevention of Motion sickness	+	0
Reduction of Gastric acid Secretion	+	+

○ **How will you maintain perioperative K homeostasis?**

Approx. total body Potassium is 40-50meq/kg. Mostly intracellular.
Kidneys are the principal organ in K homeostasis. Aldosterone, ADH and glucocorticoids increase K secretion and catecholamines decrease renal secretion.
Acute hypokalemia can be managed by KCl infusions. Hyperkalemia is managed by Calcium gluconate IV, Soda bicarb and Glucose –Insulin mixtures.
Epinephrine and Beta2 agonists decrease serum K concentrations by redistribution.

○ **Describe the features of anticholinergic syndrome and its treatment.**

Scopolamine and to a lesser degree Atropine enter the CNS and can cause this syndrome.
Symptoms range from restlessness and hallucinations to somnolence and unconsciousness. Presumably these effects are due to antagonism of central effects of ACH.
 Physostigmine 15-60 ug/kg IV is a specific treatment. Edrophonium, Pyridostigmine , and Neostigmine are not effective due to their inability to cross into the CNS.

○ **What are the clinical effects of Nalbuphine?**

It is an agonist-antagonist opioid. Equal in analgesic potential to Morphine but 1/4th potent as Nalorphine as an antagonist.
Clinical effects are: analgesia, sedation , respiratory depression and dysphoria. It is free of CVS side effects. Abrupt withdrawal can cause withdrawal symptoms milder than morphine. Antagonist effects are due to its action at mu receptors. This is useful in post operative period to reverse the ventilatory depression caused by Morphine or Fentanyl while still maintaining analgesia.

○ **What is the mechanism of action of COX-2 inhibitors?**

The cyclo oxygenase enzymes 1 & 2 are responsible for conversion of Arachidonic acid to various mediators of inflammation including prostaglandins (COX-2) enzyme is believed to be produced more in response to injury and its concentration is believed to be more in areas of inflammation. Selective inhibitors of COX 2 have preference for this enzyme hence producing selective inhibition of Prostaglandin synthesis in specific areas. This reduces some of the side effects of traditional NSAIDS especially gastric irritation.

○ **Describe the interaction of MAO inhibitors and opioids.**

MAO(Mono Amine Oxidase) is the enzyme responsible for deamination of monoamines like serotonin, dopamine , norepinehrine and epinephrine. MAO inhibitors make irreversible complex with the enzyme and as a result the Monoamine concentration increases in the CNS. Administration of opioids especially Meperidine can lead to (Type1) excitatory response (hyperpexia, agitation, skeletal muscle rigidity and headache) or a (Type2) depressive response (hypotension, depression of ventilation and coma).Derivatives of Meperidine fentanyl, sufentanil and alfentanil have been associated with similar adverse reactions though the incidence is much smaller. The opioid effects of Morphine may be potentiated but it is not associated with the above effects.

○ **Describe the toxicity related to Doxorubicin.**

Cardiotoxicity, usually in the form of congestive heart failure. Incidence of cardiotoxicity is more frequent in patients receiving total dosages of over 550 mg per square meter.Cardiotoxicity usually appears within 1 to 6 months after initiation of therapy. Cardiomyopathy has been reported to be associated with persistent voltage reduction in the QRS wave, systolic interval prolongation, and reduction of ejection fraction. It may develop suddenly and may not be detected by routine ECG. It may be irreversible and fatal but responds to treatment if detected early.

○ **What are the contraindications to the use of Ketorolac?**

Cerebrovascular bleeding (suspected or confirmed), hemophilia or other bleeding problems including coagulation or platelet function disorders, gastrointestinal bleeding (active, recent) or a history of gastrointestinal perforation, peptic ulceration, ulcerative colitis, or other ulcerative gastrointestinal disease, nasal polyp associated with bronchospasm (aspirin induced), angioedema, anaphylaxis, renal function impairment.

○ **Describe rebound hypertension caused by abrupt withdrawal of Clonidine.**

Rebound hypertension may occur but is symptomatic in only 5 to 20% of patients. It is more likely to occur after abrupt withdrawal of clonidine in patients who had been receiving doses exceeding 1.2 mg per day or if clonidine therapy is discontinued before or at the same time as concurrent beta-adrenergic blocking agent therapy. The clinical features may include: Nervousness, tachycardia, diaphoresis, abdominal pain, headache followed by Hypertension.

○ **What is the treatment of Extrapyramidal drug effects?**

Most of the acute extrapyramidal reactions respond very well to Diphenhydramine 25-50 mg IV. If severe life threatening effects occur, the complete life support measures are required.

○ **Describe the pharmacology of Physostigmine.**

Mechanism of action: Antagonizes action of anticholinergics, which block the postsynaptic receptor sites of acetylcholine, by reversibly inhibiting the destruction of acetylcholine by acetylcholinesterase, thereby increasing the concentration of acetylcholine at sites of cholinergic transmission.
Since physostigmine is a lipid-soluble tertiary amine, which (unlike the quaternary amines neostigmine and pyridostigmine) can cross the blood-brain barrier, it acts against both central and peripheral anticholinergic effects.
Easily penetrates the blood-brain barrier. Rapidly hydrolyzed by cholinesterases. Time to peak effect:
Intramuscular—20 to 30 minutes
Intravenous—Within 5 minutes .
Duration of action and elimination:
Intramuscular and intravenous—30 to 60 minutes . Very small amounts eliminated in urine; largely destroyed in body by hydrolysis.

○ **Name the drugs which have the potential to cause rebound hypertension once stopped.**

Clonidine and all beta blocking drugs. Ca channel blockers can cause coronary spasm when stopped abruptly. ACE inhibitors do not cause rebound hypertension once stopped abruptly.

O   **Describe the pharmacology of Nicardipine.**

It is a calcium-ion influx inhibitor (slow-channel blocking agent). Mainly used to treat hypertensive emergencies in small boluses or infusion. It has high cerebrovascular selectivity hence useful in neurovascular emergencies in addition.
Nicardipine is selective for vascular smooth muscle compared with myocardium and therefore acts primarily as vasodilator. Hypotensive effects are accompanied by reflex tachycardia. Available both in PO and IV form. Peak onset for IV inj. is within 1-2 minutes. Almost 95% protein bound.
Elimination: Renal 60% (less than 1% unchanged). Biliary/fecal 35%.

O   **What are the cardiovascular effects of Ketamine?**

Ketamine causes direct stimulation of the CNS leading to increased sympathetic outflow hence the cardiovascular stimulation. It is important to remember that it is a direct myocardial depressant, but indirectly causes increases in systemic and pulmonary arterial pressure, heart rate, cardiac output, cardiac work and myocardial oxygen consumption. It may increase the arrythmogenic potential of epinephrine.

O   **What are the toxic effects of Metformin?**

Lactic acidosis is the most serious side effect. This is caused by binding to mitochondrial membranes and reducing intracellular conc. of ATP hence anaerobic glucose metabolism and accumulation of lactate.
Other side effects include anorexia, nausea and diarrohea.

O   **Describe the mechanism of action of Glycopyrrolate.**

Glycopyrrolate is a quaternary ammonium compound, which causes competitive antagonism of acetylcholine at the muscarinic receptors sites. It acts on all the 3 subtypes M1, 2 and 3. These postganglionic receptor sites are present in the autonomic effector cells of the smooth muscle, cardiac muscle, sinoatrial and atrioventricular nodes, and exocrine glands. The drug is devoid of CNS activity due to its structure limiting its ability to cross the blood brain barrier.

O   **Describe the perioperative implications of ACE inhibitors and Potassium homeostasis.**

Angiotensin converting enzyme inhibitors interfere with the stimulus to release Aldosterone. This can lead to hyperkalemia especially in the presence of renal function impairment and concomitant use of K sparing diuretics.

O   **Compare the terms drug potency and efficacy.**

Potency is described as the dose required to achieve maximal response, and is represented by the dose axis on the dose response curve.
Efficacy is the maximal effect of a drug and is represented by the plateau in the dose response curve.

O   **Describe cardiac arrhythmias caused by Digitalis toxicity.**

The therapeutic dose of Digoxin is 0.5-2.0 ng/ml .It can lead to cardiac arrhythmias especially in presence of hypokalemia.
The cardiac arrhythmias an be atrial or ventricular. Initial feature may be prolongation of PR interval. The most common arrhythmia being atrial tachycardia with AV block. Ventricular fibrillation is the most frequent cause of death from digitalis toxicity.

INHALATION AGENTS

Flaming Enthusiasm, Backed Up By Horse Sense And Persistence, Is The Quality That Most Frequently Makes For Success.
Dale Carnegie

O **What is the effect of a right-to-left shunt on the speed of inhalational induction?**

Slows the rate of induction, in proportion to the size of the shunt. These effects are most marked for insoluble gases, and small or moderate with gases of intermediate solubility.

O **What is the effect of a left-to-right shunt on the rate of inhalational induction?**

Little or no effect, with normal cerebral perfusion and a normal forward flow.

O **When a vaporizer is being changed on an anesthesia machine, it is accidentally tipped. What should you do before using the vaporizer?**

Flush the vaporizer for 20-30 minutes at high flow rates of oxygen with the vaporizer set at a low concentration. In a variable bypass vaporizer, tipping may cause liquid anesthetic to spill from the vaporizing chamber to the bypass chamber, effectively creating two vaporizing chambers and increasing vaporizer output.

O **A trauma patient presents to the operating room with an undiagnosed pneumothorax and is being ventilated with a mixture of N_2O (75%) and O_2 (25%). What will happen to the size of the pneumothorax?**

The size of the pneumothorax will double in 10 minutes and equilibrate to quadruple the original size by about 30 minutes.

O **List the inhalation agents in order of increasing solubility.**

Desflurane (0.42), N_2O (0.47), sevoflurane (0.61), isoflurane (1.4), enflurane (1.91), halothane (2.3), and methoxyflurane (15). (blood/gas partition coefficients at 37°C)

O **What is the effect of inhalational agents on cerebral blood flow and cerebral metabolic rate?**

Inhalational agents increase CBF and decrease $CMRO_2$, thus uncoupling the $CBF:CMRO_2$ relationship. The mechanism of increased CBF is cerebral vasodilation, and the order of vasodilator potency is: halothane>>>enflurane>isoflurane=desflurane=sevoflurane>N_2O.

O **What is the effect of inhalational agents on evoked potentials?**

Dose-related decrease in amplitude and increase in latency of somatosensory evoked potentials (SSEP), visual evoked potentials (VEP), and brainstem auditory evoked potentials (BAEP). Decrease in amplitude is more marked than increase in latency. Evoked potentials of cortical origin (VEP & SSEP) are more readily affected by inhalation agents than those of brainstem or subcortical origin. The most sensitive are VEP, followed by SSEP, and the least sensitive are BAEP.

O **Define MAC.**

Minimum alveolar concentration of an inhalation agent at one atmosphere that prevents skeletal muscle movement in response to a standardized noxious stimulus (ie: surgical incision) in 50% of patients. It is a reflection of the partial pressure of the agent in the brain, and is a measure of the potency of the anesthetic gases.

O   **Define MAC-BAR, MAC-awake, MAC$_{95}$, and MAC-intubation.**

1.   MAC-BAR (BAR=Block Adrenergic Response) is the alveolar concentration of the agent at which the adrenergic response (sympathetic response) to a noxious stimulus is blocked. MAC-BAR = 1.5 x MAC.
2.   MAC-awake is the alveolar concentration of a given volatile anesthetic at which the patient will open their eyes to command. It is a measure of the *amnestic* potency of the agent. MAC-awake values are usually 1/2 of the respective MAC values, except for N_2O (2/3 of its MAC value).
3.   MAC$_{95}$ is the alveolar concentration at which 95% of patients will not respond to a skin incision. MAC$_{95}$=1.3 x MAC.
4.   MAC-intubation is the minimum alveolar concentration that will inhibit movement and coughing during endotracheal intubation.

O   **What is an acceptable MAC level for monitoring SSEP?**

0.5 to 1 MAC isoflurane or enflurane, and 0.5 to 0.75 MAC halothane, with 60% N_2O.

O   **Which inhalation agents cause the most myocardial depression? List them in order of most to least effect.**

Enflurane=halothane>isoflurane=desflurane=sevoflurane>>>N_2O.

O   **What is the effect of inhalation agents on the heart rate?**

Halothane causes no change or a decrease in heart rate (HR) due to impairment of the baroreceptor reflex. Isoflurane, desflurane and enflurane increase HR. The increase in HR with desflurane is more pronounced at deeper levels of anesthesia. Sevoflurane produces little to no change.

O   **List four factors that increase MAC.**

Hyperthermia, hypernatremia, chronic alcohol abuse, and increased levels of catecholamines in the CNS (MAO inhibitors, acute amphetamine intoxication, cocaine, ephedrine, levodopa).

O   **A patient is anesthetized with N2O/O2 and desflurane. His blood pressure (BP) is 140/85 mm Hg and his heart rate (HR) is 95 bpm. The anesthetist thinks that the patient is "light", and increases the inspired desflurane concentration from 3% to 10%. The BP increases to 200/110, and the HR to 130. Why?**

A sudden increase in inspired desflurane concentration causes sympathetic nervous system stimulation and increase in circulating levels of catecholamines, causing tachycardia and hypertension. This can be prevented by a more gradual increase in desflurane concentration, or by prior administration of fentanyl or a beta-adrenergic blocker (e.g. esmolol or labetalol).

O   **What happens to the vapor pressure and solubility of an inhalation agent as its temperature increases?**

The vapor pressure increases and the solubility decreases.

O   **T/F: Vapor pressure is dependent on the atmospheric pressure.**

False. Vapor pressure is dependent on the temperature and the physical properties of the inhalation agent, and independent of the atmospheric pressure.

O **What is critical cerebral blood flow (CBF)?**

As defined by Michenfelder, critical CBF is "that flow below which the majority of subjects develop ipsilateral EEG changes indicative of ischemia within 3 minutes following carotid occlusion." It varies depending on the volatile agent used. The critical CBF for halothane is 18-20 ml/100 gm/min, which is the highest of the volatile agents; whereas for isoflurane the critical CBF is 10-12 ml/100 gm/min, which is the lowest of the volatile agents.

O **Describe the effects of the inhalation agents on CSF production and reabsorption.**

Halothane: Decreases production and decreases reabsorption
Enflurane: Increases production and decreases reabsorption
Isoflurane: No effect on production and increases reabsorption

O **A female patient with hypothyroidism is scheduled for surgery. How does decreased thyroid function affect MAC in females?**

Thyroid gland dysfunction and gender of the patient have no effect on MAC.

O **What is compound A?**

It is an olefin formed by the breakdown of sevoflurane by soda lime or Baralyme. In concentrations higher than that seen in humans, it can cause renal tubular necrosis, but no case reports in humans exist. Its formation is increased in the presence of dry soda lime, low fresh gas flows (< 2L/min), higher temperatures, longer MAC hours of anesthesia, and is greater in the presence of Baralyme than soda lime.

O **Which inhalation agent is the most unstable in soda lime? Which is the most stable?**

Most unstable = sevoflurane, most stable = desflurane.

O **Is isoflurane a suitable agent for use in patients with aortic regurgitation? Why?**

Yes. The regurgitant fraction is reduced by decreasing systemic vascular resistance and increasing heart rate.

O **What is the CO_2 response curve?**

The CO_2 response curve is a graph with the $PaCO_2$ (end-expiratory PCO_2) plotted on the x-axis and the minute ventilation (alveolar ventilation of pulmonary minute volume L/min) on the y axis. This curve describes the ventilatory response to carbon dioxide. The relationship between the $PaCO_2$ and MV is nearly linear, such that in the range of 20-80 mm Hg for every 1 mm Hg increase in $PaCO_2$, the MV increases by 2 liters/min. Very high arterial $PaCO_2$ tensions depress the ventilatory response.

O **How do the inhalation agents affect the CO_2 response curve?**

As the inhalational agent is increased, the curve is shifted to the right with a decrease in the slope, indicating a decreased minute volume response to increasing hypercarbia.

O **T/F: Subanesthetic concentrations of inhalation agents do not affect the ventilatory response to CO_2, but do affect the ventilatory response to hypoxemia.**

True. The ventilatory response to hypoxemia is decreased at 0.1 MAC, and abolished at 1 MAC.

O **What is the apneic threshold?**

The maximum $PaCO_2$ that does not initiate spontaneous respiration. This is 5 mm Hg below the resting $PaCO_2$, and corresponds to the x-intercept on the CO_2 response curve at which ventilation is zero.

O   **What is the relevance of the apneic threshold to the anesthetic management of the patient?**

It limits the amount of assisted ventilation that can occur. If the patient is allowed to breathe spontaneously under anesthesia, the $PaCO_2$ will increase (e.g. to 50 mm Hg). In an effort to decrease the $PaCO_2$, the anesthetist may decide to assist the patient's respirations. But when the PaCO2 drops to 45 mm Hg, the patient will become apneic (he/she will have reached the apneic threshold which is 5 mm Hg below the resting value). Respirations will then have to be controlled rather than assisted.

O   **T/F: Isoflurane and halothane in equipotent doses produce the same degree of potentiation of nondepolarizing muscle relaxants.**

False. All inhalational anesthetics potentiate nondepolarizing blockade; isoflurane, enflurane, sevoflurane, desflurane > halothane > N_2O/O_2/narcotic. The degree of augmentation depends on the inhalational agent and the choice of muscle relaxant ie: pancuronium > vecuronium and atracurium.

O   **What is the effect of inhalation agents on uterine tone ?**

Dose-dependent uterine relaxation, with halothane, enflurane and isoflurane equally depressant at equipotent doses. The effect is modest at 0.5 MAC, but substantial at 1 MAC. N2O has little or no effect on the uterus.' At lower concentrations (less than 0.5% halothane, 1% enflurane, or 1.5% isoflurane), the uterine response to oxytocin is preserved. Furthermore, inhalational agents in low concentrations do not increase the blood loss from C/S. During vaginal delivery, 0.2 MAC appears to have minimal effect on uterine activity, duration of labor, and postpartum blood loss.
One study confirmed that sevoflurane suppress uterine activity to a lesser extent than halothane or isoflurane.

O   **T/F: The blood/gas partition coefficient is a measure of the anesthetic potency of the inhalation agent.**

False. The oil:gas partition coefficient parallels the MAC of the inhalation agent, which is a measure of its potency. MAC = 150 divided by oil:gas partition coefficient. The blood/gas partition coefficient is a measure of the relative solubility of the agent in blood, and determines the speed of onset of action of the agent. The lower the blood/gas partition coefficient, the lower is the blood solubility, and faster the onset of action.

O   **T/F: Changes in alveolar ventilation affect the rate of rise of alveolar partial pressure (P_A) of a soluble agent more than an insoluble agent.**

True. The rate of rise of P_A of a poorly soluble agent is rapid, and independent of alveolar ventilation because of its limited uptake. The uptake of a soluble agent is large, and increasing alveolar ventilation provides more agent to the lungs to offset the loss due to uptake.

O   **T/F: Changes in cardiac output affect the rate of rise of P_A of an insoluble agent more than a soluble agent.**

False. Cardiac output and alveolar ventilation influence the rate of rise of P_A of soluble agents more than insoluble agents. Increasing the cardiac output will increase the uptake of a soluble agent, slowing the rate of rise of the P_A, whereas the rate of rise of P_A of an insoluble agent is rapid regardless of changes in cardiac output.

O   **Name the inhalation agents in order of production of inorganic fluoride ions from most to least.**

Methoxyflurane>enflurane>sevoflurane>>isoflurane, desflurane, halothane (negligible release of fluoride on metabolism). 50 µmol/L is the plasma level associated with nephrogenic diabetes insipidus using methoxyflurane. Despite higher fluoride concentrations than this associated with sevoflurane, nephrogenic DI has not been reported in humans.

O   **T/F: Desflurane causes greater increases in intracranial pressure than equipotent doses of isoflurane.**

True, especially in patients with altered intracranial elastance (ie: space-occupying lesions). Desflurane increases the rate of CSF formation with no significant effect on the rate of CSF reabsorption. Induction of hypocapnia does not consistently prevent the increase in ICP. Isoflurane remains the anesthetic of choice for patients with, or at risk for, cerebral ischemia.

O   **An enflurane vaporizer is unknowingly and accidentally filled with halothane and is set to deliver 2% inspired concentration. What is the MAC of the halothane actually delivered to the patient?**

4 MAC.

The vapor pressure of enflurane is 175 mm Hg, and of halothane 245 mm Hg. That means the enflurane vaporizer will vaporize one and a half times more halothane than the concentration dialed on the vaporizer, which is calibrated only for enflurane. This will result in a halothane concentration of 3%. Since the MAC of halothane is 0.75, the MAC of the halothane delivered to the patient will be $3 \div 0.75 = 4$ MAC.

O   **What factors increase the risk for "halothane hepatitis"?**

Multiple exposures, female gender, obesity, middle age, and familial factors.

O   **What is the cause of halothane hepatitis?**

Recent evidence suggests an idiosyncratic reaction that is immunologically mediated. Liver microsomal proteins, which have been modified by trifluoroacetic acid (TFA), apparently act as triggering antigens (membrane-hapten complex) and promote the formation of antibodies which bind to hepatocytes and result in hepatic necrosis. TFA is a product of halothane metabolism by the liver.

O   **Are there any reported cases of hepatitis attributed to the newer inhalation agents?**

Enflurane has been associated with immune-mediated hepatitis (incidence of 1:800,000). There have been only a few case reports of isoflurane hepatitis. There has been a case report of fatal hepatitis occurring after exposure to desflurane, in a patient who had a halothane anesthetic several years prior. There have been no case reports of fatal hepatitis occurring after exposure to sevoflurane.

O   **How does the MAC of halothane in infants compare to that in adults?**

MAC is highest in infants 3-6 months of age. The MAC of halothane in infants approximates 1.08 at 2 months versus 0.76 at 4 years.

O   **What are the circulatory effects of the volatile anesthetics?**

Reduce contractility: enflurane > halothane > isoflurane = desflurane = sevoflurane
Reduce SVR: isoflurane = desflurane > sevoflurane > enflurane and halothane
Reduce BP: enflurane > halothane> isoflurane = desflurane>sevoflurane
Cardiac output is reduced: Halothane = enflurane, minimal change with isoflurane, desflurane or sevoflurane
Heart rate is increased: enflurane > isoflurane = desflurane >>sevoflurane, and unchanged by halothane

O   **What factors increase the concentration and production of CO during desflurane administration?**

Low flow rates (< 0.5 l/min) (concentration) and desiccation of the absorbent (production).

❍   **What are the sites of NO production?**

There are three types of nitric oxide synthases: endothelial, neuronal, and inducible. NO production is found in a variety of tissues. NO has been identified in vascular endothelium (EDRF), in the CNS (neurotransmitter), macrophages, sperm, gut wall, kidney, and uterus.

❍   **What are desflurane's essential pharmacologic characteristics?**

Desflurane has a low blood gas partition coefficient (0.42), is associated a modest decrease in blood pressure and increase in heart rate, produces some muscle relaxation and has a MAC of 6%.

❍   **Which receptors are thought to mediate the CNS effect of the potent inhaled anesthetic agents?**

GABA receptors.

❍   **What is the effect of isoflurane on ventilation?**

Isoflurane depresses the normal response to both hypoxia and hypercarbia and is associated with a decrease in tidal volume and stable respiratory rate. Increases in $PaCO_2$ as a function of inhaled agent are:
ENFLURANE > DESFLURANE = ISOFLURANE > SEVOFLURANE = HALOTHANE

❍   **What are the factors effecting the uptake of inhaled anesthetics?**

Solubility, alveolar to venous concentration gradient, and cardiac output.

❍   **What is the maximum time weighted average (TWA) limit for N_2O in the OR?**

NO 25 parts per million (PPM) is the maximum TWA for facilities using halogenated agents (maximum TWA = 2 PPM). 50 PPM is allowed when no halogenated agents are used i.e. dental facilities

❍   **What is the effect of age on the uptake of inhaled anesthetics?**

Decreased cardiac index and decreased alveolar ventilation to FRC ratio would be expected to reduce the uptake of inhaled anesthetics with advancing age.

❍   **What effects do the inhaled anesthetics have on cerebral autoregulation?**

These potent agents are cerebral vasodilators and at higher MAC levels, all will uncouple the relationship between CBF and CMR such that CBF may equal the awake CBF, despite a reduction in CMR. The relative order of dilation is halothane>> ethrane > isoflurane = sevoflurane = desflurane.

❍   **What are the effects of general anesthetics on the control of respiration.**

The potent inhalational anesthetics reduced the respiratory drive decreasing the hypoxic drive and hypercarbic drive in a dose related fashion such that the hypoxic drive is abolished at 1.1 MAC and the apneic threshold for hypercarbia is progressively increased.

❍   **What are the metabolic products of biotransformation of the inhaled anesthetics?**

Halothane is 25- 45% metabolized in the liver and transformed via the P-450 system to trifluoroacetic acid, chloride, and bromide. Reductive metabolism of halothane in the relative absence of oxygen produces bromide, fluoride, 1.1-diflouro-2-chloroethylene(CDE), 1,1,1-trifluoro-2-chloroethane (CTE) and 1,1-difluoro-2-bromo-2-chloroethylene (DBE).
Enflurane is 2-8% metabolized via P-450 to difluoro-methoxy-difluoroacetic acid fluoride (F-).
Isoflurane is 0.2% metabolized by P-450 to fluoride and trifluoroacetic acid.

Desflurane is minimally metabolized but trifluoroacetic acid has been recovered from the urine.
Sevoflurane is 1-5% metabolized by P-450 and produces hexafluoroisopropanol and increases serum fluoride concentration.
Nitrous oxide is not metabolized by human tissue but can be reductively metabolized by gut bacteria to molecular nitrogen and free radicals.

○ **What physical characteristic of inhaled anesthetics predicts potency?**

Lipid solubility (i.e. oil/gas partition coefficient) predicts MAC. The greater the lipid solubility the lower the MAC.

○ **What changes in red cell production result from chronic exposure to high concentrations of nitrous oxide?**

The inactivation of methionine synthase by N_2O results in a clinical picture of pernicious anemia, with megaloblastic hematopoiesis. 12 hours of 50% nitrous is sufficient to produce mild megaloblastic changes. The half life for (irreversible) *inactivation of methionine synthetase is shown to be 46 min* when 70% N2O is administered to patients.

○ **What physiologic effects are associated with NO?**

Selective pulmonary vasodilation (mediated by an increase in cyclic GMP), maintains coronary perfusion pressure, improves oxygenation, inhibits platelet adhesion and aggregation, modifies sickle RBC and reduces elevated P50 toward normal, reduces O_2 toxicity and increases survival during hyperoxia, decreases leukocyte activation and blunts inflammatory response to reperfusion. Discontinuation may result in rebound hypoxemia and pulmonary hypertension.

○ **What factors determine the rate of recovery after an isoflurane anesthetic?**

Most simply the rate of recovery is the reverse of uptake and is dependent upon the rate of fall of the alveolar isoflurane concentration. The rate of change is equal to the cardiac output times the solubility times the alveolar ventilation. The rate of recovery further depends upon the duration of anesthesia, the amount of drug administered ({alv} X time), patient temperature, adjuvant drug usage, the age of the patient, and the B/G partition coefficient of isoflurane.

○ **What are the effects of sevoflurane on respiration?**

Sevoflurane is associated with a decrease in tidal volume, increase in respiratory rate and an increase in PCO_2.

○ **What are the pharmacodynamic and pharmacokinetic effects of inhaled nitric oxide (NO)?**

Nitric oxide is a direct acting pulmonary vasodilator. It is administered as a gas at concentrations of 5- 100 parts per million. It reduces pulmonary vascular resistance and improves oxygenation. Its effects are evanescent. Termination of action is by binding with hemoglobin with an affinity 200,000 times that of oxygen.

○ **The blood/gas partition of desflurane is less than the blood/gas partition of nitrous oxide yet the rise in the FA/FI ratio of nitrous oxide is more rapid than desflurane. How is this possible?**

The concentration effect increases the rate of rise of the FA/FI ratio for nitrous oxide, because nitrous oxide is conventionally delivered at 10 times the concentration of desflurane. Also, the lipid solubility, as measured by the oil/gas partition coefficient partition, is higher for desflurane than it is for nitrous oxide (18.7 vs. 1.4). The rate of rise of the alveolar concentration is slower for desflurane than for nitrous oxide because desflurane has a larger volume of distribution.

○ **What is the vapor pressure of desflurane in the Tec-6 vaporizer?**

The sump of the Tec-6 vaporizer is heated to 39 degrees Centigrade. At 39 degrees, the vapor pressure of desflurane is approximately 1,300 mm Hg absolute.

O   What systemic effects are expected if beta-blockers are administered concomitantly with isoflurane?

Beta-blockers will abolish the increase in heart rate associated with isoflurane and increase its negative inotropic. The result is a stable to decreased heart rate, a decrease in cardiac output and a more significantly reduced blood pressure.

O   What factors determine the speed of induction of inhalational anesthesia in the child versus the adult?

The rate of rise of the alveolar concentration is more rapid in infants and neonates than adults. The factors speeding induction are: alveolar ventilation, solubility, tissue water and cardiac index. The alveolar ventilation to FRC ratio is 5:1 in the infant and 1.5:1 in the adult. The solubility of agent in blood is 18% less in neonates and the elderly compared to young adults. The agents are 50% less soluble in infant tissues owing to the greater water content of infants. The greater cardiac index of infants speeds the rate of equilibration of the inspired to alveolar gradient.

O   What are effects of nitrous oxide on cerebral circulation?

Nitrous oxide alone increases: CBF, ICP parallel to increased CBF and CMR. When nitrous is added to an established inhalation anesthetic, the CBF is modestly increased.

O   What is the effect of age on MAC?

MAC is usually specified for the 30 year old. MAC peaks at 6 months of age at 1.6 MAC, falls to 0.8 MAC at 60 years and is 0.6 MAC at age 80.

O   What is the effect of substituting sevoflurane for halothane, in a halothane vaporizer?

The vapor pressure of halothane is 244 mm Hg and the vapor pressure of sevoflurane is 160 mm Hg. If sevoflurane was used in a halothane vaporizer the amount of agent delivered would be 65% (160/244, the ratio of the vapor pressures) of the dial setting. Thus, if the swap were inadvertent the patient would be significantly under anesthetized.

O   What are the factors governing the production of CO by soda lime?

CO production occurs when soda is in contact with enflurane, desflurane or isoflurane. Desiccation of the absorbent and the presence of NaOH or KOH increases the production.

O   What are the B/G partition coefficients, the vapor pressures (at 20 degrees Celcius) and lipid solubilities of the inhaled anesthetics?

	B/G	VP (mm Hg)	O/G (oil/gas)
Halothane	2.5	244	224
Enflurane	1.8	172	96.5
Isoflurane	1.4	240	90.8
Desflurane	0.45	664	18.7
Sevoflurane	0.65	162	47.2
Nitrous oxide	0.47	39,000	1.4

O   Why are conventional vaporizers unsuitable for use with desflurane?

Background: Desflurane has a vapor pressure of 664 mmHg at 20 °C. The agent requires active heating to 39°C, to remain consistently vaporized, as it boils near room temperature, so small changes in temperature will produce large changes in saturated vapor pressure.

Because of the high vapor pressure (VP) of desflurane, carrier gas passing through the vaporizing chamber of a variable bypass vaporizer would entrain a much larger amount of desflurane when compared to other agents (e.g. isoflurane). For example, 100 ml of carrier gas would entrain 735 ml of desflurane (VP=669) versus 46 ml of isoflurane (VP=238). To achieve a final concentration of 1%, the bypass flow for desflurane would have to be 86 liters/min, whereas for isoflurane it is only 5 liters/min. Therefore, a special vaporizer is needed for desflurane, which takes into account its high vapor pressure. In addition, the MAC of desflurane is about four times that of the other agents, so the absolute amount of desflurane that needs to be vaporized is much higher. This can cause excessive cooling of the vaporizer and hence the need for a heated vaporizer.

O   **What factors govern rate of recovery after a sevoflurane anesthetic?**

Rate of decrease in alveolar concentration is inversely related to lipid solubility (O/G= 50), duration of administration, and B/G partition coefficient (0.63).

O   **For inhaled anesthetics, what fraction of elimination is dependent upon metabolism?**

Halothane 25- 45%
Enflurane 2-8%
Isoflurane 0.2%
Desflurane 0.02%
Sevoflurane 1-5%

O   **What effect does nitrous oxide have on air trapped in a compliant body cavity?**

Nitrous oxide will move down the concentration gradient and expand trapped air. The B/G partition coefficient of N_2O (0.47) is much greater than that of N_2 (0.015) and thus the movement of nitrous into the space is much more rapid than the movement of trapped nitrogen out. The theoretical limit of expansion for an oxygen/nitrous mixture is the reciprocal of the inspired oxygen fraction. (if the mix were 50/50 the oxygen fraction = 1/2, the reciprocal = 2, thus the volume could double, if the mix were 75% nitrous/ 25% O_2, the oxygen fraction = 1/4, the reciprocal = 4, thus the volume could quadruple)

O   **Sevoflurane is added to an isoflurane vaporizer containing some isoflurane. What is the relative concentration of agents delivered to the patient?**

The relative concentrations would be 160:240 the ratio of their vapor pressures.

NONOPIOID INTRAVENOUS ANESTHETICS

It Is The Tragedy Of The World That No One Knows What He Doesn't Know - And The Less A Man Knows, The More Sure He Is He Knows Everything.
Joyce Cary

O   **Which nonopioid intravenous anesthetic agents possess analgesic properties?**

Ketamine.

Ketamine produces profound dose-dependant analgesia and at higher doses a dissociative state. The general anesthetic effect, as well as the analgesia properties of ketamine, may be mediated by the N-Methyl-D-aspartate (NMDA) receptor. Inhibition of the dorsal horn is the probable mechanism of the spinal cord analgesia effect of ketamine.

O   **What are the effects of nonopioid intravenous anesthetic agents on somatosensory evoked potentials (SSEP)?**

A dose-dependent increase in latency and a reduction in amplitude of SSEP (with the exception of ketamine and etomidate). These changes are similar to those seen with spinal-cord ischemia but do not necessarily preclude the use of non-opioid intravenous anesthetics during SSEP monitoring. Intravenous agents have significantly less effect than equipotent doses of inhaled anesthetics.

An induction dose of thiopental (4 mg/kg) will produce a maximum affect in 4 to 6 minutes, with a return to baseline occurring after 12 minutes. When these changes are taken into account, adequate monitoring of SSEP is possible even during infusions or large IV doses of thiopental. Infusions of propofol have a similar effect on SSEP. Diazepam, 20 mg intravenously, has no effect on SSEP and midazolam 0.2 mg/kg IV bolus followed by a 5 mg/h infusion has no clinically significant effect on SSEP.

Etomidate and ketamine produce an increase in amplitude of SSEP and have been used to enhance SSEP recording in cases where reproducible responses were difficult to obtain.

O   **What is the duration and mechanism of action of thiopental?**

Thiopental induces CNS depression by an effect on the GABA receptor complex. Barbiturates both enhance and mimic the action of GABA. At low concentrations binding to the barbiturate site (one of five protein subunits), decreases the rate of dissociation of GABA from its receptor and increases the duration of GABA-activated chloride conductance through the ion channel, hyperpolarizing and reducing the excitability of the postsynaptic neuron. This results in a sedative-hypnotic effect and amnesia. At slightly higher concentrations, barbiturates directly activate chloride channels, even in the absence of GABA, which may be responsible for "barbiturate anesthesia".

O   **What are the effects of barbiturates on the central nervous system (CNS)?**

At low doses, barbiturates stimulate cerebral electrical activity. At higher doses, barbiturates produce a dose-dependent depression of the CNS. The EEG will evolve to burst suppression and finally become isoelectric. Thiopental is an effective anticonvulsant and not only does not provide analgesia but may also be hyperalgesic in subanesthetic concentration. Methohexital has a preconvulsant activity and is currently being used to induce anesthesia during electroconvulsive therapy (ECT).

Thiopental also produces a dose-dependent decrease in cerebral metabolic requirement for oxygen ($CmRO_2$), in cerebral blood flow and intracranial pressure (ICP). When the EEG becomes isoelectric the decrease in $CmRO_2$ plateaus at 55% and reflects a depression of neuronal rather than metabolic activity. A further decrease in $CmRO_2$ can only be achieved with hypothermia.

○   **What are the effects of ketamine on the CNS?**

Excitatory, with an increase in CMR, CBF and ICP.

Ketamine has an excitatory effect on the CNS thus increasing cerebral metabolism (CMR), and cerebral blood flow (CBF) which, in turn, produces an increase in the intracranial pressure (ICP). Ketamine is also a cerebral vasodilator, which will further increase the CBF and ICP. The increase in CMR and CBF can be blocked by diazepam and thiopental. The increase in ICP can be attenuated by hyperventilation as the cerebrovascular response to CO_2 is preserved with ketamine.

Ketamine can produce undesirable psychologic reactions during emergence (bad dreams and multi-sensorial illusions, which may progress to delirium).

○   **What are the effects of etomidate on the CNS?**

Hypnosis, with a reduction in CMR, CBF and ICP.

Etomidate produces hypnosis with no analgesic effect through a mechanism that is not fully understood. Since it can be reversed by a GABA antagonist, etomidate's action may be related to the GABA-adrenergic system. Induction doses of etomidate reduce $CMRO_2$ and CBF without decreasing mean arterial pressure. Etomidate also decreases ICP by up to 50% in patients with intracranial hypertension. The possibility of a neuroprotective effect is controversial.

Etomidate increases EEG electrical activity and has a pro-convulsant effect that has been proven useful for intraoperative mapping of seizures. Etomidate can also cause myoclonic movements not associated with seizure activity.

○   **What are the effects of propofol on the CNS?**

Propofol is an anesthetic agent used for sedation or for induction and maintenance of anesthesia. Propofol had gained popularity for use in surgical procedures requiring a prompt wake-up (rapid recovery profile) and early assessment of neurologic function.

Propofol may be a neuroprotective drug as it preserves cerebral autoregulation, reduces cerebral blood flow, cerebral metabolic requirement for oxygen ($CMRO_2$) and intracranial pressure. Propofol can be used to achieve EEG burst suppression, which may reduce neuronal injury following incomplete cerebral ischemia. Data concerning the effects of propofol on epileptogenic EEG activity is controversial. Propofol has been reported to both induce and treat seizure-like activity. Propofol is similar to thiopental for anticonvulsant properties, but is analgesic rather than anti-analgesic.

○   **What are the effects of benzodiazepines on the CNS?**

They have anxiolytic, hypnotic, anterograde amnestic, muscle relaxant and anticonvulsant effects.

Benzodiazepines exert their effect mainly by GABA receptor activation and potentiation of the effects of GABA throughout the nervous system. Benzodiazepines may also have other sites of action. Benzodiazepines produce a dose-dependent reduction in $CMRO_2$ and CBF. Midazolam and diazepam may provide neuroprotection during cerebral hypoxia.

○   **What are the effects of ketamine on the respiratory system?**

- Minimal effect on the respiratory drive, maintenance of spontaneous ventilation
- Bronchodilator
- Hypersalivation
- Hyperreflexia of the larynx

The response to carbon dioxide is unaltered and arterial blood gases are usually preserved when ketamine is used alone. Rarely, apnea may follow with high dose administration. In children, ketamine should be considered a respiratory depressant. It improves pulmonary compliance in patients with reactive airway diseases or bronchospasm. Bronchodilatory effects are secondary to the release of endogenous catecholamines with β_2-agonist action and a direct relaxant effect on smooth muscle of lesser significance. Pretreatment with an antisialagogue is recommended (glycopyrrolate) for hypersalivation.

O   **What are the effects of benzodiazepines on the respiratory system?**

Benzodiazepines produce dose-dependent central respiratory depression resulting in a depressed ventilatory response to carbon dioxide, reduced respiratory rate, smaller tidal-volumes and decreased minute-ventilation. Benzodiazepines and opioids may have synergistic effects. The risk and severity of apnea following benzodiazepine administration is increased in patients with chronic obstructive pulmonary disease and the elderly or debilitated.

O   **What are the effects of etomidate on the respiratory system?**

Etomidate produces minimal effect on ventilation. The incidence of apnea is lower with etomidate when compared to equivalent doses of thiopental. Depression of ventilatory response to carbon dioxide is less with etomidate when compared to equivalent doses of methohexital.

O   **What are the effects of barbiturates on the respiratory system?**

Barbiturates produce dose-dependent central respiratory depression resulting in a diminished ventilatory response to hypoxemia, reduced respiratory rate, smaller tidal volumes and decreased minute ventilation. Apnea occurs at higher doses. Barbiturates rarely produce hypersalivation, bronchospasm or laryngospasm. They can be used safely for induction of anesthesia in asthmatic patients, where the most common cause of bronchospasm is the stimulus of laryngoscopy and intubation. Laryngeal reflexes are more active with thiopental than with equivalent dose of propofol. Blunting laryngeal reflexes may require large doses of barbiturates or the use of adjuvant agents to achieve a sufficient depth of anesthesia.

O   **What are the effects of propofol on the respiratory system?**

Propofol produces respiratory depression similar to barbiturates, and only mild bronchodilation (or no significant effect on airway tone) in patients with chronic obstructive airways disease.

O   **What are the effects of barbiturates on the cardiovascular system?**

Direct venodilation and depression of myocardial contractility.

The main effect is venodilation. The myocardial depressant effect is less than that produced by volatile anesthetics. During normal induction doses systemic vascular resistance is usually unaffected, and cardiac output is reduced despite an increase in heart rate. Hypertensive patients (treated and untreated) exhibit greater hypotension for a given dose than normotensive patients.

O   **What are the effects of ketamine on the cardiovascular system?**

Increase in blood pressure, heart rate and cardiac output, which are independent of dosing.

Ketamine causes central sympathetic stimulation producing increases in blood pressure, heart rate and cardiac output, all of which are desirable during acute hypovolemic shock. This offsets ketamine's direct effects of myocardial depression and vasodilation, which are seen in patients with spinal cord transection (sympathetic blockade) or severe end-stage shock where catecholamine stores are depleted. Ketamine should be avoided in patients at risk for myocardial ischemia or right and/or left heart failure due to the indirect hemodynamic effects described and increases in pulmonary vascular resistance and myocardial oxygen demands (in excess of increases in coronary blood flow).

○   **What are the effects of etomidate on the cardiovascular system?**

Minimal. Approximately, 10% reduction in mean arterial blood pressure and peripheral vascular resistance and 10% increase in heart rate and cardiac index. Minimal changes are also observed in patients with myocardial disease. Contrary to ketamine, etomidate does not have a direct myocardial depression effect.

○   **What are the effects of propofol on the cardiovascular system?**

Induction doses of propofol produce a moderate decrease (15 to 25%) in cardiac output, stroke volume and systemic vascular resistance. The resulting 40% decrease in systemic blood pressure is caused by myocardial depression and vasodilation (direct effect on smooth muscle and reduction in sympathetic activity). Interestingly, the heart rate does not change significantly during induction.

○   **What are the effects of benzodiazepines on the cardiovascular system?**

Benzodiazepines when used alone produce a mild decrease in arterial blood pressure. Midazolam causes significantly more hypotension than other benzodiazepines, but has been reported to be safe for induction (< 0.2 mg/kg) in patients with severe aortic stenosis. A combination of benzodiazepines and narcotics may produce an exaggerated hypotensive response due to a reduction of sympathetic tone.

○   **What is the mechanism for rapid onset and short duration of action of thiopental?**

Thiopental given as an IV bolus (3 to 5 mg/kg) for induction produces a loss of consciousness within 15 seconds and maximal effect within 1 minute. Duration of action is 20 to 30 minutes with termination of the affect of an induction dose (5 to 8 minutes). Due to high lipid solubility and low ionization at physiologic pH, it quickly crosses lipid membranes into the brain producing hypnosis. Thiopental has a long elimination half-life (6 to12 hours) but a rapid initial redistribution from the central compartment to the peripheral tissues (vessel rich, muscle or lean tissues and then fat) causing the plasma concentration to quickly decline below the effective concentration. Within 1 or 2 minutes the vessel rich group will reach its peak concentration first, which will rapidly decline thereafter, the lean tissues will follow with a peak concentration between 15 and 30 minutes, and finally the fat will reach its peak around 300 minutes. At the same time, the thiopental concentration at the effect-site will rapidly decrease and the drug action will be terminated. Multiple doses, very large initial doses or a continuous infusion of thiopental will result in redistribution sites reaching equilibrium with the blood and saturation of drug-metabolizing enzymes in the liver and prolonged drug action.

○   **Does age effect IV induction dose requirements of thiopental?**

Yes, if the calculation is based on actual body weight. Doses based on lean body mass compensate for age, gender and body habitus differences. Induction doses: healthy adult 2.5 to 4.5 mg/kg; children 5 to 6 mg/kg; infants 7 to 8 mg/kg; premedicated geriatric patient 30 to 35% reduction in dose compared with younger patients.

○   **What are the determinants of the volume of distribution for barbiturates?**

Lipid solubility is the main determinant followed by protein binding and degree of ionization. The rate of delivery of the barbiturates is dependent on blood flow.

○   **Where are barbiturates metabolized?**

Liver (10 to 15% per hour). Less than 1% is excreted unchanged by the kidneys.

O **When should the calculated dose of thiopental be adjusted?**

Increased sensitivity to thiopental has been demonstrated in neonates, women, the elderly and patients in renal failure or those suffering from hypovolemia.

This increased sensitivity is due to either a change in pharmacodynamics or in early distribution pharmacokinetics. For example neonates and patients with renal failure have decreased protein binding of thiopental, which results in an increased in the free fraction available to diffuse into the brain. Sensitivity of the elderly patient has been extensively studied and remains controversial. Based on EEG analysis, there seems to be no pharmacodynamic differences between young and elderly patients. However the conclusion that this age effect can be explained by early distribution pharmacokinetic changes has been challenged.

O **List factors affecting speed of IV induction?**

Following IV administration, drugs mix rapidly within a central blood pool and are distributed by blood flow and molecular diffusion throughout the tissues of the body according to their rate of perfusion (cardiac output), affinity for the drug (lipid solubility) and the relative concentration of drug in the tissues and blood (drug concentration and protein binding).

O **What is the elimination half-life of diazepam, lorazepam and midazolam?**

Diazepam: 20 to 50 hours
Lorazepam: 11 to 22 hours
Midazolam: 1.7 to 2.6 hours

O **Define clearance, volume of distribution and elimination half-life.**

Clearance is defined as a unit of volume being completely cleared of drug per unit of time. Volume of distribution is a concept designed to describe an observed plasma concentration after a known amount of drug has been given. If an amount of drug is diluted in a volume the resulting concentration will be:

concentration = amount/volume
volume of distribution can be defined as: $Volume_D$ = amount/concentration.

Factors, such as lipid solubility, that will affect the measured plasma concentration of a drug, will effectively change the volume of distribution.

The elimination half-life is the time required for the plasma concentration to decrease by 50% due to the elimination of the drug (as opposed to the decay of the plasma concentration due to redistribution). The half-life is related to the volume of distribution and clearance according to the following equation:

Half-Life $(T_{1/2})$ = 0.693*(volume of distribution)/clearance)

O **What non-opioid intravenous anesthetic does not reduce intraocular pressure (IOP)?**

Ketamine.

In general, nonopioid intravenous anesthetics reduce IOP by relaxing extraocular muscle tone, improving outflow of aqueous humor and lowering arterial and venous blood pressure. Ketamine has been reported as either having no effect or increasing IOP. Ketamine may decrease IOP in children. Although not an anesthetic, succinylcholine transiently increases IOP and it is usually avoided in open eye injuries, although no adverse events had ever been reported in such circumstances.

O **What non-opioid intravenous anesthetic has muscle relaxant properties?**

Midazolam has muscle relaxant properties mediated by the GABA receptor. Propofol does not have intrinsic muscle relaxant properties, however good intubating conditions have been reported with propofol.

○   **What are the undesirable side effects of barbiturates?**

*   <u>Direct venodilation</u> and depression of <u>myocardial contractility</u>
*   <u>Hyperalgesia</u>
*   <u>Histamine release,</u> which is rarely of clinical importance.
*   <u>Enzyme induction</u> increasing liver microsomal protein content occurs after 2 to 7 days of sustained drug administration, of which phenobarbital is the most potent. Enzyme induction may persist for up to 30 days after drug discontinuation.
*   <u>Acute tolerance</u> may occur faster than enzyme induction and the required effective dose of barbiturate may increase six-fold.
*   <u>Intra-arterial injection</u> of thiopental results in immediate severe vasoconstriction and excruciating pain. Gangrene and permanent nerve damage may occur. Treatment must be immediate and includes leaving the intra-arterial catheter or needle in place, dilution of barbiturates by injection of saline, and injection of lidocaine, papaverine or phenoxybenzamine to produce vasodilation. If the catheter has been removed, injection of vasodilators may be attempted proximally. Direct injection of heparin has also been advocated. Other possible treatment include sympathectomy of the upper extremity with a stellate ganglion block or a brachial plexus block and urokinase.
*   <u>Anaphylactic or anaphylactoid response.</u> The estimated incidence of allergic reaction to thiopental is 1 per 30,000 patients.
*   <u>Acute intermittent porphyria.</u> Barbiturates can induce delta-aminolevulinic acid synthetase, which catalyzes the rate-limiting step in the synthesis of porphyrins, which may result in paralysis and death.

○   **What non-opioid intravenous anesthetic can cause a transient suppression of adrenocortical function?**

Etomidate.

Etomidate causes a dose-dependent reversible inhibition of the enzyme 11-beta-hydroxyse, which results in decreased production of cortisol and aldosterone. Cortisol can be restored to normal levels with vitamin C supplementation. Long term (5 days or longer) sedative infusion of etomidate was identified as the causative factor for an increased mortality in mechanically ventilated ICU patients. However following a single induction dose of etomidate, the adrenocortical suppression is not clinically significant. There is no case report of a negative clinical outcome related to a single dose of etomidate or a short term infusion. Many studies have consistently shown that cortisol levels are only slightly depressed following a single induction dose of etomidate and return to normal within 20 hours. Patients having high-stress surgery have been shown to be able to overcome the temporary adrenocortical suppression caused by etomidate.

○   **What are the other side effects of etomidate?**

Nausea and vomiting, thrombophlebitis, pain during injection, myoclonus and hiccups and enhanced neuromuscular blockade of nondepolarizing muscle relaxants.

Etomidate is associated with a high (30 to 40%) incidence of post-operative nausea and vomiting which is further increased by the addition of fentanyl. Thrombophlebitis of the vein used may occur 48 to 72 hours after etomidate injection. Pain during injection is similar to that with propofol and can be eliminated by injecting lidocaine prior to etomidate. The reported incidence of myoclonus and hiccups is variable (0 to 70%). Myoclonus may be reduced by premedication with either a narcotic or a benzodiazepine. Etomidate enhances neuromuscular blockade of nondepolarizing neuromuscular blockers.

○   **Compare the uses of propofol and ketamine.**

Propofol: IV hypnotic agent used routinely for induction and maintenance of anesthesia as well as sedation for monitored anesthetic care. Approved for neurologic and cardiac anesthesia but caution should be exercised for use in hypovolemic patients due to arterial and venous vasodilation and mild negative inotropic effects which may cause hypotension. Unlike barbiturates, it is not antianalgesic. It tends to produce a state of well-being, but hallucinations, sexual fantasies and opisthotonos have been reported. Ideal agent for ambulatory surgery patients due to antiemetic properties with more rapid recovery in cases of < 1 hour duration than barbiturates.

Ketamine: IV induction agent producing CNS depression with hypnosis, sedation, amnesia and analgesia. Ketamine is not used as a routine induction agent primarily due to its unwanted emergence reactions. Sympathomimetic activity and bronchodilating properties are unique. It stimulates the cardiovascular system, increasing heart rate, blood pressure and cardiac output. Recommended for selective use for induction in ASA IV patients with respiratory (bronchospasm) and CV disorders (cardiomyopathy, cardiac tamponade and restrictive pericarditis, right-to-left shunt congenital heart disease, sepsis or hypovolemia; excluding ischemic heart disease). Increases intracranial pressure and cerebral metabolism, so contraindicated in patients with elevated ICP. May interact with tricyclic antidepressants causing hypertension and dysrhythmias. In addition, low-dose ketamine is used as an analgesic, for sedation during off-site procedural cases in pediatric patients and as an adjunct to regional anesthesia.

OPIOIDS

Everyone Wants To Live On Top Of The Mountain, But All The Happiness
And Growth Occurs While You're Climbing It.
Andy Rooney

○   **What side effects are associated with epidural or spinal opioids?**

Respiratory depression, urinary retention, pruritus, nausea, vomiting and sedation.

○   **Which opioid is most likely to cause delayed respiratory depression after epidural or spinal administration?**

Morphine.   Morphine is hydrophilic and is more likely to diffuse to respiratory centers in the medulla.

○   **How do you treat opioid-induced biliary spasm?**

Naloxone in titrated doses and glucagon (1-3 mg IV) are both effective treatments.

○   **Which opioid should not be used in patients on MAO inhibitors?**

Meperidine. This combination can lead to excitation, convulsions, and lethal hyperpyrexia.

○   **Why is a continuous meperidine PCA infusion not recommended?**

Accumulation of its renally excreted metabolite normeperidine can cause seizures and myoclonus..

○   **If the potency of morphine is 1, what are the relative potencies of meperidine, codeine, methadone, butorphanol, hydromorphone, nalbuphine alfentanil, fentanyl, and sufentanil?**

Meperidine 0.1, codeine 0.05 to 0.1, methadone 1, butorphanol 5, hydromorphone 10, nalbuphine 1, alfentanil 10, fentanyl 100 and sufentanil 1,000. This is easily remembered as "the multiples of tens".

○   **At physiological pH, do opioids exist mainly in the ionized or unionized form?**

Ionized. The pKA values for morphine, meperidine, fentanyl, and sufentanil are 8.0,8.5,8.4, and 8.0, respectively. Alfentanil, with a pKA of 6.5, is the only commonly used opioid that is predominantly unionized. Plasma levels of morphine have the poorest correlation with analgesic effect because it is the least lipid soluble of the opioid drugs.

○   **How is morphine metabolized?**

Glucuronidation in the liver followed by renal excretion of an active metabolite (morphine-6-glucuronide).

○   **Compared to parenteral administration, how potent is oral morphine?**

One-sixth as potent. This is because of the first pass effect in the liver, with only 20-30% reaching the systemic circulation

○   **What are the times to peak analgesic effect of IV, IM, and PO morphine?**

Approximately; 20-30 min, 45 min, and 90 minutes, respectively.

O   **Morphine is an agonist for which class of opioid receptors ?**

Mu_1 receptors.

O   **What are the most prominent CNS side effects of opioids?**

Respiratory depression, nausea, vomiting, sedation, constipation, pruritus, pupillary constriction and cough suppression.

O   **To which side effects of opioid administration are patients least likely to develop tolerance?**

Constipation and pupillary constriction.

O   **What are the most prominent peripheral actions of morphine?**

Constipation, biliary spasm, pruritus, urinary retention and histamine release (vasodilation).

O   **What is the proposed site of action of neuraxial opioids?**

Mu opioid receptors in the substantia gelatinosa of the dorsal horn of the spinal cord.

O   **Do opioids affect somatosensory evoked potentials?**

Yes. They increase the latency (3 mm) and decrease the amplitude (30 to 40%). However, these changes remain stable and do NOT interfere with intraoperative monitoring.

O   **How do opioids affect the CO_2 response curve?**

The CO_2 response curve is shifted to the right.

O   **How do opioids affect hypoxic respiratory drive?**

Opioids blunt this drive.

O   **What are the potential side effects of naloxone administration?**

Tachycardia, ventricular arrhythmias, cardiac arrest, hypertension, pulmonary edema, reversal of analgesia and precipitated withdrawal syndrome.

O   **What are the characteristic withdrawal symptoms when opioids are discontinued?**

In order of increasing severity:
1: anxiety, irritability and craving for the drug
2: watery eyes, runny nose, salivation and yawning
3: dilated pupils, loss of appetite, gooseflesh, shakes, hot and cold flashes, and muscle aches
4: severe tremors, fever, high blood pressure, fast pulse, and rapid breathing
5: diarrhea, vomiting, low blood pressure, sweating, confusion, and dehydration.

O   **Does methadone produce a more severe or less severe withdrawal syndrome than morphine?**

Less severe. Methadone has a longer half-life, so symptoms develop more slowly and tend to be less intense.

O   **Which morphine metabolite is active?**

Morphine-6-glucuronide. The duration of action of M-6-G is similar to morphine and may accumulate in patients with renal failure, leading to prolonged ventilatory depression.

○   **How do opioids affect cerebral blood flow?**

If ventilation is controlled, they cause a slight decrease. There is some controversy with sufentanil, with some studies showing an increase in CBF and others demonstrating no effect.

○   **Which opioid should be used with caution in neonates?**

Morphine. The blood-brain barrier is immature in neonates, which permits higher concentrations of the polar morphine molecule to reach the brain.

○   **When is respiratory depression seen with spinal opioids?**

Early respiratory depression (within 30 minutes of administration) can be seen with lipophilic opioids, while delayed respiratory depression (3 to 10 hours) is more commonly seen with hydrophilic opioids such as morphine. Early depression is thought to be due to rapid brain penetration by lipophilic compounds, while delayed respiratory depression is due to rostral spread.

○   **What is the potency of oral propoxyphene (Darvon) compared to oral codeine?**

Propoxyphene is one-half as potent as codeine.

○   **Do spinal or parenteral opioids alter uterine blood flow?**

No. However, meperidine may increase uterine contractility.

○   **Which opioids release histamine?**

Morphine, codeine and meperidine. Fentanyl, sufentanil and alfentanil do not stimulate histamine release.

○   **What are the mechanisms of opioid-induced hypotension?**

Histamine release causing vasodilation, dose-dependent bradycardia, negative inotropic effects (meperidine) and decreased sympathetic tone.

○   **Which opioid is a cardiac depressant and increases heart rate?**

Meperidine is a negative inotrope and may elicit tachycardia due to its structural similarity to atropine.

○   **Do opioids interfere with hypoxic pulmonary vasoconstriction?**

No.

○   **What is the time to maximal respiratory depression after an IV dose of fentanyl or morphine?**

Fentanyl, 5 to7 minutes and morphine, approximately 20-30 minutes.

○   **Can short acting opioids cause delayed respiratory depression (re-narcotization)?**

Yes. This has been reported with fentanyl, sufentanil, and alfentanil, as well as with morphine and meperidine.

○   **What are the effects of opioids on cerebral metabolic rate?**

In general, opioids cause a mild to moderate decreases in CMR. This remains coupled to CBF. However, occasionally opioid-induced neuroexcitation can cause focal increases in CMR.

O   **How should opioid-induced seizures be treated?**

With barbiturates and benzodiazepines. Naloxone will generally not reverse seizure activity, especially when induced by normeperidine.

O   **Which opioid is effective in treating shivering?**

Meperidine. It is effective in treating postoperative, transfusion-related, or epidural anesthesia-related shivering.

O   **How do parenteral opioids affect the surgical stress response?**

They decrease the response, with the fentanyl class of drugs apparently more effective than morphine. Blood glucose, catecholamine, cortisol, ACTH, and growth hormone levels are all decreased. This effect appears to be short-lived, and may require sustained administration to maintain this response. Effects on postoperative outcome remain controversial.

O   **What are the effects of opioids on intraocular pressure?**

They can decrease IOP and prevent increases in IOP due to succinylcholine and intubation.

O   **Do opioids cross the placenta?**

Yes. Impaired metabolism and excretion may result in opioid effects lasting up to 3 days in the neonate.

O   **Will respiratory acidosis increase or decrease opioid respiratory depression?**

Increase. Respiratory acidosis increases the iodized fraction at the receptor site.

O   **Does alkalosis increase or decrease respiratory depression?**

Metabolic and respiratory acidosis increase opioid repiratory depression.

O   **How are opioid pharmacokinetics altered in neonates?**

Clearance is decreased, and elimination half-life is increased. Decreased protein binding may lead to enhanced effects. Intraoperative clearance of fentanyl can be quite variable in newborns.

O   **How are opioid pharmacokinetics altered in the elderly?**

Decreased clearance and increased elimination half-life. Volume of distribution and protein binding can also be less, leading to a greater opioid effect for a given dose.

O   **What is the impact of liver disease on opioid pharmacokinetics?**

Decreased clearance and longer elimination half life. Hyperbilirubinemia and hypoalbuminemia accompany liver disease, which may render patients more sensitive to opioids.

O   **Explain why patients with renal failure may be sensitive to opioid administration?**

Morphine may show an increased effect or longer duration due to decreased conjugation (40% occurs in the kidney) and decreased elimination of the active metabolite morphine-6-glucuronide. Normeperidine accumulation and toxicity can occur. Effects of drugs in the fentanyl series are not significantly altered by renal failure.

○   **How is remifentanil metabolized?**

Non-specific plasma esterases.

○   **How do opioids affect the respiratory pattern?**

Decrease in rate, tidal volume, minute ventilation and apnea at higher doses. The pattern may also be irregular.

○   **What are the toxicities of propoxyphene?**

Hallucinations, convulsions, and cardiotoxicity. The cardiotoxicity may be partly due to the metabolite norpropoxyphene, and not entirely reversible by naloxone.

○   **Which anesthetics when combined with opioids can lead to cardiovascular depression?**

Nitrous oxide, volatile anesthetics, barbiturates, and propofol. Opioids have a synergistic effect with all general anesthetics.

○   **After continuous infusion, which opioid drug level decreases most slowly: alfentanil, fentanyl, or sufentanil?**

Fentanyl.

○   **What is the mechanism of opioid-induced bradycardia?**

The dose-dependent bradycardia seen with most opioids is likely an effect secondary to direct, central stimulation of the vagal nucleus.

○   **Describe the receptors where opioids demonstrate effects.**

Mu_1: Analgesia (somatic and visceral pain).
Mu_2: Respiratory depression, bradycardia, physical dependence, euphoria and ileus.
Delta: Modulates the activity at the mu receptor.
Kappa: Analgesia (visceral pain), sedation, dysphoria and psychomimetic effects.
Sigma: Dysphoria, hypertonia, tachycardia, tachypnea and mydriasis.

○   **How does the binding of an opioid agonist with an opioid receptor produce an intracellular effect?**

Opioid receptors belong to the G protein-coupled receptor family and they signal via a secondary messenger (cyclic AMP) or an ion channel (K^+).

○   **What are the cellular effects of opioids?**

Opioids decrease calcium ion entry resulting in a decrease in pre-synaptic neurotransmitter release (e.g. substance P release from primary afferents in the spinal cord dorsal horn). They also enhance potassium ion efflux resulting in the hyperpolarization of postsynaptic neurons causing a decrease in synaptic transmission. A third mode of action is in the inhibition of GABAergic transmission in a local circuit having the net effect of exciting an inhibitory circuit.

○   **Which opioid is most suitable for the transdermal route of administration?**

Fentanyl, which has a relatively high lipid solubility compared with morphine.

○   **Describe the pharmacokinetics of transdermal fentanyl.**

The transdermal route creates a skin reservoir which results in a 12 hour delay in onset and offset. Factors that affect skin perfusion will affect the rate of absorption. The transdermal route circumvents the first pass metabolism of fentanyl in the liver.

○   **Which opioid is most suitable for continuous infusion when a rapid offset of effect is required?**

Remifentanil. The drug is extensively bound to plasma proteins (70%) and has a low volume of distribution compared with other opioids. The clearance is much greater than that of other similar drugs, as such,, remifentanil has a very short elimination half life (3-10 min). Furthermore, studies have indicated that the offset of activity following continuous infusion of remifentanil is considerably more rapid than with fentanyl or alfentanil. This can be attributed to a context-sensitive half-time of 3-5 minutes.

MUSCLE RELAXANTS

I'm A Great Believer In Luck And I Find The Harder I Work, The More I Have Of It.
Thomas Jefferson

O   **Is a Phase II block reversible with anticholinesterases?**

Often. However, the response of a phase II block to reversal is unpredictable due to a number of factors influencing development of the block. It is best not to attempt reversal.

O   **What relaxants are metabolized by the plasma cholinesterase?**

Succinylcholine and mivacurium, which are choline esters.

O   **Can the prolonged action of succinylcholine or mivacurium in patients with atypical or decreased levels of plasma cholinesterase be terminated?**

Yes, with IV administration of plasma cholinesterase, but the best action to take is to be patient and wait for recovery of the train-of-four.

Even when pseudocholinesterase activity is only 20 percent of normal the increase in duration of blockade is rarely greater than 20 minutes. Patients who are homozygous for the atypical enzyme may be paralyzed for prolonged periods. Additional doses of succinylcholine or nondepolarizing relaxants should be given only when recovery is evident. Reversal of mivacurium or succinylcholine (Phase II block) with anticholinesterase may not be effective, except when the plasma concentration of the relaxant is already low.

O   **Immediately following burn or major nerve injury, is succinylcholine contraindicated?**

No. Risk of succinylcholine-induced hyperkalemia occurs beyond the first 24 hours post injury and remains dangerous as long as the pathology of muscle degeneration and regeneration continues, for at least 1-2 years.

O   **Does Parkinson's disease predispose to hyperkalemia or malignant hyperthermia?**

No. Parkinson's disease does not usually cause hyperkalemia and is not associated with malignant hyperthermia. Parkinson's disease is a degenerative disease of the CNS characterized by loss of dopaminergic fibers in the basal ganglia. Therefore, drugs with anti-dopaminergic effects should be avoided.

O   **What are the main side effects of d-tubocurarine?**

Histamine release (most significant of all nondepolarizing muscle relaxants and frequently dose-related) which produces vasodilation and hypotension. Sympathetic ganglionic block occurs in animals, but not in the clinical dose range. Bradycardia has been reported.

O   **Are muscle relaxants contraindicated in patients with hepatorenal syndrome?**

No. Cis-atracurium (and atracurium) undergoes spontaneous breakdown at physiologic temperature and pH (Hoffmann elimination) as well as ester hydrolysis. This is the ideal agent to use in patients with end-stage liver or kidney disease. Muscle relaxants requiring significant renal excretion should be avoided (pancuronium 40%, metocurine 43%, tubocurarine 45%, doxacurium 30% and pipecuronium 38%). Vecuronium and pancuronium also have 3 OH metabolites which accumulate in renal failure. The 3 OH metabolite of vecuronium is 50% as potent as the parent compound and that of pancuronium has 2/3rd the potency of the parent compound.

Muscle relaxants that are metabolized in the liver should be avoided or administered cautiously and titrated to effect (pancuronium, vecuronium, rocuronium and pipecuronium). Vecuronium and rocuronium also have significant biliary excretion. Decreased plasma cholinesterase activity seen with liver disease may prolong the effects of succinylcholine and mivacurium.

O   **Which relaxants are nearly totally dependent on the kidneys for excretion?**

Gallamine is excreted unchanged in urine. Alcuronium, doxacurium and pipecuronium use bile as a secondary pathway but are primarily excreted unchanged in urine. Pancuronium is 80% excreted renally.

O   **Is succinylcholine contraindicated in patients who have a pacemaker?**

No. Fasciculations produced by the administration of succinylcholine may be interpreted by the pacemaker sensor as an intrinsic cardiac impulse, which may then inhibit the pacemaker from firing (depending on the type of pacer). Precautions to minimize this risk include: reprogramming the pacemaker to an asynchronous mode or "defasciculating" the patient with a small dose of nondepolarizing muscle relaxant prior to the administration of succinylcholine. With current bipolar pacemakers, where electrical activity is sensed between two cardiac sensors, this is less of a concern. If a patient has a unipolar pacemaker, then fasciculations should be expected to be a problem, as only one sensor is located in the myocardium and the ground sensor is outside the heart.

O   **Is succinylcholine-induced masseter muscle spasm diagnostic of malignant hyperthermia susceptibility?**

No. There is evidence that this symptom could be a harbinger of malignant hyperthermia, but all cases of masseter spasm do not progress to MH.

Masseter muscle spasm is an exaggerated contractile response causing rigidity or trismus of the jaw muscles. Clinical presentation follows the administration of succinylcholine with complete neuromuscular blockade, and then intense difficulty in opening the patient's mouth. This can happen in all patients, especially children (1% incidence, of which 50% may prove to be MH-susceptible by muscle biopsy). Both myotonia and MH can cause masseter spasm, which should be differentiated from incomplete jaw relaxation, which is very common. It is controversial whether to cancel elective surgery or continue using a nontriggering general anesthetic. If the patient is susceptible to MH; a full-blown episode typically occurs 20 to 30 minutes after the onset of masseter spasm.

O   **Is open globe injury of the eye a contraindication to using succinylcholine?**

Not unless the anterior chamber is open, where there is a theoretical risk (never reported clinically) of extrusion of vitreous through the wound. Succinylcholine increases IOP 5 to 10 mm Hg for 5 to 10 minutes after administration, through contracture of the extraocular muscles. Prior administration of a defasciculating dose of nondepolarizing muscle relaxant may prevent the increase in 10P.

This is nowhere near the magnitude of increase seen in IOP with "bucking" on an endotracheal tube or squinting (increases IOP 25 mm Hg). Factors which increase IOP include: coughing, straining, bucking, laryngoscopy and intubation, hypercarbia, airway obstruction, "light general anesthesia", pupillary dilatation, venous congestion of the head and neck (Trendelenburg and prone positioning), pressure on the eye, retrobulbar hemorrhage and hypertension.

O   **Name two common qualitative tests for plasma cholinesterase?**

Dibucaine number, fluoride number.

O   **What is the dibucaine number?**

Normal plasma cholinesterase can be effectively inhibited by dibucaine in vitro. In the presence of 10^{-5} M of dibucaine, its activity is reduced by 80%, whereas the homozygous and heterozygous atypical enzymes are inhibited by only 20% and 60%, respectively. The dibucaine numbers are then 80, 20, and 60. It is the dibucaine-susceptible enzyme, which functions in vivo.

○ **Is pseudocholinesterase a true enzyme?**

Yes, it is plasma cholinesterase. Likewise, tissue or RBC cholinesterase is also called true cholinesterase.

○ **T/F: Plasma cholinesterase is stable in banked blood.**

True.

○ **How often do you expect markedly prolonged duration of action of mivacurium?**

As is with succinylcholine, patients with homozygous atypical plasma cholinesterase (1:2500) will remain paralyzed for hours, with twice the normal duration of block seen in patients who are heterozygous. In contrast to succinylcholine, with return of a twitch response to nerve stimulation, recovery from mivacurium blockade will be facilitated by the administration of cholinesterase inhibitors.

○ **Will the duration of action of cisatracurium be prolonged in patients with atypical plasma cholinesterase? Why?**

No. Cisatracurium, like atracurium, does not depend on plasma cholinesterase for its breakdown. It is eliminated by Hoffmann degradation and hydrolysis by non-specific esterases.

○ **Which relaxants are potential histamine releasers?**

d-Tubocurarine >>atracurium, mivacurium and doxacurium (ie: benzylisoquinoline compounds). Cisatracurium is also a benzylisoquinoline, but up to $8xED_{95}$ has no significant histamine release.

○ **Do muscle relaxants cause allergic reactions?**

Yes. Succinylcholine is the worst offender. After that, metocurine (hypersensitivity to iodide) and pancuronium (hypersensitivity to bromide) cause the most allergic reactions. The histamine-releasing side effects of muscle relaxants may cause hypotension which can confuse a diagnosis, as histamine related effects are clinical manifestations of anaphylaxis in the anesthetized patient.

○ **What is the main difference between atropine and glycopyrrolate?**

Glycopyrrolate is quaternary, and does not penetrate the blood-brain barrier. Atropine is a tertiary amine and does cross the blood-brain barrier. Atropine has been implicated as a rare cause of central anti-cholinergic syndrome.

○ **What are the main differences in the mechanism of action of edrophonium and neostigmine?**

Both drugs possess positively charged quaternary ammonium groups but edrophonium lacks a carbamate and ester group and relies on non-covalent electrostatic binding to attach to the anionic site of the acetylcholinesterase enzyme. Edrophonium's onset is 2 minutes (probably due to presynaptic release of acetylcholine) and duration of action 45 to 60 minutes. Neostigmine has a carbamate group which binds to the esteratic site of the enzyme and acts as a competitive substrate for acetylcholine. Onset is 7 minutes and duration of action 60 to 90 minutes. In equipotent doses edrophonium has less muscarinic effect, requiring only one half the amount of anticholinergic drug to prevent bradycardia. The anticholinergic drugs are chosen to match the onset of action of each anticholinesterase ie: glycopyrrolate with neostigmine and atropine with edrophonium.

O   **What is the clinical dose of edrophonium?**

Usually 0.5 to 1 mg/kg. Maximum dose is 1-1.5 mg/kg.

O   **What is the main determinant of reversibility of neuromuscular blockade?**

The main determinant is the presence of at least a single twitch on the train of four monitors, but preferably two. There are many factors: depth of block at the time of antagonism, dose of antagonist used, choice of antagonist, rate of spontaneous recovery expected from muscle relaxant, capability of metabolic clearance (organ dysfunction or hypothermia), presence of conditions/drugs such as inhaled anesthetics or aminoglycoside antibiotics known to potentiate muscle relaxants, and presence of certain abnormalities of electrolyte concentrations.

O   **How do the twitches in a train-of-four pattern with peripheral nerve stimulation relate to the reversibility of paralysis?**

The sequential disappearance of train-of-four twitches correlates with the extent of blockade (fourth twitch disappears at 70-75% block, third at 85% block and second at 94% and the last twitch at 99%). Surgical relaxation requires 75 to 95% neuromuscular blockade (only one or two twitches present). A train-of-four count of 4 twitches generally correlates with clinical reversibility with any NMB. A train-of-four count of 2 or 3 twitches indicates reversibility, but satisfactory reversal will require more time or a larger dose of anticholinesterase drug. With the presence of a single twitch, most patients will be reversible, but any complicating factor in NMB metabolism or presence of potentiating drugs could prevent complete and timely reversal.

O   **If you have no IV access, how can you administer a muscle relaxant to break laryngospasm?**

IM or sublingual route. The muscle relaxant most suitable for intramuscular injection is succinylcholine.

O   **After prolonged use of muscle relaxants in the intensive care unit (one week) how will neuromuscular transmission recover?**

The most important determinant of duration of action is depth of blockade. If the TOF indicates 1 or 2 twitches, which corresponds to an 85-95% receptor blockade, recovery will be seen within hours of discontinuing the drug. In the ICU, drug choice is important due to the impact of liver and kidney dysfunction on drug metabolism and clearance, and the possibility of accumulation of active metabolites (pancuronium and vecuronium). In addition, drugs or clinical conditions may prolong neuromuscular blockade. This includes: class I antiarrhythmics, magnesium, streptomycin, polymyxin, neomycin, lithium, corticosteroids and calcium channel blockers, respiratory acidosis, metabolic alkalosis, hypothermia and hypercalcemia. Close monitoring of neuromuscular function is essential.

O   **Explain the clinical significance of upregulation of the acetylcholine receptors?**

Any condition that significantly decreases/eliminates motor nerve activity causes a proliferation of extrajunctional neuromuscular receptors. The cell is essentially "searching" for an acetylcholine signal by putting out more receptors. These receptors are abnormal and extend beyond the normal boundary of the endplate. Hyperkalemia, predisposing to ventricular arrhythmias or cardiac arrest, may result from depolarization of these receptors by succinylcholine, which causes a massive outpouring of intracellular potassium into the plasma. Conditions include: burns, muscular dystrophies, spinal cord injuries, closed head injuries, upper and lower motor neuron disease, prolonged immobility, hemiparesis or intra-abdominal sepsis (debatable as cause but reportedly associated). It usually takes at least 24 hours for extra-junctional receptors to present.

O   **What is the response of burn patients to nondepolarizing muscle relaxants?**

Resistance. Burned patients require 2 to 5 times the normal dose of nondepolarizing muscle relaxant as an increased number of extrajunctional receptors in burns patients means more receptors to block and these receptors appear to be not very sensitive to non depolarizering muscle relaxants. Acetylcholine and succinylcholine depolarize extrajunctional receptors more easily in these patients.

○   **How do pregnant patients respond to succinylcholine?**

Normally. From the 10th week of pregnancy until 6 weeks postpartum, they have a 25 to 30% reduction in plasma cholinesterase activity. This decrease has little clinical significance.

○   **How do parturients differ from nonpregnant patients in dose requirements for nondepolarizing relaxants?**

Their dose-response curve is not significantly altered.

○   **How do the antibiotics potentiate the nondepolarizing muscle relaxants?**

They enhance neuromuscular blockade by inhibiting acetylcholine formation (pre-junctional mechanism).

○   **How is aminoglycoside-induced paralysis best managed?**

With assisted mechanical ventilation until satisfactory recovery of neuromuscular transmission occurs. A dose of neostigmine (maximum IV dose of 70 mcg/kg, to avoid nicotinic effects) may be tried.

○   **How does stereochemistry improve therapeutic indices of anesthetic drugs?**

Different isomers have been evaluated in hopes of decreasing drug-induced toxicity. Cisatracurium causes less histamine release than atracurium. L-bupivacaine may be less cardiotoxic than bupivacaine.

○   **How does the pharmacokinetics of rocuronium differ between young and elderly patients?**

Elderly patients have a similar speed of IV onset, but a prolonged duration of action attributed to decreased hepatic clearance. The pharmacodynamic effects of rocuronium do not differ between these two age groups.

○   **How do you calculate the IV dosage of muscle relaxants in the obese patient?**

Nondepolarizing muscle relaxants are ionized compounds that have a volume of distribution equal to that of the extracellular fluid. Since they are hydrophilic, they are poorly distributed to adipose tissue. In obesity, the volume of distribution, elimination half-lives, and clearance for muscle relaxants is not significantly different from that of nonobese individuals. Thus, when dosing nondepolarizing muscle relaxants, the patient's ideal body weight or 20% more than ideal body weight should be used for dose calculations.

Obese patients have higher levels of pseudocholinesterase activity than healthy subjects. Dosing succinylcholine at 1.2-1.5 mg/kg is recommended.

○   **Why is IV succinylcholine routinely not used for relaxation to facilitate abdominal closure after reversal of neuromuscular blockade with neostigmine?**

The duration of the subsequent block is unpredictable. Succinylcholine at intubating doses (1.5 mg/kg) normally provides 5-10 minutes of neuromuscular blockade. After administration of neostigmine, a dose of succinylcholine will cause neuromuscular blockade for up to 60 minutes. The mechanism of increased duration of neuromuscular blockade is due to the inhibition of pseudocholinesterase.

○   **How is mivacurium metabolized?**

Mivacurium is hydrolyzed by plasma cholinesterase (pseudocholinesterase) at 80-90% of the rate of succinylcholine.

○   **What drugs or disease states can prolong the duration of action of mivacurium?**

Patients with reduced plasma cholinesterase activity: those heterozygous or homozygous for the atypical plasma cholinesterase gene, pregnancy, liver or kidney disease, malignant tumors, infection, burns, anemia, decompensated heart disease, peptic ulcer or myxedema.

Drugs that reduce plasma cholinesterase activity include: oral contraceptives, glucocorticoids, monoamine oxidase inhibitors and irreversible inhibitors of plasma cholinesterase (eg: echothiophate or organophosphate insecticides). Extended neuromuscular blockade with mivacurium following pancuronium has been documented, presumably due to inhibition of plasma cholinesterase.

○   **How is the reversal of neuromuscular blockade assessed?**

Sustained head lift for 5 seconds, recovery of train-of-four, sustained tetany, and effective abdominal and intercostal muscle activity.

Clinical assessment includes: the ability to maintain head lift for 5-10 seconds, arm lift for 45 seconds, ability to lift legs off the table, and inspiratory effort of < 40-50 cm H2O. Adequacy of recovery of respiratory and upper airway function from nondepolarizing NMB is suggested by a TOF ratio of 0.9 or more at the adductor pollicis. Tetany (50 or 100 Hz) with a sustained contraction for 5 seconds indicates adequate, but not necessarily complete reversal.

○   **Do all inhaled anesthetics potentiate nondepolarizing muscle relaxants?**

Yes, but to varying degrees.

Inhaled anesthetics produce CNS depression with a generalized decrease in muscle tone and decrease in sensitivity of the postjunctional membrane to depolarization. In addition, isoflurane may increase blood flow to skeletal muscle, effectively delivering more drug to the receptor sites. In general, ether-type inhaled anesthetics (isoflurane and enflurane) have a greater dose-dependent effect on augmenting the block than halothane. Halothane has a greater effect than nitrous oxide-barbiturate-narcotic or propofol anesthesia. This effect is most significant with pancuronium.

○   **How do antibiotics potentiate nondepolarizing muscle relaxants?**

Aminoglycosides (neomycin, streptomycin, gentamicin and netilmicin) are notorious for potentiating the effects of nondepolarizing NMB. They exert their effects by inhibiting acetylcholine formation on the pre-junctional side of the neuromuscular junction. Other antibiotic groups known to potentiate nondepolarizing muscle relaxants include polymixins and lincosamines (clindamycin and lincomycin). Clindamycin prolongs the effect of pancuronium and vecuronium even in the absence of evidence of NMB. At clinically relevant doses the penicillins, cephalosporins, tetracyclines and erythromycins are devoid of effects at the NM junction.

○   **Do local anesthetics impact the recovery from nondepolarizing neuromuscular blockade?**

Yes. Small doses can augment the blockade produced by non-depolarizing muscle relaxants, while large doses can completely block neuromuscular transmission. The mechanism for local anesthetic augmentation of blockade includes the interference with pre-junctional release of acetylcholine, the stabilization of post-junctional membranes and the direct depression of skeletal muscular fibers.

○   **What other drugs can interact with nondepolarizing muscle relaxants?**

Cardiac antidysrhythmics: lidocaine (enhance), quinidine (enhance)

Diuretics: lasix (enhance)
Electrolytes: calcium (antagonize), magnesium (enhance)
Others: -Lithium (enhance)
        -Carbamazepine (antagonize)
        -Phenytoin (antagonize)
        -Cyclosporine (enhance)
        -Azathioprine (antagonize)
        -Dantrolene (enhance)
        -Calcium Channel Blockers (enhance)
        -Trimethaphan (enhance)

○ **What effect does magnesium have on the potency of nondepolarizing muscle relaxants? depolarizing muscle relaxants?**

Magnesium increases the potency of both depolarizing (mechanism unknown) and nondepolarizing MR (decreased pre-junctional release of acetylcholine and decreased sensitivity to acetylcholine).

○ **What are some other potential causes of prolonged neuromuscular blockade (NMB)?**

The more intense the neuromuscular blockade, the more likely that adequate time will be needed for complete resolution of neuromuscular blockade. Other factors that could impact reversal of NMB include acid-base disorders, electrolyte disturbances and hypothermia. Impairment of renal or hepatic function may significantly impact the clearance of muscle relaxants and their active metabolites.

○ **Do non-depolarizing muscle relaxants easily cross the placenta?**

Non-depolarizing muscle relaxants do not cross the placenta at detectable levels that are considered to be clinically significant due to quaternary ammonium groups that are highly ionized at physiologic pH and limit lipid solubility.

○ **Do depolarizing muscle relaxants cross the placenta?**

Depolarizing muscle relaxants do not cross the placenta at detectable levels when given in routine intubating doses. There are multiple case reports of neonatal neuromuscular blockade at birth involving either neonatal pseudocholinesterase deficiency or extremely large IV doses of succinylcholine given to the mother (300 mg).

○ **What are the EKG findings of succinylcholine induced hyperkalemia?**

ECG abnormalities and arrhythmias typically do not appear until the serum potassium level is greater than 6.5 mEq/L. Common ECG signs include: widened QRS, peaked T-waves, prolonged PR interval, loss of P waves, or atrial systole. ST-segment elevation may mimick acute myocardial infarction. First degree block may ultimately lead to complete heart block. Late signs include prolonged QRS complex that can lead to sine wave ventricular arrhythmia, ventricular fibrillation or asystole.

○ **What is the treatment for succinylcholine induced hyperkalemia?**

Direct cardiac antagonism, intracellular shift, and removal of potassium from the body.

Arrhythmia and hypotension are treated with either calcium gluconate or calcium chloride (10 ml of a 10%). Intracellular shifting of potassium can be accomplished by administering sodium bicarbonate (50-100 meq IV), glucose and insulin (25-50 g of dextrose with 10-20 units regular insulin IV) and hyperventilation ($PaCO_2$ 25-30 mm Hg). Kayexalate, furosemide, peritoneal dialysis, or hemodialysis can all decrease the total body potassium level.

○ **What is the definition of ED_{50}?**

The mean dose of a muscle relaxant producing a 50% suppression of the single twitch response at the adductor pollicis.

○   **What is the significance of ED$_{95}$?**

ED$_{95}$ is the mean dose of a muscle relaxant producing a 95% suppression of the single twitch response at the adductor pollicis. Most commonly, it is used to describe the relative potency of NMB in a nitrous oxide-barbiturate-opioid anesthetic. 2 x ED$_{95}$ of a muscle relaxant is routinely used for comparison of onset and duration between different muscle relaxants.

○   **What are the characteristics of a phase I block using a peripheral nerve stimulator?**

(1) Single-twitch, train-of-four and tetanus amplitudes are decreased in relation to the degree of blockade
(2) No fade in response to repetitive stimuli
(3) No post-tetanic facilitation
(4) Augmentation of neuromuscular blockade after administration of an anticholinesterase drug
(5) Describes depolarizing NMB

○   **What causes a phase II (desensitization) block?**

A phase II block is due to ionic and conformational changes in the cell membrane after large doses or a continuous infusion of succinylcholine. It is clinically similar to the block that is present after the administration of nondepolarizing muscle relaxants. However, the response to the reversal by acetylcholinesterase inhibitors is unpredictable.

○   **What are the characteristics of a phase II block?**

1. Decreased contraction in response to a single twitch stimulation
2. Fade of the muscle response with repetitive stimulation
3. TOF ratio of <0.3,
4. Post-tetanic facilitation
5. Antagonization of neuromuscular blockade after administration of an anticholinesterase drug
6. Describes nondepolarizing NMB

○   **What are the most common cardiovascular effects of succinylcholine?**

Cardiac muscarinic cholinergic receptor stimulation may cause sinus bradycardia, progressing to asystole, especially in children or after a second IV dose. Elevation in heart rate and blood pressure can occur as succinylcholine mimics the effects of acetylcholine on the autonomic ganglia.

○   **Why is succinylcholine the ideal drug for rapid sequence induction of anesthesia?**

Succinylcholine has the fastest onset (30-60 sec) and recovery (4-10min), compared to other muscle relaxants.

○   **Which muscle relaxant is traditionally used for ECT therapy? Why?**

Succinylcholine 0.5-1 mg/kg. Muscle relaxants are routinely used during electroconvulsive therapy to prevent injury to the patient. Succinylcholine is chosen for its quick onset and short duration. Other potential options include mivacurium, atracurium and cis-atracurium.

○   **Is Na$^+$ an intracellular or extracellular ion at the neuromuscular junction?**

Na$^+$ is an extracellular ion, while K$^+$ is an intracellular ion. This unequal distribution of ions causes a transmembrane potential of -90 mV to exist across the membrane.

○   **How does the train-of-four (TOF) correlate with diaphragmatic paralysis?**

Different muscles have different sensitivities to muscle relaxants of which the diaphragm and vocal cords are most resistant. The adductor pollicis (ulnar nerve) is routinely used for twitch monitoring. A stimulus delivered at 2 per second (2 Hz) for a total of 4 stimuli is known as a TOF. Surgical relaxation usually requires a 75-95% neuromuscular blockade. When the adductor pollicis is 90% blocked by rocuronium, the diaphragm is only 25% blocked. The diaphragm has a greater ED_{50}, ED_{95} and faster recovery of the twitch height than does the adductor pollicis when rocuronium is used. It has also been found that atracurium and vecuronium exhibit a similar degree of sparing of the diaphragm.

○   **Do muscle relaxants have the same effect on the larynx, diaphragm, adductor pollicis, and orbicularis oculi muscles?**

Neuromuscular blockade at the larynx and the diaphragm is less intense than at the adductor pollicis muscle. The laryngeal adductors (vocal cords), corrugator supercilia (superciliary arch), diaphragm, and abdominal rectus are more resistant and recover from neuromuscular blockade sooner than does the thumb (adductor pollicis) and eyelid (orbicularis oculli). The masseter, and pharyngeal muscles are most sensitive.

○   **Which muscle relaxants are ideal for patients with end-stage renal disease?**

Cis-atracurium and mivacurium. The duration of action of atracurium is independent of renal function, but laudanosine (metabolite) may accumulate due to a prolonged elimination half-time. Cisatracurium also produces laudanosine but because of the greater potency of cisatracurium, laudanosine quantities produced by Hofmann elimination are 5-10 times lower than in the case of atracurium. The clearance of vecuronium and rocuronium is slowed in patients with renal disease. Approximately 30% of rocuronium and 40% of vecuronium appears in the urine as unchanged drug during the first 24 hours. The duration of action is less predictable, with multiple or large doses resulting in a prolonged effect.

○   **Is renal failure a contraindication to succinylcholine?**

Only with pre-existing hyperkalemia, as succinylcholine increases the serum potassium concentration 0.5-1 meq/L or in the presence of uremic neuropathy where exaggerated.

○   **What implication does myasthenia gravis have on your choice of muscle relaxants?**

Patients with myasthenia gravis are very sensitive to nondepolarizing muscle relaxants and theoretically resistant to succinylcholine. Short or intermediate-acting muscle relaxants without active metabolites (mivacurium and cis-atracurium) may be given, starting with 1/10 the normal dose, and titrating to effect.

○   **What IM dose of succinylcholine is used for intubation in the neonate?**

Succinylcholine 4 mg/kg.

○   **What IV dose of succinylcholine is indicated for a RSI or intubation in the neonate?**

Succinylcholine 2 mg/kg.

○   **Explain the increase in succinylcholine dosing for neonatal intubation.**

The neonatal response to neuromuscular blockers is affected by immaturity of the neuromuscular junction and an increase in extracellular fluid and volume of distribution. Therefore, initial dosing of non-depolarizers is similar to that of adults. The dosage of succinylcholine, however, is increased to as much as twice the adult dosage.

○   **Should succinylcholine be used for routine intubation in pediatric patients?**

This is a controversial issue. The "black box warning" indicates that there are rare reports of ventricular dysrhythmias and cardiac arrest secondary to acute rhabdomyolysis with hyperkalemia in apparently healthy children who received succinylcholine. Many of these children were subsequently found to have a skeletal muscle myopathy whose clinical signs were not obvious. Since it is difficult to identify which patients are at risk, it is recommended that the use of succinylcholine in children should be reserved for emergency intubation or where immediate securing of an airway is necessary.

PHARMACOGENETICS

Education Without Values, As Useful As It Is, Seems Rather To Make Man A More Clever Devil.
C.S. Lewis

○ **Characteristics of Familial Dysautonomia (Riley-Day syndrome) include generalized diminished sensation, emotional lability and sympathetic denervation. What are the best drug choices for these patients?**

Diazepam or midazolam is used to treat a dysautonomic crisis triggered by stress (hypertension, tachycardia, abdominal pain, diaphoresis and vomiting). Fluids and direct-acting vasopressors (phenylephrine) are indicated for hypotension, as these patients may elicit denervation hypersensitivity with unpredictable responses to sympathomimetic drugs. Most patients are chronically hypovolemic, so vasodilatory or cardiopressant drugs may cause profound hypotension. Spinal and epidural anesthesia may be poorly tolerated.

○ **What type of IV fluids should be avoided in patients with the hypokalemic variant of familial periodic paralysis?**

Paralysis can be precipitated by high sodium or carbohydrate loads and exposure to cold temperatures. Glucose-containing solutions should be avoided as they may exacerbate the hypokalemia and muscle weakness.

○ **Which muscle relaxant should be avoided in the hyperkalemic variant of familial periodic paralysis?**

Succinylcholine (myotonia and hyperkalemia).

○ **Which reversal agent is contraindicated in myotonia congenita?**

Neostigmine. Myotonia congenita is characterized by generalized and persistent contraction of skeletal muscle after stimulation. This disorder may be exacerbated by the nicotinic effects of neostigmine.

○ **In myotonic muscular dystrophy, what effect do nondepolarizing muscle relaxants have on myotonic contractions?**

None. The contractions are not relieved by regional anesthetics, nondepolarizing muscle relaxants or deep anesthesia.

○ **What effect does succinylcholine have in patients with myotonic dystrophy?**

It produces sustained muscle contraction causing trismus and respiratory muscle rigidity which may make ventilation of the lungs and tracheal intubation difficult or impossible. Deterioration of skeletal, cardiac and smooth muscle function is progressive. In the presence of minimal or no weakness or atrophy, succinylcholine-induced hyperkalemia should not be a risk.

○ **Duchenne's muscular dystrophy is the most common and severe form of muscular dystrophy. This is a sex-linked recessive disease with an incidence of 3 in 10,000 births. Which muscle relaxant is contraindicated and why?**

Succinylcholine. Patients with Duchenne's muscular dystrophy have increased extra junctional acetylcholine receptors. Succinylcholine may cause massive rhabdomyolysis, hyperkalemia, dysrhythmias and cardiac asystole.

○   **What are the major clinical features of muscular dystrophy?**

1.   Degeneration of cardiac muscle which may lead to reduced contractility or mitral regurgitation.
2.   Restrictive lung disease due to degeneration of ventilatory muscles.
3.   Degeneration and atrophy of skeletal muscle.
4.   Gastrointestinal tract hypomotility, gastroparesis and impaired swallowing resulting in an increased aspiration risk.

Death is due to congestive heart failure or pneumonia.

○   **What percentage of normal children develop myoglobinemia after a single dose of intravenous succinylcholine?**

Approximately 40%.

○   **What genetic disorders are of concern when succinylcholine is used?**

Pseudocholinesterase deficiency (prolonged apnea), muscular dystrophy (especially unrecognized Duchenne's muscular dystrophy causing hyperkalemia), and myotonic dystrophy (muscle contracture).

○   **Which drugs can precipitate a hemolytic crisis in glucose-6-phosphate dehydrogenase deficiency?**

Prilocaine, lidocaine, sulfa drugs, quinidine, antimalarial drugs, aspirin (antipyretic drugs), non-narcotic analgesics (phenacetin), vitamin K, methylene blue and perhaps sodium nitroprusside. The common denominator is metabolism to a compound requiring G6PD for detoxification. Oxidant stressors include methemoglobin, glutathione and hydrogen peroxide.

○   **What is the usual time course for drug-induced hemolytic anemias?**

Drug-induced hemolytic anemias are immune-mediated. Therefore, a crisis usually begins 2-5 days after drug administration and generally ceases when drug therapy ends.

○   **What is the most common clinical presentation of pseudocholinesterase deficiency?**

Prolonged paralysis after succinylcholine administration.

○   **Which drugs are contraindicated in pseudocholinesterase deficiency?**

Succinylcholine, mivacurium and ester-linked local anesthetics (tetracaine, procaine, 2-chloroprocaine).

○   **What is the incidence of pseudocholinesterase abnormalities?**

Homozygous for atypical pseudocholinesterase, 1 in 2500. Heterozygous, 1 in 50.

○   **What is the pathophysiology of prolonged paralysis after succinylcholine administration in pseudocholinesterase deficiency?**

Inability to metabolize succinylcholine, which continues to depolarize the acetylcholine receptors.

○   **What is the treatment for prolonged paralysis secondary to succinylcholine?**

Continued ventilatory support, whether due to pseudocholinesterase deficiency or phase II block.

❍ **What is the dibucaine number? What are the clinical implications?**

The dibucaine number is a *qualitative* measurement of plasma cholinesterase activity. Dibucaine inhibits normal plasma cholinesterase by 80% and atypical plasma cholinesterase by 20%.

Dibucaine number 80: Normal enzyme, normal succinylcholine (SCh) metabolism.

Dibucaine number 40 to 60: Heterozygous for atypical plasma cholinesterase; moderately prolonged block with SCh.

Dibucaine number 20: Homozygous for atypical cholinesterase; very prolonged block with SCh.

❍ **Esmolol and remifentanil are metabolized by esterases. Does pseudocholinesterase deficiency affect dosing?**

No. Esmolol is hydrolyzed by RBC esterases with an elimination half-life of 9 minutes. Remifentanil is hydrolyzed by blood- and tissue-nonspecific esterases with a $t_{1/2}$ β of 5 to 8 minutes.

❍ **Discuss CATCH-22 syndrome [DiGeorge Sequence].**

CATCH-22 syndrome occurs with an incidence of 1 in 5000, and is highly pleiotropic involving cardiac, metabolic, and airway effects. The primary defect alters structures derived from the third and fourth pharyngeal pouches and the fourth branchial arch. Hypocalcemia is the primary metabolic defect. Sterility for intravenous catheters and invasive monitors must be maintained, because these patients may have thymic hypoplasia with low T-lymphocyte counts and relative immunodeficiency.

❍ **List the hepatic porphyrias which can cause life-threatening neurologic abnormalities.**

Acute intermittent porphyria, variegate porphyria and hereditary coproporphyria. Porphyria cutanea tarda causes photosensitivity, liver disease, and does not incur neurologic sequelae.

❍ **What are the symptoms of an acute porphyria crisis?**

Severe colicky abdominal pain and neurotoxicity (autonomic instability, psychiatric disorders and lesions of the lower motor neuron that can progress to bulbar paralysis).

❍ **In patients with hepatic porphyria, what should the pre-anesthesia physical examination specifically document?**

A complete neurological exam indicating peripheral neuropathies, autonomic dysfunction and cranial nerve involvement with impaired swallowing and respiratory muscle weakness.

❍ **What are "safe" drugs for administration to a patient with acute intermittent porphyria?**

Anticholinergics, anticholinesterases, depolarizing and nondepolarizing, muscle relaxants, droperidol, opioids, nitrous oxide, volatile anesthetics and propofol. Those of questionable safety include: etomidate and ketamine. Drugs considered "unsafe" induce the enzyme ALA synthetase and exacerbate the disease process. These include barbiturates, diazepam, phenytoin, corticosteroids and pentazocine.

❍ **Which synthetic process and enzyme activity is involved in an acute intermittent porphyria crisis?**

Heme synthesis pathway with a block at the conversion of porphobilinogen to uroporphyrinogen I and III with aminolevulinic acid and porphobilinogen present in the urine.

❍ **What is the mechanism by which barbiturates precipitate a porphyria crisis?**

Barbiturates induce the enzyme ALA synthetase which stimulates heme production and in the presence of a functional enzyme deficit results in the overproduction of porphyria compounds and their precursors.

○   **What is the pharmacologic treatment for an acute porphyria crises?**

The acute attack should be treated with glucose infusion, opioids (pain), beta antagonist (autonomic dysfunction: hypertension and tachycardia), intubation and mechanical ventilatory support (oxygenation and ventilation, prevent aspiration) and nasogastric suctioning (ileus and gastroparesis). Hyponatremia, hypokalemia, and hypomagnesemia should be treated. Pyridexine and hematin have been valuable in some cases. Prevention includes: avoiding starvation, dehydration, sepsis and triggering drugs.

○   **What species of hemoglobin are contained in adult blood?**

Oxyhemoglobin, reduced hemoglobin, methemoglobin and carboxyhemoglobin.

○   **What is the definition of methemoglobinemia?**

Greater than 1% methemoglobin.

○   **What effect does methemoglobin have on the pulse oximeter reading (SpO_2)?**

In the presence of methemoglobin, SpO_2 overestimates arterial oxygen saturation (SaO_2) (ie: at low levels of SaO_2 the SpO_2 is falsely high) and the pulse oximeter becomes less sensitive to SaO_2 as the levels of metHb increase with SpO_2 approaching 80% to 85%.

○   **How does pharmacologic induction of methemoglobinemia occur?**

Medications may oxidize the iron in hemoglobin from the ferrous to the ferric state resulting in methemoglobin. Methemoglobin reductase will convert methemoglobin back to hemoglobin.

○   **Which classes of drugs are implicated in causing methemoglobinemia?**

*   Local Anesthetics: prilocaine, benzocaine; lidocaine (questionable).
*   Nitrates, nitrites, sodium nitroprusside, nitroglycerin, amyl nitrite, and silver nitrite.
*   Antimalarials: chloroquine.
*   Antileprosy: dapsone.
*   Miscellaneous: phenacetin, sulfonamides, aniline dyes, chlorates, and nitrobenzenes.

○   **How do you diagnose acute drug-induced methemoglobinemia?**

Central cyanosis unresponsive to O_2 therapy without a cardiac or pulmonary explanation. A reddish brown venous blood sample, unchanged in color when exposed to air, is diagnostic.

○   **What is the drug treatment for inherited methemoglobinemia?**

Methylene blue 1mg/kg IV. Ascorbic acid is given mainly for cosmetic reasons. Homozygous patients are able to tolerate higher methemoglobin levels, although high levels of metHb may cause symptoms due to diminished oxygen-carrying capacity as well as a shift in the oxyhemoglobin dissociation curve. Avoidance of drugs known to induce methemoglobinemia is prudent.

○   **What is the incidence of malignant hyperthermia?**

1:4,500 to 1:60,000 general anesthetics. MH is rare in infants, and the incidence decreases after 50 years of age with up to a five fold greater incidence in males. Fifty percent of MH-susceptible individuals have had a previous triggering anesthetic without developing MH.

○ **What disorders have been associated with malignant hyperthermia?**

MH has been clearly associated with central core disease. Other disorders such as neuroleptic malignant syndrome, Duchenne muscular dystrophy, myotonia congenita, King syndrome, osteogenesis imperfecta, sudden infant death syndrome and sudden death in adults are controversial.

○ **What is the genetic transmission of malignant hyperthermia?**

Autosomal dominant with highly variable expression.

○ **Which drugs are considered triggering agents in malignant hyperthermia?**

Succinylcholine, all volatile anesthetics and potassium (possible retriggering agent).

○ **What are the clinical signs of malignant hyperthermia?**

The earliest signs of MH include tachycardia, tachypnea (in an unparalyzed patient) and increased end-tidal CO_2 levels, all reflecting a fulminant state of increased metabolic activity. MH has been reported to occur as late as 24 hours postoperatively.

Whole body muscle rigidity, rhabdomyolysis, increased temperature (delayed onset), metabolic and respiratory acidosis and increased sympathetic activity (tachycardia, arrhythmias, sweating and hypertension) are seen. Masseter spasm causing trismus following inhalation induction and succinylcholine is associated with an incidence of MH of approximately 50%.

○ **Which receptor is defective in malignant hyperthermia?**

The ryanodine receptor (calcium release channel) on the terminal cisternae of skeletal muscle sarcoplasmic reticulum.

○ **What is the cellular pathophysiology in malignant hyperthermia?**

The ryanodine receptor allows free unbound ionized calcium to be released from the sarcoplasmic reticulum. The calcium pumps attempt to restore homeostasis, which results in ATP utilization, increased aerobic and anaerobic metabolism and finally acidosis and cellular death. Rigidity occurs when unbound myofibrillar calcium approaches the contractile threshold.

○ **How does dantrolene ameliorate acute malignant hyperthermia?**

It inhibits the sarcoplasmic reticulum from releasing calcium.

○ **What medications are considered safe in malignant hyperthermia and how do you prepare an anesthesia machine?**

Safe drugs include: barbiturates, narcotics, local anesthetics, benzodiazepines, nitrous oxide and nondepolarizing muscle relaxants (all of the drug components necessary for total intravenous anesthesia). Remember that the anesthesia machine is safe when the vaporizers have been removed, the soda lime and circle system with reservoir bag changed and the system flushed with high-flow oxygen for 10 minutes to prevent patient exposure to trace gas contamination.

○ **What test is diagnostic for malignant hyperthermia and what are the two positive phenotypes?**

Muscle biopsy halothane-caffeine contracture testing.

The H-Type phenotype develops hypercontracture to caffeine and halothane alone; they are definitely susceptible to malignant hyperthermia.

The K-type phenotype exhibits only hypercontracture to halothane and caffeine combined. The degree of susceptibility to malignant hyperthermia of these patients is unclear.

○   **Epidermolysis bullosa is a rare hereditary disorder of the skin characterized by bullae formation, especially when lateral shearing forces are applied to the skin. What factors contribute to drug selection for anesthesia?**

Drug selection may be influenced by an increased incidence of porphyria. Succinylcholine is acceptable.

○   **T/F: Appropriate management of laryngeal edema seen in patients with Hereditary Angioedema includes epinephrine, antihistamines and steroids.**

False. The symptomatology mimics anaphylaxis but is recalcitrant to epinephrine, antihistamines or steroids. Hereditary angioedema is characterized by an absence of C1 esterase inhibitor in the plasma (uncontrolled activation of the complement system) with resultant episodic painless edema of the skin (face and limbs) and mucous membranes (respiratory and gastrointestinal tract) from release of vasoactive mediators that increase vascular permeability. Preoperative prophylaxis includes danazol (anabolic steroid), transfusion of FFP or purified preparation of C1 esterase inhibitor. Long-term prophylaxis treatments include antifibrinolytic therapy and anabolic steroids. During an acute attack no specific treatment is reliably effective. The airway must be secured with an endotracheal tube.

○   **What is the effect of cyclophosphamide on pseudocholinesterase?**

Cyclophosphamide is an inhibitor of pseudocholinesterase and as such may prolong the apneic response to succinylcholine. Its suppressive effect may be dose-dependent.

○   **A patient on echothiophate for treatment of glaucoma needs an emergency appendectomy. She was slow to recover from succinylcholine. Diagnosis?**

Echothiophate inactivates plasma cholinesterase, thus prolonging actions of succinylcholine.

○   **A healthy baby presents with increased temperature during hernia repair. He was induced with halothane, nitrous oxide and O2. Intubation was facilitated by atropine and succinylcholine and was maintained on halothane, N2O and O2. Most likely diagnosis?**

MH until proven otherwise. Looking for an increase in CO2 is appropriate as the first sign. In the face of normocarbia, the rise in temperature is most likely due to the anticholinergenic effect of atropine on sweat glands or overbundling.

○   **What are the effects of nitrous oxide on DNA synthesis?**

Nitrous oxide oxidizes cobalamin, a cofactor for the enzyme methionine synthase. Methionine synthase (MS) is the key enzyme of one-carbon transfer reactions needed to synthesize thymidylate. MS is a critical enzyme for DNA replication and cell growth because it is the only de novo source of thymine nucleotide precursors for DNA synthesis.

○   **What is the treatment for an acute malignant hyperthermia episode?**

*   Discontinue volatile anesthetics and triggers
*   Hyperventilate use100% O_2 with portable tank (see below for reuse of anesthetic equip)
*   Give dantrolene 2.5 mg/kg every 5min until symptoms subside
*   Cool patient with packed ice, cold IV fluids and gastric lavage
*   Maintain adequate volume with diuretics (mannitol and furosemide)
*   Monitor arrhythmias

- Initiate continuous electrolyte monitoring: treat hypocalcemia, hyperkalemia (insulin and glucose) and metabolic acidosis.

After successful treatment, dantrolene is continued at 1mg/kg IV every 6 hours for 24 to 48 hours to prevent recrudescence of symptoms. The Malignant Hyperthermia Association of the United States should be notified.

○ **Regional plexus and conduction anesthesia for extremity procedures in epidermolysis bullosa patients is an acceptable technique. What modifications in the regional technique are recommended for these patients?**

- Skin preparation should be with poured antibacterial solution
- Scrubbing should be avoided
- When testing for level of blockade, avoid trauma to the skin and mucous membranes
- Tracheal intubation with minimal frictional trauma to oropharynx
- Avoid tape when securing the endotracheal tube
- Supplemental O_2 may be given with nasal prongs or face mask lubricated with steroid ointment
- Catheters should be sutured or held in place with gauze wrap.

○ **How is dantrolene prepared?**

Dantrolene is prepared by mixing 20 mg of dantrolene with at least 60 ml of sterile water. Sodium chloride as the diluent will cause precipitation. Preparation is tedious as dantrolene dissolves slowly into solution. Therefore, you will need to call for help.

○ **Is cerebral palsy predictive of malignant hyperthermia?**

No.

LOCAL ANESTHETICS

Thanks To Modern Medicine We Are No Longer Forced To Endure Prolonged Pain, Disease, Discomfort And Wealth.
Robert Orben

○ **What is the most important property determining the potency of a local anesthetic?**

Lipophilicity. The greater the lipophilicity, the greater the potency. Alteration of molecular structure can also increase potency (e.g. the addition of a four-carbon chain to procaine to create tetracaine and the replacement of the methyl on the tertiary amine of mepivacaine with a butyl group to create bupivacaine).

○ **What is the mechanism of action of local anesthetics?**

They reversibly block the sodium ion channels at the neuronal membrane, which inhibits neuronal transmission. In addition, they block calcium and potassium channels in addition to NMDA receptors.

○ **Do other agents bind and block sodium channels?**

General anesthetics, substance P inhibitors, alpha 2 agonists, tricyclic antidepressants and nerve toxins also bind and inhibit sodium channels. The latter two classes of drugs have been tested as possible replacements for local anesthetics.

○ **Which regional block site is associated with the highest peak serum level of local anesthetic?**

The absorbance of local anesthetics is highest from the intercostal space. This is followed in descending order by the caudal epidural space, the remainder of the epidural space, the brachial plexus, the lower extremity peripheral nerves and subcutaneous tissue.

○ **What is primary route of metabolism of amide local anesthetic?**

The liver. Ester anesthetics are metabolized by plasma cholinesterases. The duration of action of esters may be prolonged in patients with pseudocholinesterase deficiency.

○ **A patient states she had a severe allergic reaction to an unknown anesthetic. What class of local anesthetic is most likely responsible?**

The overall incidence of true allergic reactions to local anesthetics is very low, the majority being esters. The common metabolite of esters, para-aminobenzoic acid, is frequently present in the chemical environment and prior exposure may lead to sensitization. Alternatively, intravascular injections in the dentist's office associated with epinephrine induced side effects (tachycardia and arrhythmias) and tinnitus may be reported as an "allergic reaction."

○ **What compound is responsible for the majority of allergic reactions to the amide class of local anesthetics?**

Methylparaben, the preservative in multi-dose vials. Preservative-free amides should be used in patients who are allergic to ester local anesthetics.

○ **A 32-year-old male has been administered a prilocaine epidural anesthetic for an ORIF of the femur. One hour after surgery starts, the patient's pulse oximetry begins to slowly decrease to 85%. What is the most likely cause and what is the treatment?**

The metabolites of prilocaine (O-toluidine) are potent oxidants, transforming the iron in hemoglobin from ferric to ferrous state and creating methemoglobin. Reversal occurs by enzymatic reduction. At doses greater than 600 mg cyanosis may develop, but the reduction in oxygen carrying capacity is rarely symptomatic unless the cardiopulmonary reserve is limited. Treatment is to administer 100% oxygen, send a blood gas sample for methemoglobin level, and rule out other causes. If the methemoglobin level is elevated, the treatment is methylene blue, 1-2 mg/kg intravenously.

Benzocaine and lidocaine have also been implicated as causes of methemoglobinemia.

○ **What are the premonitory symptoms associated with toxic blood levels of a local anesthetic?**

The patient may complain of ringing in the ears, difficulty hearing, a metallic taste in the mouth, numbness around the lips and a general feeling of restlessness or impending doom.

○ **While performing an axillary block, 15 cc of 0.25% bupivacaine was accidentally injected intravascularly. What signs and symptoms should you look for?**

Systemic administration may produce both central nervous and cardiac toxicity. Initially there may be CNS excitation (light-headedness, peri-oral numbness, dizziness, blurred vision) followed rapidly by disorientation, drowsiness, generalized convulsions and respiratory depression/arrest. Cardiovascular collapse may occurs when the heart sees a high plasma concentration either through very large IV administration, or a high concentration returning to the heart as a bolus (as in an injection of 0.75% bupivacaine traversing the route from the epidural veins to azygos veins and then directly to the heart).

○ **Do ropivacaine or levobupivacaine reduce the risk of toxicity.**

Ropivacaine and levobupivacaine both have an improved safety profile compared to bupivacaine particularly with respect to cardiac toxicity. However there are numerous recent reports of both cardiac and CNS toxicity to these agents. Commercial bupivacaine is a 50:50 racemic mixture of both the S- and R-enantiomers. Ropivacaine and levobupivacaine are the pure S- form of the drug which is less cardiotoxic than the R-isomer. All currently available LA are racemic mixtures (50:50) with the exception of lidocaine (do not have asymmetry), ropivacaine (S-enantiomer), levobupivacaine (S-enantiomer).

○ **What are the factors which contribute to CNS and cardiotoxicity from local anesthetics?**

Amount of available drug (overdosage, decreased protein binding, speed of injection, direct inadvertent intravascular injection, site of injection: i.e. 0.25 cc into the vertebral artery = seizures) and systemic absorption. More potent agents are usually more toxic: (i.e. 0.75 % bupivacaine). Bupivacaine is also the most cardiotoxic because of its slow dissociation from myocardial sodium channels resulting in refractory cardiac depression. Hypoxia, hypercarbia, acidosis, and pregnancy all potentiate systemic toxicity.

○ **How does hypercarbia increase toxicity to local anesthetics?**

Hypercarbia reduces the seizure threshold to local anesthetics. Elevation of the $PaCO_2$ increases cerebral blood flow and delivery of the agent to the CNS. Decrease in pH decreases the amount of protein binding of local anesthetics increasing the free plasma fraction.

○ **Which local anesthetic is associated with a low risk of systemic toxicity?**

2-chloroprocaine. It is rapidly metabolized by pseudocholinesterase (plasma half-life less than 30 seconds), allowing doses of up to 12 mg/kg.

○ **In choosing a local anesthetic, the anesthetist desires a drug with a pKa closest to physiologic pH. What would be the anesthetic of choice?**

Mepivacaine with a pKa of 7.6. Lidocaine (pKa of 7.8) and bupivacaine (pKa of 8.1) would be alternate choices. As the pKa of the drug decreases the percentage in the nonionized form increases. It is this form that crosses the nerve cell membrane.

O   **What role does ionization play in the effect of local anesthetics?**

The concentration of the nonionized portion is significant because this is the amount available to pass through the lipophilic membrane. However, once inside the membrane, it is the ionized portion which then blocks the sodium channels.

O   **A newly discovered local anesthetic was found to have a pKa of 7.4. What percent of the anesthetic will be unionized in the plasma?**

50%. The pKa of a drug is the pH at which 50% of the drug is ionized and 50% is nonionized.

O   **What effect does sodium bicarbonate have when mixed with a local anesthetic?**

The bicarbonate raises the pH of the solution. This alkalization increases the nonionized fraction of the anesthetic and speeds onset.

O   **What steps can you take to make a local anesthetic more alkaline and thus have more molecules in the nonionized state?**

You can add bicarbonate to the solution. The ratio for lidocaine is 1cc bicarb to 9 cc of lidocaine. The ratio for bupivacaine is 0.1 cc of bicarb for each 9.9 cc of bupivacaine. Also, select solutions which do not have epinephrine commercially added. These solutions typically have a starting pH of 3-5.0.

O   **Cimetidine administration will likely increase plasma levels of which class of local anesthetics?**

Cimetidine decreases hepatic clearance of amide anesthetics. Ester metabolism is independent of hepatic blood flow and cytochrome P450 action.

O   **Why have anesthesia providers been cautious with the intrathecal use of 2-chloroprocaine?**

2-chloroprocaine has been associated with cauda equina syndrome. Although follow-up studies have implicated the preservatives or additives (Bisulfite, EDTA) as the true etiology of the neurotoxicity recent animal studies have demonstrated opposite effects. Intrathecal administration of chloroprocaine induced significant functional impairment and histologic damage, whereas bisulfite did not. In addition, coadministration of bisulfite reduced injury induced by chloroprocaine.(sodium bisulfite scapegoat for chloroprocaine neurotoxicity? Regardless of the anesthetic chosen, only preservative free solutions should be used in the intrathecal space.

O   **A 22-year-old female complains of severe back pain 2 days after having a labor epidural with 2-chloroprocaine. What may be a likely explanation?**

Epidural 2-chloroprocaine has been associated with severe muscle spasm and back pain. The mechanism may involve the preservative EDTA chelating calcium in the paravertebral muscle.

O   **What are the anesthetics which can be applied topically?**

Tetracaine, lidocaine, cocaine and EMLA cream (Eutectic Mixture of Local Anesthetics). Attention to maximum dosages must be closely observed to avoid systemic toxicity.

O   **What are the active ingredients in EMLA topical cream?**

EMLA 5% cream is made from a 2.5% lidocaine – 2.5% prilocaine mixture. Its onset time is approximately 45 to 60 minutes.

○ **Toxicity after the use of EMLA cream has been associated with what systemic effects?**

Because of the prilocaine present in EMLA, methemoglobinemia can occur with the use of EMLA cream. Usually there is minimal plasma absorbance, but toxic blood levels are possible with prolonged application or when applied to abnormal skin.

○ **Which topical anesthetic is associated with intense vasoconstriction?**

Cocaine is an intense vasoconstrictor and is beneficial in topicalization of the nasopharynx.

○ **Which neuronal membranes are blocked first by local anesthetics and why?**

B fibers, which are the preganglionic sympathetic fibers, are the first to be blocked. Large, myelinated fibers which are the motor fibers, appear to be the most resistant to blockade. Traditional texts often state that small-diameter axons, such as C fibers, are more susceptible to local anesthetic blockade than larger-diameter fibers are. However, when careful measurements are made of single-impulse annihilation in individual nerve fibers, exactly the opposite differential susceptibility is seen. There is evidence that large myelinated fibers are more sensitive to LA blockade than the smaller unmyelinated fibers. Neverthless, placement of local anesthetic solutions in the subarachnoid space produces conduction blockade of small diameter nerve fibers first, because the anatomy of the dorsal nerve root is such that small diameter nerve fibers are close to the nerve root surface. (This shortens the diffusion. distance of the local anesthetic). The diffusion path to the large diameter nerve fibers, which are situated deeper in the dorsal nerve roots, is longer, making it appear that the small diameter nerve fibers are more sensitive to local anesthetic blockade than the larger diameter nerve fibers.

○ **Are local anesthetic solutions which contain epinephrine more acidic or more alkaline when compared to similar solutions without epinephrine?**

Commercially prepared solutions containing epinephrine are more acidic. For example, lidocaine hydrochloride has a pH of 5.0 – 5.5 whereas premixed with epinephrine the pH is 2.0 – 2.5. The latter prevents the spontaneous hydrolysis of the solution. The greater acidity leads to less nonionized drug immediately available and slows onset. This is why 'fresh' epinephrine is added to local anesthetic solutions just prior to administration.

○ **Which local anesthetic's duration of action is most affected by the addition of epinephrine?**

The addition of epinephrine to the relatively short acting lidocaine significantly increases the clinical duration of action. This enhancement is due to epinephrine's ability to counteract the vasodilatory effects of lidocaine and keeps the drug from being absorbed systemically.

○ **When comparing plain solutions of lidocaine and mepivacaine, which agent has a greater duration of action?**

Mepivacaine has a greater duration of action even though other local anesthetic characteristics are similar.

○ **Which class of local anesthetics is more rapidly metabolized – esters or amides?**

In general, the esters are more rapidly metabolized.

○ **What is the amide local anesthetic with the shortest half-life?**

Prilocaine. It has a short half-life because it also is metabolized in the lung and kidney.

○   **What is the average time to two segmental dermatome regression after placement of 20 cc of 2% lidocaine in the epidural space?**

60 to 90 minutes.

○   **What local anesthetics provide the best differential blockade?**

Ropivacaine and bupivacaine provide the best differential blockade. Lower concentrations of these drugs can provide reliable sensory blockade with minimal motor blockade.

○   **A patient with end-stage liver disease is most susceptible to local anesthetic toxicity from which class of agents?**

Amides

○   **An 18-month-old 12 kg child presents for hypospadias repair. A single injection caudal blockade is planned for postoperative pain relief. What is the maximum recommended dose of bupivacaine?**

The maximum dose is 2 mg/kg. In this scenario, one could use 0.25% bupivacaine plain, 9.5 cc (24 mg) total.

○   **In which of the following instances is using 0.75% bupivacaine contraindicated: axillary block, spinal anesthetic, labor epidural, retrobulbar block or sciatic nerve block?**

0.75% bupivacaine is not recommended for labor epidurals because of the risk of cardiac arrest with an inadvertent intravenous bolus injection.

○   **The nurse anesthetist is preparing to perform an awake fiberoptic intubation on a 40 kg patient. How much 4% cocaine can she use to aid in topicalization of the airway?**

3 cc or 120 mg. The maximum dose for topical cocaine is 3 mg/kg.

○   **A spinal anesthetic was placed for a cesarean section. In what order will the differential blockade occur?**

The first modality blocked is the sympathetic fibers. This is followed by loss of sensation (temperature first, then pain, touch and proprioception). The last nerves blocked are the motor fibers.

○   **What is the expected clinical duration of a single dose of epidural 2-chloroprocaine?**

30 to 45 minutes.

○   **After an interscalene block is performed, it is noted that the patient developed anesthesia in the shoulder earlier than in the fingers. Why?**

Peripheral nerve blockade proceeds from a proximal to distal distribution. The nerve mantle contains fibers to distal areas in the core and fibers to proximal areas along the outer edge of the mantle.

○   **While performing an intercostal block, the patient suddenly seizes. Describe appropriate management.**

CNS toxicity can occur from intravascular injections. Management of the airway is the first step. Hyperventilation is helpful to decrease local anesthetic levels in the brain and to increase the PaO_2 of the patient during the seizure. Benzodiazepines or small doses of barbiturates should be administered to terminate the seizure. The patient should be carefully monitored for hemodynamic instability and treated as appropriate with iv fluids, vasopressors and ACLS protocols.

○   **What effect does protein binding have on the duration of action of local anesthetics?**

Highly protein bound local anesthetics have a prolonged duration of action. For example, procaine is poorly protein bound (6%) and accordingly has a very short duration of action.

○   **After performing a field block with 10 cc of 0.5% bupivacaine for an incision and drainage of an abscess, the surgeon notes that the patient is still very uncomfortable. What might explain this?**

Local anesthetics are less effective in acidic environments such as infected tissue. This is due to the low tissue pH increasing the ionized portion of the anesthetic, making less nonionized anesthetic base available to cross the lipophilic membrane.

○   **Which local anesthetic is associated with inhibition of norepinephrine re-uptake?**

Cocaine inhibits norepinephrine re-uptake, resulting in frequent episodes of hypertension and tachycardia.

○   **What are the possible reasons to avoid epinephrine in labor epidurals?**

Epinephrine, when absorbed systemically, may decrease uterine blood flow due to the alpha-adrenergic effects and worsen hypertension in a preeclamptic patient. The beta agonist effect may also cause uterine relaxation and prolong labor. Furthermore, resistance to beta-adrenergic effects may mean an intravascular "test dose" injection will not reliably produce the diagnostic tachycardia indicative of intravascular injection.

○   **A patient allergic to PABA should not be given which type of anesthetic?**

Allergic reactions to para-aminobenzoic acid has been associated with cross reactivity to ester anesthetics. The preservative methylparaben may also cross react with PABA and methylparaben is commonly found in small dosages in multi-dose vials of amide anesthetics. In general, any patient allergic to PABA should be given an amide local anesthetic from a single-dose vial.

○   **What class of nerve fibers are the first to be blocked by local anesthetics?**

B fibers which are the preganglionic autonomic fibers.

○   **What is the maximum recommended dosage of epinephrine used in peripheral nerve blocks?**

Maximum recommended dosage is 200 to 250 micrograms.

○   **After placement of an axillary block with 40 cc of 2% lidocaine with epinephrine 1:100,000 the patient develops multiple PVC's. Explain.**

A 1:100,000 solution contains 10 micrograms of epinephrine per cc of solution. This patient received a total of 400 micrograms of epinephrine and the PVC's are a symptom of possible systemic toxicity.

○   **What is the one factor most influencing the onset of a local anesthetic?**

The pKa. The closer the pKa is to pH of 7.4, the more rapid the onset. An exception to this rule is 2-chloroprocaine. It has a pKa of 8.1. However, it has a rapid onset because it is used in such high concentrations (3%).

○   **What are the common ester local anesthetics?**

Procaine, 2-chloroprocaine, cocaine and tetracaine. Only one '*i*' in the name. Am*i*no Am*i*des typically have 2 '*i*'s in the name. i.e. Bup*i*vaca*i*ne.

○   **How do local anesthetics given intravenously affect MAC?**

MAC is decreased.

○   **Do local anesthetics cross the placenta?**

Yes. More protein bound agents (bupivacaine, etidocaine) have less delivery to the fetus. Ester local anesthetics also reach the fetus to a lesser extent because of their short plasma half life.

○   **Does fetal acidosis affect fetal transfer of local anesthetics?**

Yes. Higher fetal concentrations of amide local anesthetic (ionized fraction) are detected during fetal acidosis (ion trapping).

○   **How is lidocaine metabolized?**

Lidocaine is metabolized in the liver by mixed-function oxidases and amidases. Metabolism is reduced by drugs that reduce hepatic enzyme activity (i.e. propranolol, cimetidine). Drugs such as barbiturates that induce microsomal enzymes in the liver may slightly increase lidocaine metabolism.

○   **Does lidocaine cause TNS (Transient Neurologic Symptoms)?**

Intrathecal lidocaine has been implicated as a cause of TNS. Use of the lithotomy position may be a contributory factor.

○   **What is the antiarrhythmic drug of choice in treating bupivacaine cardiotoxicity?**

Amiodarone now seems to be the drug of choice for treatment of bupivacaine induced ventricular arrhythmias.

CHRONIC PAIN MANAGEMENT

The Worst Pain A Man Can Suffer: To Have Insight Into Much And Power Over Nothing.
Herodotus

○ **What areas in the CNS are involved in pain generation and perception?**

Afferent pathways, CNS and efferent pathways.

Nociceptors transmit pain sensation to the dorsal horn of the spinal cord (substantia gelatinosa, laminae) across to the contralateral spinal cord and through spinothalamic tracts to the thalamus. There are two spinothalamic tracts: neospinothalamic tract for acute pain (transmits pain sensations to midbrain, postcentral gyrus and cortex) and paleospinothalamic tract for dull and burning pain (transmits pain sensations to the reticular formation, limbic system and midbrain). Stimulation of the periaqeductal gray site in the midbrain results in activation of efferent pathways which inhibit pain impulses.

○ **What are the indications for sympathetic blockade?**

Diagnosis and treatment of sympathetically-mediated acute or chronic pain, prevention of neuropathic pain; postherpetic neuralgia (no evidence, may be beneficial); treatment of CRPS (effective); acute/chronic vascular insufficiency (may be beneficial), hyperhidrosis, miscellaneous: stellate ganglion block for Bell's palsy, quinine toxicity, retinal artery occlusion and certain types of hearing loss.

○ **What is Complex Regional Pain Syndrome (CRPS)?**

Chronic disorder usually occurring at the site of an injury (most commonly arms and legs) simultaneously affecting the nerves, skin, muscles, blood vessels, and bones. Symptoms include: severe burning pain, pathological changes in bone and skin (warm, shiny red skin turns bluish and cool), excessive sweating, tissue swelling and extreme sensitivity to touch. The pain is out of proportion to the severity of the injury and gets worse over time. Eventually disuse atrophy of the skin, muscles, and joints results. There are two types: CRPS 1 (without nerve injury, replaces the term reflex sympathetic dystrophy) and CRPS2 (with identifiable nerve injury, replaces causalgia).

○ **Describe options for pain management related to pancreatic disease.**

Medical management (opioids, antidepressants, anticonvulsants, antiarrythmics), *acupuncture, radiographically guided injections* (celiac plexus block, peripheral nerve block, neuraxial blocks, interpleural blocks), *behavioral* (psychotherapy, relaxation, biofeedback), *intravenous infusions* (lidocaine, phentolamin, IV regional sympathetic block), *neuromodulation* (spinal cord stimulation, transcutaneous electric nerve stimulation), *intrathecal drug delivery systems*.

○ **Are NSAIDs indicated for the treatment of acute low back pain?**

They are the mainstay of drug therapy. Benefit from the combined analgesic and anti-inflammatory properties of NSAIDs s or acetaminophen is seen within seven days of the onset of symptoms. If no medical contraindications are present, a two- to four-week course of acetaminophen or NSAIDs is indicated. The use of benzodiazepines (Valium®) does not appear to offer any significant benefit.

○ **What are Waddell signs?**

Nonorganic signs indicating the presence of a functional component of back pain.
• Superficial, nonanatomic tenderness
• Pain with simulated testing (axial loading or pelvic rotation)
• Inconsistent responses with distraction

- Nonorganic regional disturbances (nondermatomal sensory loss)
- Overreaction

○   **Phantom limb pain is frequently intractable and chronic. Are there any effective therapies available?**

Medical treatments, nerve blocks, regional blocks, intrathecal/epidural opioids, sympathetic blocks, electrical nerve stimulators and ablative surgical procedures (brain or spinal cord) have limited effectiveness. Sensory discrimination training, mirror visual feedback, restoring motor cortex activity with illusory movements of the paralysed limb and using an electrical prosthetic limb moved by signals from the patient's muscle may reverse the sensory cortex to its original state of nerve transmission and reduce pain.

○   **Is botulinum toxin (BTA-A) effective in the treatment of myofascial pain?**

Several studies have shown that BTX-A may be effective in reducing pain in myofascial disorders. Compared to 1% lidocaine, steroids, marcaine and placebo, the BTX-S groups showed greater improvement in subjective pain scores.

○   **What is breakthrough pain and how is it managed?**

Supplemental opioids (morphine, hydromorphone, oxycodone), short-acting oral immediate-release or transmucosal opioids (fentanyl). Intra-nasal delivery systems are being developed. If higher dosages of fixed schedule opioids are maintained at all times as a prophylactic strategy, unacceptable side effects may result.

In 1990, Portenoy and Hagen proposed a standard definition of breakthrough pain as a transient increase in the intensity of moderate or severe pain, occurring in the presence of well-established baseline pain. It is rapid in onset (within 3 minutes) and a short duration (median 30 minutes). The American Pain Society definition 2002: "intermittent exacerbations of pain that can occur spontaneously or in relation to specific activity; pain that increases above the level of pain addressed by the ongoing analgesia; includes incident pain and end-of-dose failure."

○   **What are the clinical features of lumbar radicular pain?**

Lumbar radicular pain ("sciatica") is caused by irritation of the sensory root or dorsal root ganglion of a spinal nerve (disc prolapse is the commonest cause, but spinal stenosis is more likely in the elderly). The pain is sharp, shooting and is typically felt as a narrow band down the length of the leg, both superficial and deep, but does not follow the corresponding dermatomes and it is the sensory loss that indicates the affected segment. It may be associated with sensory and/or motor dysfunction (radiculopathy) and may coexist with spinal or somatic referred pain.

○   **Define hyperalgesia.**

Abnormal hypersensitivity to noxious mechanical or thermal stimulation, which is a symptom of neuropathic pain.

○   **Discuss the medical and surgical management of trigeminal neuralgia (TN).**

TN is a pain syndrome characterized by intermittent often lancinating pain which is typically one-sided in the distribution of the trigeminal nerve (typically maxillary V2 or mandibular V3 areas). The annual incidence of trigeminal neuralgia is estimated at 2 to 5 per 100,000 and prevalence increases with age, in 90% of cases beginning after the age of 40 years and more common in women than men. The goal of drug therapy is to reduce pain. Carbamazepine (Tegretol) is the most effective medical therapy, with selected patients benefiting from phenytoin, baclofen, gabapentin, Trileptol and Klonazepin. Surgical options include: peripheral nerve blocks or ablation, gasserian ganglion and retrogasserian ablative procedures, craniotomy with microvascular decompression and stereotactic radiosurgery (Gamma Knife®).

O **What is sympathetic-mediated peripheral nerve pain?**

Type I complex regional pain (sympathetic dystrophy) and type II complex regional pain (causalgia).

O **List treatment options for non-malignant neuropathic pain.**

There is no proven treatment to prevent or cure neuropathic pain. Treatment has traditionally been through a combination of medications and nerve blocks, implantable devices, physical therapy, TENS and psychological/occupational therapy. Amitriptyline (up to 150 mg daily) is the first choice (especially for diabetic neuropathy or postherpetic neuralgia), while gabapentin may be better tolerated. Carbamazepine is indicated for trigeminal neuralgia. Topical capsaicin, lamotrigine, baclofen, and opioids may also relieve pain in some patients.

O **What are the signs and symptoms of RSD (reflex sympathetic dystrophy)?**

In a prospective study of 829 patients (Lancet 1993) the early phase of RSD was characterized by an exaggerated regional inflammatory response to injury or operation. Pain, hypoaesthesia and hyperpathy were common. With time, tissue atrophy, involuntary movements, muscle spasms, pseudoparalysis, tremor and muscular incoordination were evident.

Traditionally, RSD has been described as *three consecutive phases of disease (acute, dystrophic and atrophic)* with the early symptoms those of a disturbance of sympathetic function.
Acute stage during the first 1-3 months: burning pain disproportionate to the degree of injury, extreme sensitivity to touch, skin color and temperature changes.
Dystrophic stage at 3 to 6 months involves constant pain and swelling, increased muscle tone, stiffness, and wasting, and early bone loss.
During the *atrophic phase* of skin, muscle and bone, the skin becomes cool and shiny, with muscle stiffness, weakness, spasm and tremor, and symptoms may spread to another limb. Depression and anxiety may be present.

O **What is chronic pain?**

Somatic, visceral or neuropathic pain lasting more than 3 months.

O **What is post-thoracotomy pain syndrome?**

Chronic pain resulting from surgical trauma or fibrosis of the intercostals nerves which is typically neuropathic, usually in the distribution of the affected intercostal nerve. Management of the pain includes the use of tricyclic antidepressants and anticonvulsants. Repetitive local anesthetic and steroid blocks may be useful. For terminal cancer patients, implantation of an epidural catheter for continuous infusion has been beneficial.

O **During labor does a basal infusion for PCEA (patient-controlled epidural analgesia) enhance analgesia?**

The use of basal infusions of local anesthetics and fentanyl in obstetrics (in addition to on-demand dosing) remains controversial. The few studies that control for basal infusions generally find that they increase total drug use without significantly enhancing analgesia.

O **List the complications of celiac plexus block.**

Rapid absorption of the drug leading to systemic toxicity, subarachnoid injection and resulting block, sympathetic blockade leading to hypotension, bleeding, infection and punction of an abdominal viscous (mainly kidney).

O **What are the diagnostic criteria for *fibromyalgia syndrome*?**

American College of Rheumatology 1990 Criteria for the Classification of Fibromyalgia

1. History of widespread pain in all four quadrants of their body for a minimum of three months. Pain is considered widespread when all of the following are present: pain in both sides of the body, pain above and below the waist, axial skeletal pain must also be present (cervical spine, anterior chest, thoracic spine or low back pain). Low back pain is considered lower segment pain.
2. Pain in 11 of 18 tender point sites on digital palpitation which cluster around the neck, shoulder, chest, hip, knee and elbow regions.

○   **T/F: The goal of treatment of reflex sympathetic dystrophy is pain control through drug therapy and immobilization of the affected limb.**

False. The goal of treatment is pain control (NSAID for inflammation, tramadol for noninflammatory, antidepressants such as amytriptyline, doxepin, nortriptyline and trazodone for pain that disrupts sleep, anticonvulsants such as carbamazapine and gabapenitn for suddent sharp pain, and opiods such as propoxyphine, codeine and morphine for generalized, severe pain) and mobilization of the affected limb with physical therapy. Muscle cramps and stiffness can be treated with clonazepam and baclofen, localized pain related to nerve injury has been treated with Capsaicin® cream, and medications that block selected actions of the sympathetic nervous system (clonidine oral or patch formulations) may be useful. Sympathetic nerve blocks, TENS and spinal cord stimulators

○   **What is the cause of hyperalgesia in neuropathic pain?**

Primary hyperalgesia is caused by sensitization of C-fibers which occurs immediately within an area of injury. C fibers (small unmyelinated afferents) penetrate directly and generally terminate no deeper than lamina II. After peripheral nerve injury there is a prominent sprouting of large afferents dorsally from lamina III into laminae I and II. After peripheral nerve injury, these large afferents gain access to spinal regions involved in transmitting high intensity, noxious sisgnals, instead of merely encoding low threshold information.

○   **Describe the pathophysiology of phantom limb pain.**

There is no agreement as to the mechanism, all have supporting data and it is likely that the cause is multifactorial. The theories are divided into: peripheral causes (sensation due to a loss of previously present peripheral nerve activity, regeneration of the nerves that were injured/cut, neuroma formation with resulting painful nerve activity, alteration in ion channel activity at the site of injury), spinal causes (deafferentation), and central causes (changes in parts of the cortex and thalamus). Stress and depression may contribute to the syndrome.

○   **What is the anatomy of the celiac plexus block?**

The celiac plexus surrounds the celiac artery at the level of L1, anterior to the aorta. Blockade involves preganglionic fibers from the greater and lesser splanchnic nerve, postganglionic sympathetic fibers, preganglionic parasympathetic fibers, afferent visceral nociceptive fibers and branches of the right vagus. The results in dennervation of the stomach, liver, gall bladder, pancreas, kidneys, gut to the transverse colon, diaphragm, spleen and abdominal aorta.

○   **Is fentanyl useful in the treatment of chronic pain?**

Fentanyl is an ideal agent for delivery via the transdermal therapeutic system due to its low molecular weight, high potency and lipid solubility. These systems release the drug into the skin at a constant rate ranging from 25 to 100 ug/hour. Compared with oral opioids, the advantages of transdermal fentanyl include a lower incidence and impact of adverse effects (constipation, nausea and vomiting, and daytime drowsiness), a higher degree of patient satisfaction, improved quality of life, improved convenience and compliance resulting from administration every 72 hours and decreased use of rescue medication. Therapeutic blood levels are attained 12-16 hours after patch application and decrease slowly with a half-life of 16 to 22 hours following removal.

O   **What are the complications of stellate ganglion block?**

CNS toxicity (intra-arterial injection of local anesthetic into the vertebral artery), vaso-vagal reactions, Horner's syndrome (unilateral meiosis, ptosis and enophthalmos), brachial plexus blockade, phrenic nerve block, spinal or epidural injection, recurrent laryngeal nerve palsy with hoarseness. Pneumothorax is possible is the needle is inserted in a caudad direction. Intercostal neuralgia has been described manifesting as severe chest wall pain. Bilateral stellate ganglion blocks are contraindicated.

O   **What is the risk of administering cocaine for local anesthesia and constriction of nasal mucosa prior to inhalational anesthesia?**

Increased risk of ventricular fibrillation or other severe ventricular arrhythmias, especially in patients with pre-existing heart disease. Inhalational anesthetics such as halothane (chloroform, cyclopropane and trichloroethylene), more than isoflurane and to an even lesser extent enflurane sensitize the myocardium to the effects of sympathomimetics.

O   **Describe the pharmacokinetic properties of cocaine.**

Cocaine is readily absorbed from all mucous membranes. Due to its local vasoconstrictive effect, measurable quantities have been reported to remain in the nasal mucosa for 3 hours after application. The is a significant risk of systemic toxicity due to rapid absorption with an onset of action in less than 1 minutes, 5 minutes to peak effect and elimination half-life of 1 to 1.5 hours. Duration of action is approximately 30 to 60 minutes (average 20 to 40 minutes). Cocaine is hydrolyzed by plasma and hepatic cholinesterases. The primary metabolites (benzoylecgonine and ecgonine methyl ester) and 10 to 20% of the unchanged drug are renally eliminated.

O   **What are the systemic effects of cocaine?**

Tachycardia (increase in heart rate of 20 to 50%), hypertension, ventricular arrhythmias and fever due to excessive sympathetic stimulation. When low doses are administered tachycardia may initially be preceeded by bradycardia due to central vagal stimulation. Signs and symptoms of systemic toxicity occur in three phases: early stimulation (cardiovascular; CNS: agitation, excitement, dysphoria, headache; abdominal pain, nausea, sweating; unusually large pupils), advanced stimulation (ventricular arrhythmias, CNS hemorrhage, CHF, convulsions, myocardial ischemia) and depression (loss of reflexes, flaccid paralysis, fixed dilated pupils, loss of consciousness, pulmonary edema, cardiac arrest).

O   **What is postherpetic neuralgia?**

Postherpetic neuralgiz results from reactivation of the varicella-zoster virus from the dorsal root ganglia which remains dormant after the primary "chickenpox" infection. Herpes zoster presents with a classic dermatomal rash and burning pain which preceeds the rash and may persist well after the resolution of the rash. The pain may be very debilitating and require narcotics for adequate pain control. Tricyclic antidepressants, anticonvulsants, capsaicin, lidocaine patches and nerve blocks have been used in selected patients.

O   **What is the difference between unilateral right versus left stellate ganglion blockade on left ventricular function?**

With TEE assessment, blood pressure and heart rate are not significantly changed. Following right stellate ganglion blockade there are no significant differences in systolic and diastolic function. Left stellate ganglion block results in denervation of the left ventricle without a change in systolic function, but relaxation is prolonged. LVEDV (left ventricular end-diastolic volume) and LVESV (end-systolic volumes) are significantly increased. In patients without cardiovascular disease (ASA I), these effects are not clinically significant as the heart responds with a small stroke volume increase to offset the simultaneous decrease in afterload.

O   **What is the difference between fibromyalgia (FMS) and myofascial pain syndrome (MFP)?**

Myofascial pain syndrome (MPS) is a painful muscloskeletal condition characterized by the development of trigger points in muscle or junction of the muscle and fascia and "referred pain". MPS presents as local pain with fatigue and morning stiffness uncommon. Prognosis is good, with resolution with treatment. FMS is chronic pain syndrome characterized by diffuse pain, fatigue, morning stiffness, tender points, with a poor prognosis.

O   **What is some of the therapies for the treatment of myocascial pain syndrome?**

Trigger Point Therapy (myofascial release therapy, myotherapy, medical massage therapy)
Spray and Stretch Technique (vapocoolant spray on the trigger point and then PT-directed stretch therapy)
Trigger Point Injections (local anesthetic injected directly into the trigger points)
Dry Needling (the use of a needle to disrupt the trigger point with no injection)
Chiropractic manipulation
Cranioscral therapy
Exercise
Improvement of nutrition
Changing sleeping habits
TCA in low doses
Elimination of stress, biofeedback, counseling for depression
For MPS there is no role for injected steroids

O   **What are the complications of regional pain syndrome 1 (RSD)?**

The signs and symptoms of sympathetic nervous system involvement are discussed above. In addition, signs of motor system dysfunction include: difficulty starting movement, increased muscle tone, muscle spasm, tremor and weakness. Additional problems are infections, migraine headache, excessive sweating, fatigue, dermatitis, eczema, depression and anxiety. Skin, muscle and bone atropy with reduced function of the limb are frequent.

O   **Describe the use of autonomic nerve block for chronic non-malignant pain originating in the pelvis.**

It has been claimed that some chronic perineal pain syndromes respond to bilateral lumbar sympathetic block and superior hypogastric block has been used for chronic non-malignant pelvic pain syndromes.

O   **Describe the efficacy of neurolytic blocks in the treatment of chronic pelvic pain associated with cancer.**

The pain of rectal tenesmus due to pelvic carcinoma may be helped with celiac plexus block. Neurolytic superior hypogastric plexus blocks have been used for chronic pelvic pain and block of the ganglion impar at the inferior end of the sacrum has been used for perineal pain in cancer.

O   **What are the diagnostic criteria for CRPS Type I (Merskey and Bogduk 1994)?**

1.   The presence of an initiating noxious event, or cause of immobilization;
2.   Continuing pain, allodynia, or hyperalgesia in which the pain is disproportionate to any inciting event;
3.   Evidence at some time of edema, changes in skin blood flow or abnormal pseudomotor activity in the region of the pain;
4.   No other conditions that would account for the degree of pain and dysfunction should be present.

Criteria 2-4 must be satisfied.

O   **What are the diagnostic criteria for CRPS Type II?**

1. The presence of continuing pain, allodynia, or hyperalgesia after nerve injury, not necessarily limited ot the distribution of the injured nerve;
2. Evidence at some time of edema, changes in skin blood flow or abnormal sudomotor activity in the region of the pain;
3. No other conditions would account for the degree of pain and dysfunction should be present.

All 3 criteria must be satisified.

○ **Describe diagnostic and neurolytic lumbar sympathetic block.**

Diagnostic block uses 2-5 cc of bupivacaine 0.5 % at each level. Therapeutic local anesthetic injections of 5-10 cc of bupivacaine may be given at a single level. Some authors recommend a prognostic block with a continuous catheter for up to 5 days as a prerequisite to neurolytic block. Neurolytic injections are made with aqueous pheol 6%, or a stronger solution, dissolved in x-ray contrast medium. A volume of 1-10cc is the recommended range. The needle should be flushed with local anesthetic before withdrawal to avoid leaving a track of phenol through the more superficial tissues. The lumbar sympathetic trunk is situated in the retroperitoneal connective tissue anterior to the vertebral bodies and the medial margin of psoas muscle. Blocks for the lower limb are performed in the prone or lateral position, usually targeting the anterior edge of the vertebral body of L3 and L4, with a block at L1 indicated for renal pain.

○ **What are C fibers?**

Small-caliber, pain-mediating fibers representing roughly 70% of the peripheral nerve system. C fibers are the slowest and smallest and mediate the sensation of warmth and are the main component responsible for the sensation and transmission of pain, at a conduction velocity less than 2 m/sec. In addition, C fibers subserve most of the autonomic peripheral functions.

PERIPHERAL NERVE BLOCKS

Continuous Efforts, Not Strength Or Intelligence, Is The Key To Unlocking Our Potential
Winston Churchill

○ **What's the major landmark for an interscalene block?**

Identification of the interscalene groove between the anterior and middle scalene muscles at the level of the cricoid cartilage.

○ **What frequently marks the level of the cricoid cartilage in the interscalene groove?**

The external jugular vein traversing the anterior triangle of the neck. At the level of the cricoid cartilage it intersects with the posterior border of the sternocleidomastoid muscle, overlying the interscalene groove.

○ **How does an interscalene brachial plexus block progress, proximal to distal or vice versa?**

Proximal to distal.

○ **List the major complications of interscalene brachial plexus block.**

CNS toxicity (even with minimal arterial injection), local anesthetic toxicity, nerve and spinal cord damage, epidural and intrathecal injections, pneumothorax in addition to the effects of blockade of the phrenic (raised hemidiaphragm), vagus and recurrent laryngeal (hoarseness) nerves. It is not infrequent for patients to develop Horner's syndrome (miosis, ptosis and enophthalmos).

○ **Name the components of the brachial plexus?**

Starting from their origin and progressing distally they are named *r*oots, *t*runks, *d*ivisions, *c*ords and *b*ranches. (*R*andy *T*ravis *D*rinks *C*old *B*eer).

○ **Is an interscalene brachial plexus block ideal for hand surgery?**

No. Interscalene brachial plexus blocks provide consistent anesthesia of the shoulder, arm and elbow. With this approach there is frequently ulnar nerve sparing (a branch of the lower trunk). More distal approaches to the plexus such as infraclavicular or axillary are more appropriate for hand surgery.

○ **How do you perform a radial nerve block at the elbow?**

Insert the needle in the intermuscular groove between the brachioradialis and the long head of the biceps tendon 2 cm proximal to the flexor skin crease. Using an insulated needle and nerve stimulator, advance the needle in the direction of the radial nerve until initial muscle contractions become visible. Reduce current and optimize needle position until visible muscle contractions occur at lower current levels (< 0.5 mA). Following needle aspiration for blood, inject the local anesthetic drug in incremental doses. The patient should be fully monitored and receive sedation and supplemental oxygen with resuscitation equipment and suction immediately available.

○ **Is the brachial artery medial or lateral to the median nerve at the elbow?**

The brachial artery is medial to the median nerve at the elbow.

○   **With an axillary block of the brachial plexus what nerves are frequently missed?**

Nerves which are no longer encased within the sheath. Frequently the musculocutaneous nerve, the median cutaneous nerve and the intercostobrachial nerve will be missed.

○   **The axillary block of the brachial plexus is best for procedures located where relative to the elbow?**

It's best for procedures distal to the elbow, innervated by the terminal nerves of the plexus.

○   **How can the musculocutaneous nerve be blocked to augment an axillary brachial plexus block?**

An injection into the coracobrachialis muscle will often block the musculocutaneous nerve. Forearm flexion (biceps) in response to peripheral nerve stimulation can be used to locate the nerve.

○   **What important blood vessel runs in the interscalene groove, just below the brachial plexus?**

The subclavian artery runs in the interscalene groove, forming the notch on the superior surface of the first rib.

○   **Following neurologic injury to peripheral nerves, how much time must elapse before the nerve conduction study (NCS) demonstrates an abnormality?**

The process of degeneration may take 10 to 14 days to be completed. NCS performed during this period may be interpreted as normal, despite significant injury.

○   **How are nerve injuries classified?**

Classically, there are 3 groups representing the degree of neuronal disruption: neurapraxia (local myelin injury), axonotmesis (axonal disruption with endoneurial preservation) and neurotmesis (complete severing of the entire nerve). Neurapraxia has the greatest chance of functional recovery.

○   **What is the relation of the femoral nerve to the femoral artery at the inguinal ligament?**

The femoral nerve is approximately 1cm lateral to the femoral artery (sometimes posteriolateral to the artery), invested within its own fascia and deep to the fascia lata. Penetration of the two fascial layers are discerned as distinct 'pops' when using a blunt needle. This technique is used when performing a fascia iliac block.

○   **What nerves must be blocked to provide lower limb anesthesia?**

The lower limb is supplied by both the lumbar plexus and the sacral plexus. While a single central neuraxial injection (epidural or spinal) can result in anesthesia, no single peripheral nerve block can reliably block both nerve plexus.

○   **What are the major branches of the lumbar plexus?**

The lumbar plexus arises from the ventral rami of T_{12} to L_4 and has six main nerves. The three important branches for lower limb anesthesia/analgesia are the femoral nerve (and its saphenous nerve branch which continues below the knee), lateral femoral cutaneous and the obturator nerve. The other 3 nerves are the iliohypogastric, ilioinguinal and genitofemoral nerves.

○   **What is the largest branch of the lumbar plexus?**

The femoral nerve.

○   **What muscle does the lateral femoral cutaneous nerve supply?**

None. It is purely a sensory nerve.

○   **Can blockade of the obturator nerve be assessed by checking sensation on the medial aspect of the thigh?**

In many people the obturator nerve has no cutaneous nerve supply to the thigh.

○   **What are the major branches of the sacral plexus?**

The sacral plexus arises from the ventral rami of L_4 through S_4. The main branches are the sciatic nerve (tibial & common peroneal components), the pudendal nerve, posterior femoral cutaneous nerve and the superior and inferior gluteal nerves. When a proximal sciatic nerve block is performed both the sciatic and the posterior femoral cutaneous nerves are blocked.

○   **What is a "3-in-1" block?**

A large volume of local anesthetic (20 to 30 ml) is injected at the site of the femoral nerve block and proximal (retrograde) spread within the fascial sheath blocks the femoral, lateral femoral cutaneous and obturator nerves within the psoas muscle. In practice, while femoral nerve blockade is reliable actual blockade of all 3 nerves occurs less frequently.

○   **Which nerve is most likely to be missed in a "3-in-1" block?**

The lateral cutaneous nerve. It is often invested in its own fascial sheath, whereas the femoral and obturator nerves often share a common sheath.

○   **Which peripheral nerve blocks are required to provide regional anesthesia for a total knee replacement?**

Both blockade of the lumbar plexus and sciatic nerve are required. A posterior approach to the lumbar plexus more reliably blocks the 3 nerves (femoral, lateral femoral cutaneous and obturator nerves) compared to the femoral '3 in 1' approach. The sciatic nerve must be blocked separately.

○   **What are the components of the sciatic nerve?**

The sciatic nerve consists of 2 separate nerve trunks, the tibial nerve and the common peroneal nerve on the lateral side. These 2 nerves diverge about 7 cm proximal to the popliteal crease. In the popliteal fossa the sciatic nerve lies lateral and superficial to the popliteal artery.

○   **Does blockade of the sciatic nerve in the popliteal fossa result in complete distal extremity anesthesia?**

No. Cutaneous innervation of the medial leg below the knee is provided by the saphenous nerve, a superficial terminal extension of the femoral nerve.

○   **What stimulus will be typically elicited by stimulation of the tibial nerve in the popliteal fossa?**

Planter flexion and inversion of the foot. While common peroneal nerve stimulation results in dorsiflexion and eversion.

○   **Does performing an ankle block include blocking a branch of the lumbar plexus?**

Yes. The saphenous nerve is a sensory branch of the femoral nerve. Except for this branch, an ankle block largely involves blockade of the terminal branches of the sciatic nerve (posterior tibial, sural, deep peroneal and superficial peroneal nerves).

O   **What is Hilton's Law?**

Hilton's law states that a nerve supplying motor innervation to a muscle responsible for joint movement will also supply sensory innervation to that joint and the skin overlying the joint. In general, any nerve traversing a joint will also supply it. For example, the hip joint is innervated by the femoral, sciatic and obturator (mixed function), as well as lateral cutaneous (sensory only) nerves.

O   **When using a peripheral nerve stimulator, how should the leads be configured?**

The positive lead connected to the patient (ground electrode) and the negative to the needle.

O   **What is an acceptable current when using a peripheral nerve stimulator?**

Pulsed, synchronous movement at a current less than 0.5 mA when using an insulated needle usually indicates that the tip of the needle is 2 to 3 mm away from the nerve.

O   **What is the difference between a retrobulbar and peribulbar block?**

The position of the needle tip in relation to the cone formed by the extra-ocular muscles. Peribulbar involves depositing local anesthetic outside the cone and has a slower onset of action.

O   **What is the most common complication of retrobulbar block?**

Hematoma formation, especially in the vicinity of the point at which the ophthalmic artery crosses the optic nerve. The risk can be minimized by using needles shorter than 35 mm. Other complications include intravascular and subarachnoid injections, optic atrophy, optic nerve injury, globe penetration and ocular muscle paresis.

O   **What is the occulocardiac reflex?**

Traction on the eye or ocular muscles resulting in bradycardia, asystole or arrhythmias. The afferent pathway involves transmission via the ciliary ganglion to the ophthalmic division of the trigeminal nerve while the efferent pathway is the vagas nerve.

O   **What is the sympathetic chain?**

It is a ganglionated nerve chain extending from the base of skull to the coccyx, lying 2 to 3cm lateral to the vertebral column. Inferiorly, the two chains unite and terminate on the anterior surface of the coccyx.

O   **Where is the stellate ganglion?**

It is formed by the fusion of the lower cervical and first thoracic ganglions (cardiothoracic ganglion), present in 80% of individuals. It lies on the anterior surface of the seventh cervical transverse process.

O   **What features indicate a successful stellate ganglion block?**

The development of a unilateral Horner's syndrome: partial ptosis, meiosis, apparent enophthalmos, lack of sweating and nasal congestion. Sympathetic blockade in the upper extremity should also be evident.

O   **List the potential complications of stellate ganglion block?**

Intravascular injection (vertebral artery) resulting in seizures, epidural and subarachnoid spread of drug, hematoma and pneumothorax. Other side effects include hoarseness and dysphagia (recurrent laryngeal block), Horner's syndrome and brachial plexus block.

❍ **What are the three principal cranial nerves innervating the airway?**

Trigeminal (nasopharynx), glossopharyngeal (pharynx, tonsillar pillars, soft palate and posterior third of the tongue) and vagus (mucosa from the epiglottis to distal airways: superior and recurrent laryngeal nerves).

❍ **How can the superior laryngeal nerve be blocked?**

The greater cornu of the hyoid is identified. A needle is placed inferiorly and 2 ml of local anesthetic injected.

❍ **What does the celiac plexus innervate?**

The celiac plexus innervates most of the abdominal viscera, including the stomach, liver, bilary tract, spleen, kidneys, omentum, small bowel and large bowel to the level of the splenic flexure.

❍ **Does the celiac plexus supply the pelvic organs?**

No. The hypogastric plexus supplies the pelvic organs.

❍ **What are the complications of celiac plexus block?**

Neuraxial block, puncture of the aorta and tracking of neurolytic solution to lumbar nerve roots, pneumothorax, retroperitoeal hematoma. Orthostatic hypotension also frequently occurs due to decreased sympathetic tone.

❍ **What's the toxic dose of lidocaine in peripheral nerve blocks?**

Approximately 7-8 mg/kg is considered the maximum dose of lidocaine with epinephrine (plain lidocaine 5 mg/kg). Recommendations are based on subcutaneous administration and apply only to single-shot injections.

CAUDAL, EPIDURAL AND SPINAL ANESTHESIA

The roots of education are bitter, but the fruit is sweet.
Aristotle

○ **What is the subdural space?**

A potential space located between the dura mater and the arachnoid.

○ **What structures are traversed (midline approach) in sequence by a needle as it is passed, starting dorsal and moving ventral, toward the dura?**

Skin, subcutaneous tissue, supraspinous ligament, interspinous ligament, ligamentum flavum, epidural space and finally, the dura mater.

○ **At what level does the spinal cord proper end in an adult?**

The spinal cord descends caudally in the spinal canal and changes in conformation from a solid structure to a strand-like continuation of the nerves referred to as the cauda equina (horse's tail), usually at the level of the first or second lumbar vertebral body. The conus medullaris usually lies about the level of the L_1/L_2 inter-vertebral disc, although this is variable.

○ **At what level does the spinal cord end in a neonate?**

Anywhere from T_{12} to L_3, lower than the normal level in adults. During the first year of life, the spinal cord recedes to the L_1 adult level.

○ **What is the largest vertebral interspace?**

The largest interlaminal interspace of the vertebral column is the L_5/S_1 interspace.

○ **What is the Taylor approach to the subarachnoid space?**

Lumbosacral subarachnoid approach described by Taylor in 1940. The technique is a variation of the paramedian approach carried out at the L_5/S_1 interspace. The lowermost prominence of the posterosuperior iliac spine is identified and the skin entered 1cm medial and 1 cm caudad to this point. The needle is directed medially and cephalad to enter the subarachnoid space at L_5/S_1.

○ **Define density.**

The density of a substance is the ratio of its mass to its volume under specified conditions of pressure and temperature. The dimensions of density are weight per unit volume.

○ **Define specific gravity.**

Specific gravity is the ratio of the mass of a substance compared with a standard (mass of an equal volume of distilled water at 4 degrees Celsius or air or hydrogen) under prescribed conditions of temperature and pressure.

○ **Define baricity.**

Baricity is analogous to specific gravity, but the ratio is between the densities of local anesthetic solutions and cerebrospinal fluid (specific gravity 1.003-1.008 at 37 degrees Celsius). Baricity is a relevant term because it indicates how the solution will "behave" after subarachnoid injection.

○   **What is meant by the terms hyperbaric, hypobaric and isobaric?**

The density of CSF at 37 degrees C is 1.001-1.008 gm per ml. Local anesthetic solutions with densities (at 37 degrees C) greater than 1.008 are termed hyperbaric. Solutions with densities between 0.998 and 1.007 are considered to be isobaric. Solutions with densities less than 0.997 are termed hypobaric. Specific gravities of commonly used agents: bupivacaine 0.5% in 8.25% dextrose = 1.0278, in water = 1.0058; lidocaine 2% 1.0066; lidocaine 5% in 7.5% dextrose 1.0333.

○   **How does the baricity of a local anesthetic affect the level of anesthetic?**

An isobaric solution tends to remain in the immediate area of injection. It is not significantly affected by patient position. A hypobaric solution tends to move away from the dependent area in the CSF. A hypobaric solution is useful when administered in positions such as prone jackknife. A hyperbaric solution tends to move by gravity to a lower site and is useful for a saddle block.

○   **How is caudal anesthesia related to epidural anesthesia?**

Caudal anesthesia is a form of epidural anesthesia in which the injection is made at the sacral hiatus (S_5) through the sacrococcygeal ligament. Because the dural sac normally ends at S_2, accidental spinal injection is rare. Caudal anesthesia is primarily used in children for postoperative analgesia for hernia repair or urologic procedures.

○   **What is a postdural puncture headache (PDPH)?**

This is a headache thought to be from a persistent leak of spinal fluid through the dural puncture site. Depletion of CSF, which acts as a cushion for the spinal cord and brain, is believed to allow stretching of the supporting structures activating stretch-sensitive nociceptors. Pain may also result from distention of the blood vessels; which, because of the fixed volume of the skull, must compensate for the loss of CSF volume. The characteristic spinal headache occurs 6-12 hours after the spinal anesthetic has regressed, being worse in the upright posture.

○   **What is the classic presentation of a dural puncture headache?**

The defining feature of a dural puncture headache is a severe pounding headache that worsens as the head is elevated. The pain typically begins in the occipital area and spreads to the frontal area, and radiates to the neck and shoulders. Dizziness, nausea, vomiting, photophobia, diplopia, tinnitus, deafness and abducens nerve palsy are less common symptoms.

○   **What are the risk factors for a dural puncture headache?**

Risk factors for dural puncture headache include parturients, younger patients (less than 50 years of age), obese, women, use of needles with large-bore, cutting needles (Quincke or diamond point) rather than conical point (Greene, Whitacre, Sprotte) and multiple punctures. Inserting a needle with the bevel perpendicular to the longitudinal dural fibers, and glucose-containing local anesthetics can also increase the risk of spinal headache. Continuous spinals and timing of ambulation do not increase the incidence of PDPH.

○   **What is the incidence of dural puncture headache with a 24-gauge Sprotte needle?**

The 24-gauge Sprotte needle has been reported to cause a 0.02% incidence (or less than 1%) of dural puncture headache.

○   **When is a dural puncture headache most likely to occur?**

The headache may occur immediately after a dural puncture but usually occurs 24-48 hours later.

○   **Name three commonly accepted treatments for a postdural puncture headache.**

Infusion of epidural saline, intravenous or oral caffeine and epidural blood patch. Intravenous hydration has not been shown to be an effective treatment. Intravenous ACTH or cosyntropin (synthetic ACTH analogue) and sumatriptan have been reported to be efficacious.

○   **By what mechanism does caffeine relieve a dural puncture headache?**

Caffeine probably relieves the headache by reversing the reflex vasodilatation of cerebral vessels.

○   **How does epidural saline or blood patch relieve headache?**

Epidural blood patch or saline infusion either stops the transdural leak of CSF or re-establishes the normal CSF pressure.

○   **How effective is epidural saline for treatment of a dural puncture headache?**

Though proponents claim it is effective in up to 90% of patients, a high relapse rate limits the technique.

○   **When performing an epidural blood patch, what is an appropriate amount of blood to inject?**

Fifteen to 20 cc of the patient's own blood is injected into the epidural space at the same level as the original dural puncture until fullness is either felt at the needle or the patient reports symptoms such as fullness in the ears or pressure in the head.

○   **What is meant by the term 'multi-orifice' catheter?**

The distal end of the catheter can be either open (single port) or closed (multi-port). A closed tip catheter has three orifices at 1/2 cm intervals, starting 1/2 cm from the tip. The orifices are each orientated at 120° to the axis of the catheter in order to facilitate spread.

○   **What would you do if a catheter tip sheared off when placing an epidural catheter?**

Any attempt to withdraw a catheter through a needle with an angled bevel may produce shearing or complete transection of the plastic catheter. No direct harm usually results from this since the materials used are non-irritating and "tissue-implantable." The patient should be informed of the foreign body present, but surgical removal is usually not required.

○   **How does spinal curvature affect the level of spinal anesthesia?**

Anatomic configuration of the spinal column has a minor effect. Severe kyphosis or kyphoscoliosis, with a decreased volume of cerebrospinal fluid, can be associated with a higher than expected level of block using hypobaric techniques or rapid injection.

○   **What are the common side effects with neuraxial opioids?**

Respiratory depression, urinary retention, pruritus, nausea and vomiting. Early respiratory depression is associated with the highly soluble drugs e.g. fentanyl, whereas delayed respiratory depression (up to 24 hours) is associated with poorly soluble drugs e.g. morphine.

○   **What dose of fentanyl is commonly added to intrathecal injection?**

15 – 25 mcg is frequently used in combination with the shorter acting local anesthetics in the ambulatory surgey setting in order to extend the sensory block without increasing the duration of motor block or time to micturition.

○   **How much 1:1,000 epinephrine must be added to 20 ml of a local anesthetic solution to obtain a 1:200,000 concentration of epinephrine?**

A 1:1,000 solution contains 1,000 µg/ml of epinephrine. A 1:200,000 solution contains epinephrine 5 µg/ml. A 20 cc solution contains 100 µg or 0.1 cc of epinephrine 1:1,000.

○   **What is the dermatome level of the nipple?**

T_4.

○   **What is the dermatome level of the inguinal ligament?**

L_1.

○   **What is the dermatome level of the xiphoid?**

T_6.

○   **What are the dermatomes that supply to the knee?**

The anterior knee is supplied by the saphenous nerve, or L_{-1-4}. the posterior knee is supplied by the posterior tibial nerve, or L_{4-5}, S_{1-3}.

○   **What is the dermatome that supplies the umbilicus?**

T_{10}.

○   **What is the sacral hiatus?**

The sacral hiatus is due to non-fusion of the fifth sacral vertebral arch immediately cephalad to the coccyx and is covered by the sacrococcygeal ligament (an extension of the ligamentum flavum).

○   **What is the sacral cornu?**

The large bony processes on each side of the sacral hiatus.

○   **At what level does the dural sac (spinal dura mater) terminate?**

The dural sac usually terminates at the level of the second sacral vertebra, where the filum terminale blends with the periosteum on the coccyx.

○   **For what types of surgical procedures is caudal anesthesia used?**

Caudal blocks can be used for most of the indications recommended for lumbar block. However, there is often difficulty getting the local anesthetic to spread high enough, so the technique is usually reserved for procedures that require a blockade of the sacral nerves (cystoscopy or perineal surgery).

○   **What is the disadvantage of using commercially prepared solutions of local anesthetics with epinephrine added?**

Commercial preparations are more acidic (pH approximately 4.0) because epinephrine is rapidly inactivated in an alkaline solution. In such an acidic medium, very little local anesthetic is available in the unionized form for penetration of neural tissue; therefore, onset of analgesia is slower with commercial products.

○   **What are the factors that affect the level of anesthesia when performing a spinal anesthetic?**

Factors that are documented to have a major affect on the height of a spinal anesthetic block include; drug dosage, drug baricity and patient position. Factors probably unrelated include added vasoconstrictor, coughing or straining, barbotage, rate of injection (except hypobaric), needle bevel (except Whitacre needle), gender and weight.

○   **What recommendations should be made concerning the postoperative initiation of LMWH therapy in a patient who has had a neuraxial block technique?**

This is determined by the proposed LMWH regimen. For single daily dosing the first dose of LMWH may be given 6-8 hours postop, with the second dose withheld for a further 24 hours. For twice daily dosing regimens the first dose should be given no sooner than 24 hours postop. Any concomitant medications with effects upon hemostasis may increase the risk of spinal hematoma.

○   **Can LMWH be administered in the presence of an indwelling epidural catheter?**

Catheters can be used for postoperative analgesia during LMWH therapy. More specifically, the timing of the catheter removal represents the highest risk of spinal hematoma. For single daily dose regimens, the catheter should be removed a minimum of 10-12 hours after the preceding dose of LMWH and an interval of at least 2 hours before the subsequent dose of LMWH. For twice daily dose regimens, the catheter must be removed on postop day 1 prior to the start of LMWH, with at least 2 hours before the first dose of LMWH.

○   **Blood is seen in the needle during the difficult placement of an epidural catheter. What actions should be taken?**

Surgery should not be postponed by traumatic needle or catheter placement. There is an increased risk of spinal hematoma and LMWH therapy should be delayed for 24 hours.

○   **Where do epidural opioids principally act?**

Epidurally administered opioids must cross the dura and arachnoid mater through the CSF to the spinal cord to reach the opioid receptors in the dorsal horn.

○   **Do epidural opioids only act at the spinal cord?**

No. Depending on the physicochemical properties of the opioid, the amount reaching the spinal cord may be small and its effect may largely be due to systemic uptake and redistribution to the brain. Considerably more morphine than the more lipid soluble fentanyl reaches the spinal cord when administered epidurally.

○   **Is fentanyl the ideal epidural opioid?**

No. Investigators have shown that a continuous intravenous infusion of fentanyl produced the same quality of analgesia and side effects as compared to a similar dose of epidural fentanyl by continuous infusion.

○   **You are called to evaluate a patient 12 hours after a spinal anesthetic for a cesarean section. She is complaining of a non-positional headache. Is this a postdural puncture headache?**

Probably not. Postdural puncture headaches are characteristically positional in nature, worse when the patient is upright and improved when the patient is recumbent. In addition, spinal headaches usually occur 1-2 days after dural puncture. Patients typically complain of pain in the frontal and occipital regions.

❍   **In the recovery room, a patient has full motor and sensory recovery after spinal anesthesia. She is unable to void, and the surgeon is blaming the anesthetic. Could the surgeon be correct?**

Yes. Urinary retention has been described with longer acting local anesthetics and neuraxial narcotics. On emergence from spinal anesthesia, the bladder is last to regain function and urinary retention is not uncommon.

❍   **Why did the Sprotte needle design initially lead to many reports of "failed spinal anesthetics"?**

The Sprotte needle has an elliptical opening, much longer than any other spinal needle. The length of this opening could allow the hole to be only partially through the dura. During injection, it would be possible for some of the anesthetic to exit into the epidural space rather than the subarachnoid space. Also, dural puncture can be more difficult with a Sprotte needle compared to a sharper Quincke needle.

❍   **How does a spinal anesthetic cause bradycardia directly?**

The mechanism is multifactorial. Unopposed vagal tone from a high sympathectomy (T_{2-5}), blockade of the cardioaccelerator fibers (T_1 to T_4), and the Bezold-Jarisch reflex (slowing of the heart rate secondary to a drop in venous return). Other considerations include ancillary drug effects (fentanyl, remifentanil), vagal maneuvers (peritoneal traction, bladder distension, vaso-vagal reaction) and disease processes (hypoxia, myocardial ischemia, sinus node disease).

❍   **What factors are most influential in the distribution of a spinal anesthetic?**

The most significant is the amount or dose (not volume) of local anesthetic.

Other factors include: 1) baricity of the local anesthetic, 2) position of the patient in the first five minutes after injection of the spinal anesthetic (hypobaric solution rises: hyperbaric solution sinks with gravity), 3) patient factors (height, gender, intra-abdominal pressure and configuration of the lumbar spine), 4) type of needle, site of injection and direction of needle, 5) volume of CSF in the spinal canal (reduced with ascites or pregnancy).

❍   **Upon placing an interscalene block, the patient develops a high spinal. Explain.**

Subarachnoid injection can occur two different ways; 1) inadvertent needle placement into the spinal canal and 2) injection through the dural sheath which at the cervical level extends out the foramina to cover the nerve root.

❍   **If air or clear fluid is aspirated after needle insertion during a caudal block, should you proceed with the caudal block?**

No. Aspiration of air or fluid indicates improper needle placement. Aspiration of air may indicate entrance of the needle into the peritoneum. The "clear fluid" may be cerebrospinal fluid if the needle has advanced past the S_2 level.

❍   **Is ambulatory surgery a contraindication to use of a spinal anesthetic?**

Absolutely not. If appropriate local anesthetics are chosen based on the anticipated length of surgery, these patients can be discharged in a similar time course as those patients who have had a general anesthetic. In addition, regional anesthesia can result in less nausea and vomiting than general, resulting in shorter PACU stays.

❍   **Does the bevel direction of an epidural needle influence the catheter direction?**

No. There is no correlation between the two.

❍   **In performing a thoracic epidural in an anesthetized patient using the hanging drop technique, does it matter if the patient is under controlled or spontaneous ventilation?**

Yes. The hanging drop technique depends on the negative pressure of the epidural space to "suck " in the drop once the epidural space has been entered. This pressure is increased with controlled ventilation. The safest approach would be to place the epidural catheter in an awake patient.

❍   **Four hours after your last dose of 2% lidocaine into a lumbar epidural catheter, your patient is in the recovery room with full motor and sensory blockade. She has no discomfort. What should you do?**

Inform the surgeon and order a STAT MRI of the thoracolumbar spine (upper cuts must correspond to spine segments above the catheter tip).

2% lidocaine (plain) has an expected duration of sensory and motor block of 60 to 90 minutes.   The sensory block can be augmented by the addition of epidural opioids. Addition of epinephrine to 2% lidocaine will prolong the anesthetic effect. The diagnosis of epidural hematoma is extremely rare, but in the presence of leg weakness should be excluded as this represents a neurosurgical emergency.

❍   **Five minutes after starting an "easy" labor epidural, the patient has complete pain relief with no motor block, but a sensory level on the left-side at T_1 and right-side at T_{10}. What is your diagnosis?**

Subdural catheter placement.

This diagnosis presents with a very rapid onset of pain relief and an unusually variable presentation of sensory block. An inadvertent subarachnoid (spinal) injection would also present with rapid pain relief, but the patient would have motor blockade and little discrepancy in sensory levels between sides. The catheter should be removed and certainly never be used in the event of an emergency cesarean section.

❍   **After using 3% 2-chloroprocaine for your epidural anesthetic, the surgeon requests epidural duramorph. What is your response?**

Duramorph has been shown to be ineffective after the use of epidural 3% 2-chloroprocaine. In addition, one of 2-chloroprocaine's metabolites, 4-amino-2-chloroprocaine, may impair the action of bupivacaine if used concurrently.

❍   **How far should an epidural catheter be advanced into the epidural space?**

Approximately 2 to 5 cm. If you advance the catheter greater than 6 cm the catheter tip is likely to exit the central axis via a neural foramina. Placement at 4-5 cm has been shown to be most efficacious

❍   **You use 5 cc of normal saline in a "loss of resistance" technique to identify the epidural space. You remove the trocar and several drops of fluid run out. Is this CSF?**

Probably not. A 17 gauge needle which penetrates the dura usually runs like a faucet. To be certain, you can check the temperature (warm if it is CSF) and glucose content (positive test with a urine dip stick).

❍   **How much does a spinal anesthetic affect the glomerular filtration rate?**

A spinal anesthetic to at least the T_{11} level will reduce the glomerular filtration rate proportionally to decreases in arterial pressure due to its effects on autoregulation.

❍   **If a patient has a spinal anesthetic to the C_8-T_1 level, how much will this block affect her inspiratory capacity?**

It will be decreased by as much as 20%.

○   **What spinal level is most dependent in the supine position? What is its significance?**

The T_4-T_6 level is most dependent in the supine position. Following placement of a hyperbaric spinal, when the patient is repositioned supine, the anesthetic will flow cephalad and may produce a T_4-T_6 level. The associated sympathetic block (2 levels above sensory) may affect the cardiac accelerators (T_1-T_4) and intercostal muscle function.

○   **Does the baricity of a spinal anesthetic impact its duration of action?**

Yes. An isobaric solution has a clinically longer duration of action than a hyperbaric or hypobaric spinal solution. The limited spread of the local anesthetic with an isobaric solution produces a higher concentration in the CSF and thus increases the time until the minimally effective concentration is reached.

○   **Hypotension frequently follows placement of a subarachnoid block. What is the etiology and treatment?**

Decreased vascular resistance and diminished cardiac output.

Hypotension may be ameliorated by prior administration of intravenous fluids and is treated with volume expansion or sympathomimetic agents (ephedrine, phenylephrine and/or atropine).

Factors that increase the incidence and severity of hypotension include:
- Hypovolemia
- Sensory level greater than T_4
- Baseline systolic blood pressure less than 120 mm Hg
- Level of needle insertion at or above L_{2-3}
- Addition of epinephrine to the local anesthetic solution
- Use of a combined spinal-general anesthesia technique

RESPIRATORY PHYSIOLOGY AND ANESTHESIA

To Laugh Often And Much: To Win The Respect Of Intelligent People And The Affection Of Children, To Earn The Appreciation Of Honest Critics And Endure The Betrayal Of False Friends; To Appreciate Beauty, To Find The Best In Others, To Leave The World A Bit Better Whether By A Healthy Child, A Garden Patch, Or Redeemed Social Condition; To Know Even One Life Has Breathed Easier Because You Have Lived. This Is To Have Succeeded.
Ralph Waldo Emerson

○ **What constitutes anatomic dead space?**

Volume of the regions of the airway that histologically cannot participate in gas exchange: upper airways (oral cavity, nasopharynx, larynx), cartilagenous airways (trachea, bronchi, membranous bronchioles). Can be calculated from the single breath nitrogen washout test (Fowler's method). Approximately 2 ml/kg, ideal body weight.

○ **What is the relationship between asthma and PEEP?**

Patients with bronchospasm can develop intrinsic auto-PEEP due to incomplete expiration. Addition of extrinsic PEEP may exacerbate this effect with resultant hemodynamic compromise and no improvement in respiratory function.

○ **How do you treat intraoperative bronchospasm due to asthma?**

Bronchodilation with beta 2 agonists (i.e.: albuterol), anticholinergics (i.e. ipratropium), deepen the level of anesthesia with propofol and/or inhaled agents, and initiate steroids (i.e. methylprednisolone; antiinflammatory with no immediate effect). Consider ketamine, intravenous epinephrine, theophylline/aminophylline, and intravenous magnesium (smooth muscle relaxation).

○ **What causes an increase in dead space?**

Increase in anatomic deadspace: neck extension, anticholinergic drugs.

Increase in alveolar dead space (West zone 1) due to decreased perfusion: upright position, positive pressure ventilation, PEEP, hypotension, low cardiac output, pulmonary embolism.

Increase in V/Q mismatch: ARDS, general anesthesia and age, emphysema, COPD, pulmonary fibrosis, smoking, increased gas density.

○ **Is there a change in the CO diffusing capacity in patients with COPD?**

Yes, it is decreased in proportion to the severity of the emphysema and is the best functional predictor for the severity of the disease. However, it is not a sensitive test for young smokers or mild emphysema.

○ **What are the components of functional residual capacity?**

Expiratory volume, ERV, RV, (equal to the lung volume at end of normal exhalation).

○   **What conditions extend the volume of Zone 1 of the pulmonary circulation?**

Decreased perfusion: upright position, hypotension, low cardiac output, pulmonary embolism.

Increased alveolar pressure: positive pressure ventilation, PEEP.

Decreased vasculature: age, emphysema, COPD, pulmonary fibrosis, smoking.

○   **How do you diagnose intrathoracic airway obstruction?**

Utilizing direct bronchoscopy, radiographic imaging, CT, flow volume loops, and pulmonary function tests.

○   **What is the definition for hypoventilation?**

Reduced alveolar ventilation resulting in an increase in arterial PCO_2.

○   **What is diffusion hypoxia and how do you prevent it?**

Hypoxemia seen on recovery from general anesthesia due to the outpouring of large volumes of (very soluble) nitrous oxide into the alveoli, thereby displacing alveolar oxygen and diluting alveolar and arterial carbon dioxide and decreasing respiratory drive. Prevented by high inspired fractions of oxygen and adequate ventilation during the postoperative washout period.

○   **What are the effects of PEEP?**

Pulmonary effects: improved oxygenation through redistribution of extravascular water and increased FRC through distention and recruitment of alveoli, and decreased shunt. *Cardiovascular effects*: diminished cardiac output due to decreased venous return to right heart, right ventricular dysfunction, and alterations in left ventricular distensibility.

○   **What are the effects of smoking cessation on respiratory complications after anesthesia?**

Postoperative pulmonary complications are four fold more common in current smokers versus never smokers. A two month smoke free interval reduces the risk to that of non smokers. Reduction in smoking or cessation less than two months prior to surgery is associated with a seven fold higher risk versus no reduction. The beneficial effects of smoking cessation such as a decrease in airway secretions and reactivity take 2-4 weeks to manifest. The short term cessation (48-72 hours) increases secretions and causes hyperactive airways, but the major benefit appears to be the decrease in carboxyhemoglobin content and better oxygen availability to the tissues.

○   **What is the etiology of hypoxemia?**

- Low mixed venous PO_2 (increased oxygen consumption, low cardiac output)
- Decreased alveolar PO_2 (high altitude, low FiO_2, high partial pressure of alternate gas, hypoventilation)
- Increased (A-a) O_2 gradient (cardiac shunt, pulmonary shunt, V/Q mismatch, diffusion limitations)
- Decreased oxygen carrying capacity (low or abnormal hemoglobin, carbon monoxide toxicity)

○   **What is a flow-volume loop and how do you interpret the information?**

Most helpful in the anatomical localization of airway obstruction. Lung volume is plotted on the x axis, expiratory (above) and inspiratory flow (below) is plotted on the y axis as the subject inhales fully to total lung capacity (negative flow), performs an FVC maneuver (positive flow) and then inhales back to TLC. The curves are highly effort dependent. A fixed obstruction decreases inspiratory and expiratory flow creating a plateau effect; a variable extrathoracic obstruction above the sternal notch decreases flow which flattens the inspiratory loop; a variable intrathoracic obstruction decreases flow and flattens the expiratory loop.

O   **What are the normal values for PaO_2 in newborns?**

Neonatal PaO_2 50 -70 mmHg, as a result of an (A-a) O_2 gradient mostly due to shunting.

O   **What information is obtained from spirometry?**

A spirogram illustrates expiration of a vital capacity breath recorded over 4 or 5 seconds. The most clinically useful measurements are: forced vital capacity (FVC), forced expiratory volume in one sec (FEV_1), and flow between 25% and 75% of the FVC ($MMMF_{25-75}$). Calculation of the FEV_1/FVC ratio is an indicator of the severity of obstructive airway disease. Spirometry does not provide information about lung volumes and capacitites or indicate the cause of airway obstruction.

O   **How does postobstructive pulmonary edema (POPE) occur and how is it treated?**

There are two recognized types of POPE. Type I may be associated with any cause of acute airway obstruction (ie: postextubation laryngospasm) and type II develops after surgical relief of chronic upper airway obstruction in patients otherwise not at risk for pulmonary edema (ie: post-tonsillectomy/adenoidectomy). The pathogenesis of POPE I is multifactorial. High negative intrathoracic pressure generated by forceful inspiratory attempts against an airway obstruction are transmitted to the lung interstitium, creating decreased perimicrovascular hydrostatic pressure, which effectively sucks fluid into the lungs. Venous return is increased, cardiac output is decreased and fluid transudates into the alveolar spaces. POPE II results from sudden removal of PEEP produced by the obstructing lesion which leads to interstitial fluid transudation and pulmonary edema. POPE generally resolves with release of the obstruction, but may require supplemental oxygen, intubation and low levels of PEEP, positive pressure ventilation, and diuresis.

O   **Is arterial oxygenation age dependent?**

Yes. The transition from fetal circulation leads to a decrease in shunt with a PaO_2 of 50-70 mmHg in the newborn. In infants the alveolar-arterial oxygen gradient is slightly larger than the 5-6 mmHg measured in adolescents; it increases with age up to 30 mmHg, likely due to an increase in closing capacity.
$PaO_2 \approx 102 - 0.3$ age.
A-a gradient = 0.21 (age + 2.5)

O   **What is the effect of PEEP on arterial PO_2?**

Improves arterial PO_2 through alveolar distention, alveolar recruitment, redistribution of extravascular lung water.

O   **What is optimal PEEP in ARDS?**

PEEP level that provides maximum oxygen delivery and lowest dead space ventilation. Clinically this is the PEEP level that will result in adequate perfusion and a PaO_2 of 60 mmHg or greater, with an adequate hemoglobin level at an FiO_2 of less than 50%.

O   **How can pulmonary function testing distinguish between obstructive disease states?**

Decreased FEV_1 for upper airways obstruction, decreased FEV 25-75% for midsize airways obstruction (effort independent), response with and without bronchodilators for distinguishing between reactive airways disease (ie asthma) and structural airways disease (i.e., emphysema).

O   **What are the findings of pulmonary function tests in restrictive vs obstructive lung disease?**

A reduction in vital capacity to less than 80% predicted is indicative of restrictive lung disease. A reduction in

FEV_1/FVC to less than 70% indicates mild, less than 60% moderate, and less than 50% severe obstructive disease.

○   **Calculate physiologic dead space ventilation.**

Can be derived from Bohr's equation:
total volume of expired gas = volume of alveolar gas + volume of dead space

$$V_D = (PaCO_2 - P_ECO_2) \, V_E \, / \, PaCO_2$$

Where P_ECO_2 is mixed expired CO_2 tension and assuming alveolar CO_2 partial pressure is equal to arterial CO_2 partial pressure. Physiologic dead space ventilation includes anatomic and alveolar deadspace ventilation.

○   **What is the status of PaO_2 and $PaCO_2$ when V_A/Q is 0.01?**

As V/Q ratio decreases (increased right-to-left shunting), PaO_2 decreases rapidly and progressively. $PaCO_2$ increases gradually at first and then quite rapidly.

○   **What are the distinguishing features of pressure support ventilation?**

Augments every breath during spontaneous breathing. Practically, a breath is initiated by the patient's respiratory effort and supported with rapid flow until a preset pressure is reached. Inspiration then ceases and the exhalation valve is opened allowing expiration. Advantages over intermittent mandatory ventilation (IMV) include increased tidal volume and decreased work of breathing. Methods of setting pressure include: (a) maximum inspiratory pressure (pressure = maximum inspiratory pressure / 3) and (b) proximal airway pressure (pressure = peak pressure – plateau pressure).

○   **Is there a role for intravenous epinephrine in severe bronchospasm?**

Yes.

○   **List causes and effects of surfactant deficiency.**

Pulmonary surfactant deficiency can result from destruction of type II pneumatocytes or from the destruction or inactivation of surfactant. Genetic deficiencies have been described. Surfactant lines the alveolus to provide a host defense barrier and reduces alveolar surface tension preventing collapse (adhesive atelectasis). Deficiency produces diffuse loss of lung volume, shunt, and the influx of interstitial fluid resulting in impaired gas exchange. ARDS, hyaline membrane disease, pneumonia, interstitial lung diseases, alveolar proteinosis, obstructive lung disease, smoke inhalation, coronary artery bypass graft surgery, uremia and prolonged shallow breathing are conditions which frequently produce generalized surfactant deficiency. Pulmonary embolism and radiation pneumonitis have a similar effect localized to the affected segment of lung.

○   **How is tidal volume determined on a ventilator?**

By the ventilator mode: in volume preset modes the tidal volume is selected, in pressure preset modes the set pressure limit determines the end of each inspiration and tidal volume.

○   **What are the effects of increased V/Q mismatch?**

Increased dead space ventilation, increased shunt fraction. Thus, arterial hypoxemia, and increased carbon dioxide levels, even though this is compensated for to a large extent by hyperventilation. Also, change in the rate of uptake of anesthetic gases with the effect depending on the mismatch and solubility of the agent.

○   **Which factors affect the VD/VT ratio?**

Position, age, pulmonary disease, perfusion abnormalities, anticholinergic drugs, general anesthesia, ventilation parameters.

○ **What is the best ventilation strategy for asthmatics?**

Providing adequate expiratory time to avoid incomplete exhalation and auto-PEEP: low respiratory rate, low I:E ratio. Permissive hypercapnia.

○ **List differential diagnosis for wheezing during anesthesia.**

The machine, the endotracheal tube or the patient.

Examples: endobronchial intubation, pulmonary embolism, bronchospasm, pulmonary edema, mucus secretions, cuff herniation, bronchial flow disturbance by tumor, infection, swelling, foreign body aspiration, pneumothorax, chest tube.

○ **Which conditions activate HPV (hypoxic pulmonary vasoconstriction)?**

Alveolar PO_2 less than 100 mmHg, maximal response at PO_2 30 mmHg. Elevations in arterial hydrogen ion concentration or alveolar PCO_2 may augment pulmonary vasoconstriction.

○ **Which conditions inhibit HPV?**

Inhaled anesthetic agents including nitrous oxide, direct vasodilating drugs (NTG, SNP, isoproterenol), and hypocapnia directly decrease HPV. Conditions that increase pulmonary arterial pressure will decrease HPV: mitral stenosis, volume overload, a progressive increase in the amount of diseased lung, thromboembolism, hypothermia, vasoactive drugs. Selective application of PEEP to nondiseased lung can divert flow back to diseased lung.

○ **What are your options for improving oxygenation during one lung ventilation?**

Ensuring adequate minute ventilation, clearing secretions from airways, avoiding malposition of double lumen tube, increasing FiO_2, applying selective CPAP to non dependent lung, increasing PEEP to dependent lung, clamping pulmonary arterial blood flow to non dependent lung, intermittent two lung ventilation.

○ **Which pharmacologic agents worsen hypoxemia?**

Agents that decrease ventilation, increase pulmonary shunt, inhibit HPV, inhibit oxygenation of hemoglobin by causing methemoglobinemia, increase oxygen consumption. Examples: opiates, hypnotics, neuromuscular blocking agents, nitrates, nitroglycerin, sodium nitroprusside, inhaled anesthetic agents, prilocaine, antimalarials, sulfonamides, catecholamines.

○ **List signs of intraoperative pulmonary embolism.**

Increased pulmonary arterial pressure, increased central venous pressure, right ventricular strain, decreased cardiac output with decreased PCWP and decreased end-tidal PCO_2, increased arterial PCO_2 due to hypoventilation (increased dead space), hypoxemia, pulmonary edema and bronchoconstriction with wheezing. Signs may be subtle or can present with cardiocirculatory collapse depending on size and location of pulmonary embolus.

○ **List signs of intraoperative asthma.**

Wheezing, prolonged exhalation, incomplete exhalation with developing auto-PEEP, upward slope on the end tidal CO_2 trace, hypotension due to decreased venous return with increasing intrathoracic gas volume, and hypoventilation. Changes in arterial blood gases: progressive hypoxemia, initial normocarbia then respiratory alkalosis deteriorating to respiratory acidosis.

O   **What is the etiology of the alveolar to end-tidal PCO_2 gradient?**

Mixing of exhaled gases from the physiologic deadspace with gases from the alveoli causes a dilution of alveolar (equal to arterial) PCO_2. The alveolar fraction of CO_2 is exhaled last and represented in peak end tidal CO_2 with complete exhalation. With incomplete exhalation alveolar CO_2 is not represented on the expiratory CO_2 trace.

O   **List causes of increased end-tidal to arterial PCO_2 gradient.**

Usually, $ETCO_2$ is less than arterial PCO_2 due to increased alveolar to arterial gradient and/or increased end-tidal to alveolar gradient. Pulmonary hypoperfusion due to hypotension, pulmonary (air) embolus, low cardiac output, hypoventilation, sampling error due to esophageal intubation, circuit disconnection, kinked endotracheal tube, or airleak around endotracheal tube. During heavy exercise $ETCO_2$ can overestimate arterial PCO_2.

O   **List causes of increased end-tidal to alveolar PCO_2 gradient.**

$ETCO_2$ less than alveolar PCO_2 is caused by increased deadspace fraction, incomplete exhalation with $ETCO_2$ not representative of alveolar PCO_2, leakage of alveolar gas prior to sampling site (ETT leak, obstruction, circuit disconnect), artifact through high sampling rate of sidestream capnograph in the face of elevated fresh gas flow.

O   **List causes of increased alveolar to arterial PCO_2 gradient.**

Arterial PCO_2 greater than alveolar PCO_2 is caused by unventilated areas of perfused lung (e.g. atelectasis, infection) with high regional arterial PCO_2 and low alveolar PCO_2. Increased alveolar PO_2 in hypoxic patients will shift the CO_2 dissociation curve (Haldane effect) contributing to the rise of arterial PCO_2.

O   **What is the distribution of pulmonary blood flow in the upright lung?**

Pulmonary blood flow is distributed according to gravity with the lowest flow in the apical aspects of the lung and maximal flow in the basilar regions.

O   **What are the effects of gravity on respiratory physiology?**

Pulmonary blood flow is gravity dependent, leading to the definition of West Zones I, II, and III. Pulmonary ventilation is higher in the dependent alveoli in an awake spontaneously breathing person because the basal alveoli are in the steeper portion of the compliance curve of the alveoli due to the increase in pleural pressure. Due to increase in pleural pressure, basal alveoli are ¼ volume of the apical alveoli and therefore more compliant. Apical alveoli are maximally inflated and relatively noncompliant.
The V/Q ratio decreases rapidly at first then more slowly into the dependent lung regions.

O   **What distinguishes the basilar regions of the lungs?**

Highest rate of perfusion, least distended alveoli at end-expiration, majority of tidal volume generation, lowest V/Q ratio, regional hypoxemia and hypercarbia.

O   **List compensatory mechanisms for respiratory acidosis.**

Augmented ventilatory drive occurs via feedback to the brain and the medullary respiratory control center, mediated by central and carotid body chemoreceptors. Metabolic buffering through decreased hepatic HCO_3 uptake and shift of HCO_3 from red blood cells to plasma, carbonate release from bone, decreased urea and lactic acid production (which utilizes HCO_3). Acutely HCO_3 increases 0.8 mmol/l for each 10 mmHg of CO_2 greater than 40. Longterm increase in $PaCO_2$ induces renal compensation with decreased chloride and phosphate reabsorption, increased HCO_3 reabsorption and increased H^+ secretion. Chronically, HCO_3

increases 5 mmol/l for each 10 mmHg of $PaCO_2$ greater than 40.

○ **What causes a decrease in end-tidal CO_2?**

Hyperventilation, decrease in CO_2 production (e.g. hypothermia), decrease in alveolar CO_2 due to higher fraction of second alveolar gas (increased alveolar nitrous oxide or oxygen), pulmonary hypoperfusion due to hypotension, pulmonary (air) embolus, low cardiac output, cardiac arrest, sampling error, esophageal intubation, circuit disconnection, kinked endotracheal tube, or air leak around endotracheal tube.

○ **What is the difference in work of breathing for infants vs adults?**

The work of breathing is increased for infants due to reduced lung compliance and increased airway resistance. The components of work of breathing include: elastic work (lung elastic recoil, chest wall compliance), frictional work (air-flow resistance) and inertial work (tissue frictional resistance which is negligible in healthy subjects).

○ **What are the effects of respiration on blood pressure readings?**

Most noticeable in central venous pressure tracings: with positive pressure ventilation, during inspiration intrathoracic pressure increases resulting in an increase in central venous pressure reading; with spontaneous negative pressure breathing, intrathoracic pressure decreases during inspiration with a concurrent decrease in the CVP pressure tracing. CVP pressure readings are routinely obtained at end-expiration.

○ **What are causes of atelectasis?**

Obstruction of major airways and bronchioles (secretions or tumor), compression of the lung from fluid or air in the pleural space, infection, surfactant deficiency (adhesive atelectasis), high alveolar PO_2 (absorption atelectasis), or hypoventilation especially in areas with low V/Q.

○ **What are the physiologic effects of hypoxemia/hypoxia?**

Cardiovascular effects: catecholamine and renin-angiotensin release cause excitatory and vasoconstrictive effects mediated via aortic and carotid chemoreceptor, baroreceptor and central cerebral stimulation. Direct local hypoxemic effects are inhibitory and vasodilatory and occur late. The response depends on the degree of hypoxemia: $SaO_2 > 80\%$: increased heart rate, stroke volume, cardiac output, inotropy. SaO_2 60-80%: decrease in blood pressure and SVR with vasodilation. $SaO_2 < 60\%$: slow pulse, low blood pressure, shock, cardiac dysrhythmia. Also: increased cerebral blood flow due to cerebral vasodilation, increased ventilatory drive, increased pulmonary artery pressure, increased hemoglobin in chronic hypoxemia with right shifted oxyhemoglobin dissociation curve.

ENDOCRINE

Estimated Amount Of Glucose Used By An Adult Human Brain Each Day, Expressed In M & Ms: 250
Harper's Index, October 1989

○ **What happens to serum concentrations of ADH and aldosterone after surgery?**

ADH, aldosterone, renin and angiotensin increase resulting in sodium and water retention and a secondary expansion of the extracellular space.

○ **Where is aldosterone produced and what is its stimulus for secretion?**

Aldosterone is a mineralocorticoid secreted from the zona glomerulosa of the adrenal gland. Its secretion is stimulated by pituitary ACTH, angiotensin II (renin-angiotensin system) and increased serum potassium concentration. Hypovolemia, hypotension, congestive heart failure and surgery also increase aldosterone levels.

○ **Where does aldosterone exert is primary effect and what is this effect?**

Aldosterone secretion enhances sodium reabsorption in the distal nephron of the kidney in exchange for potassium and hydrogen ions. The net effect is fluid retention and expansion of the extracellular fluid space, with a reduction in serum potassium concentration and metabolic alkalosis.

○ **What are the effects of alpha and beta adrenergic stimulation on insulin and glucagon secretion?**

Beta islet cells (insulin secreting) have both alpha and beta adrenergic receptors. The stimulation of the alpha-receptors inhibits insulin secretion while stimulation of the beta-receptors increases insulin release. The alpha islet cells (glucagon secreting) only have beta-receptors which lead to an increase in glucagon release when stimulated.

○ **What are the precursors of epinephrine?**

Epinephrine is produced by the conversion of phenylalanine (phenylalanine hydroxylase) to tyrosine, tyrosine (tyrosine hydroxylase) to DOPA, DOPA (DOPA decarboxylase) to dopamine, dopamine (dopamine β-hydroxylase) to norepinephrine, and finally norepinephrine (phenylethanolamine-N-methyltransferase) to epinephrine.

○ **What enzymes and organs are involved in the production of angiotensin II from its precursors?**

Renin (from kidneys) converts angiotensinogen (from liver) to angiotensin I. Angiotensin I is then rapidly converted, primarily in the lungs, by angiotensin-converting enzyme to angiotensin II. Kidney, liver and lungs are involved.

○ **Which has a more potent effect during stress, angiotensin I or II and what are these effects?**

Angiotensin II; a potent direct vasoconstrictor, potentiates the actions of norepinephrine and increases the secretion of aldosterone, while directly increasing sodium reabsorption in the proximal renal tubules.

○ **What are the signs/symptoms of hypothyroidism?**

The signs and symptoms of hypothyroidism are nonspecific and difficult to diagnose. These include: fatigue, decreased mental acuity, depression, somnolence, cold intolerance, constipation, dry skin, brittle hair, menorrhagia, and weight gain. Physical exam reveals hypothermia, periorbital edema, decreased or absent deep tendon reflexes, sinus bradycardia, and hoarseness. Myxedema coma is characterized by hypoventilation, hypothermia, hypotension, congestive heart failure, hyponatremia, hypoglycemia, obtundation and adrenal insufficiency. This condition is frequently fatal and often seen in patients with severe long-standing unrecognized hypothyroidism who are subjected to cold exposure, surgery, trauma, infection or antidepressants.

○   **What happens to the cardiac output in hypothyroidism?**

Cardiac output is decreased due to a reduction in heart rate and stroke volume. In addition, decreased blood volume, baroreceptor reflex dysfunction and pericardial effusion make the patient susceptible to the cardiodepressant effects of anesthetic agents.

○   **What laboratory findings (excluding abnormal thyroid function tests) are characteristic in hypothyroidism?**

Hyponatremia, hypoglycemia, hypercholesterolemia and a normochromic normocytic anemia. Chest x-ray may show an enlarged heart secondary to pericardial effusion and the EKG characteristically shows sinus bradycardia, low voltage and a prolonged QT interval.

○   **How would you treat refractory hypotension in myxedema coma?**

IV thyroid supplement (T_3 or T_4) and steroid replacement (hydrocortisone 100 mg IV q8 h) should be given until the hypothalamic-pituitary-adrenal axis can be evaluated.

○   **What are the signs/symptoms of hyperthyroidism?**

Signs include: goiter, tachycardia, proptosis, alopecia, pretibial myxedema, arrhythmias, mitral valve prolapse, congestive heart failure and unexplained atrial fibrillation in patients over 60 years of age. Common symptoms include: anxiety, fine tremors, insomnia, diarrhea, emotional lability, pruritis, heat intolerance, fatigue, weight loss and proximal muscle weakness.

○   **What are the hemodynamics of thyroid storm?**

Extreme tachycardia with a high cardiac output, tachyarrhythmias, peripheral vasodilatation and possibly profound hypotension.

○   **What are the ocular signs in hyperthyroidism?**

Exophthalmos from an infiltrative process involving the retrobulbar fat and eyelids, lid sag, lid retraction and periorbital swelling. The extraocular muscles, cornea and optic nerve are also involved.

○   **What are the associated laboratory findings in hyperthyroidism?**

Hypercalcemia, hypokalemia, hyperglycemia, hypocholesterolemia, mild anemia, thrombocytopenia, lymphocytosis, granulocytopenia, hyperbilirubinemia and increased alkaline phosphatase.

○   **What is the differential diagnosis of thyroid storm?**

Symptoms usually present 6 to 18 hours following surgery and include: hyperthermia, tachycardia, congestive heart failure, dehydration, hyperglycemia, change in level of consciousness, shock and death.

Differential diagnosis includes: sepsis, pheochromocytoma, cocaine/amphetamine overdose, a neuroleptic malignant syndrome in those receiving antipsychotic medications and malignant hyperthermia.

○ **What is the initial treatment of thyroid storm?**

First, treat life-threatening changes in vital signs. Then, make the diagnosis, correct precipitating causes and treat high circulating levels of thyroid hormone and resulting effects with β-blockers (maintain heart rate < 90 beats/min), IV fluids for volume replacement, cooling and acetaminophen (antipyretic), and antithyroid drugs: propylthiouracil via nasogastric tube (PTU 600 to 1000 mg, followed by 200 to 400 mg q 8 hourly), followed one hour later by an iodide preparation.

Hydrocortisone (100 to 200 mg q 8 hourly) has been reported to increase survival. The duration of storm averages 3 days. Supportive therapy may be needed for fever, tachycardia, hypotension, volume depletion, hyperglycemia and altered consciousness.

○ **What are the CNS manifestations of myxedema?**

Depression, memory loss, ataxia, frank psychosis and ultimately coma.

○ **What is the mechanism of hyponatremia in hypothyroidism?**

Although previously thought to be secondary to SIADH, it is currently thought to be a function of impaired water excretion related to decreased delivery of sodium and volume to the distal renal tubules as a result of decreased renal blood flow.

○ **Describe the pulse pressure in thyrotoxicosis.**

Widened, reflecting increased flow and vasodilation.

○ **How is thyroid storm different from thyrotoxicosis?**

Thyroid storm is a severe and life-threatening exacerbation of thyrotoxicosis usually precipitated by a non-thyroidal illness such as an infection, surgery, withdrawal of iodine therapy, diabetic ketoacidosis, vigorous palpation of the thyroid gland, radioactive iodine therapy.

○ **Are thyroid function tests necessary prior to the initiation of treatment for thyroid storm?**

No. This is a medical emergency that requires immediate and aggressive management. Presumptive diagnosis is made on the basis of history and clinical findings.

○ **What is the percentage of cortisol that is not protein bound?**

5-10%.

○ **Primary adrenal insufficiency refers to disruption of which component of the hypothalamic-pituitary-adrenal axis?**

Adrenal gland.

○ **Secretion of which adrenal hormone is not impaired by secondary adrenal insufficiency?**

Aldosterone.

Secondary adrenal insufficiency is caused by inadequate ACTH secretion by the anterior pituitary. The adrenal cortex produces cortisol and aldosterone. Aldosterone secretion is regulated by the renin-angiotensin system (angiotensin II).

○ **What is the characteristic hemodynamic pattern of adrenal insufficiency?**

Refractory hypotension due to decreased systemic vascular resistance and to a lesser degree, decreased cardiac contractility, hypovolemia and electrolyte disturbances.

O   **Which sedating agent used for prolonged periods has been shown to increase mortality in critically ill patients by inducing primary adrenal insufficiency?**

Etomidate.

In induction doses, etomidate is a selective inhibitor of adrenal 11β-hydroxylase, the enzyme that converts deoxycortisol to cortisol. Mortality rates may be increased when etomidate is used as a long-term continuous infusion for sedation in mechanically ventilated critically ill patients.

O   **Is there any evidence to support the use of corticosteroids in septic shock?**

No.

Only animal studies have shown improved survival with steroid treatment in sepsis. Human trials have shown no overall benefit, with a higher mortality rate in patients with renal insufficiency.

O   **In which disease states have randomized prospective trials shown improved outcome with the use of corticosteroids?**

Bacterial meningitis, acute spinal injury, typhoid fever, pneumocystis carinii pneumonia and possibly, treatment of the fibroproliferative phase of acute respiratory distress syndrome.

O   **How much cortisol is produced per day in patients undergoing minor and major surgery?**

The adrenal cortex normally produces 20 to 30 mg of cortisol per day. The amount increases in response to minor stress (50 mg) and major stress (75-100 mg). Production rates of cortisol seldom exceed 200-300 mg/day. Current dosing recommendations for supplemental corticosteroids in patients with suspected adrenal insufficiency are:

Minor stress   25 mg hydrocortisone
Moderate stress   50-75 mg/day or 25 mg intraoperatively, followed by IV infusion 100 mg over 24 hours
Major stress   100-150 mg/day or 200 to 300 mg/70kg in divided doses/day

O   **Should all individuals with chronic unexplained alveolar hypoventilation be tested for hypothyroidism?**

Yes.

O   **Is obstructive sleep apnea common in hypothyroidism?**

Yes. Both conditions have decreased ventilatory response to increased CO_2 and decreased O_2 with some degree of baseline hypoventilation. Contributing factors in the hypothyroid patient include obesity, enlarged tongue causing intermittent upper airway obstruction and myopathy.

O   **What other endocrine disorder is associated with an increased frequency of sleep apnea?**

Acromegaly. Sleep apnea may be central or obstructive in origin.

O   **What type of malignancies are commonly associated with hypercalcemia?**

Breast cancer is the most common cause. Others include lung cancer, squamous cell carcinomas of the head, neck and esophagus, gynecologic tumors, renal cell carcinoma and multiple myeloma. The secretion of humoral mediators by solid tumors (PTH-like substances, cytokines or prostaglandins) may produce hypercalcemia through increased bone osteoclastic activity, even without bony metastases.

O   **What are the pulmonary manifestations of polycythemia?**

Pulmonary embolism related to hyperviscosity of blood and intravascular thrombosis and pulmonary hemorrhage associated with an increased bleeding tendency. This rarely occurs at hemoglobins less than 18 gm/dl, and is probably more important in primary versus secondary polycythemia.

O   **What are the two types of diabetes insipidus (DI)?**

Central (insufficient ADH secreted by the anterior pituitary) and nephrogrenic DI (renal tubules do not respond to ADH).

Urine is dilute despite high serum osmolarity. Central DI may result from head injury, or diseases or surgery to the pituitary. Nephrogenic DI can result from electrolyte abnormalities, illnesses such as sickle cell anemia, myeloma, renal insufficiency or uropathy, or drugs such as lithium. While both types of DI are treated with fluid resuscitation (usually with normal saline), only central DI is treated with DDAVP.

O   **How is the syndrome of inappropriate ADH secretion (SIADH) diagnosed?**

ADH (also known as vasopressin) is stored in the posterior pituitary and regulates plasma osmolarity. SIADH occurs when ADH continues to be secreted despite hyponatremia. The diagnosis is made on the basis of the urine being inappropriately concentrated (plasma osmolality < 280 mOsm/kg, urine osmolality > 100 mOsm/kg, urine sodium >20 mEq with serum sodium <130 mEq/L) with the patient adequately volume replaced and no evidence of renal, cardiac, liver, adrenal of thyroid dysfunction.

O   **How is hyponatremia treated?**

Water restriction is the first treatment of hyponatremia, with sodium-containing fluids used if sodium is <120 mEq/L. Correction of sodium > 0.5 meq/hour may cause central pontine myelinolysis.

O   **What is the anatomy and physiology of carcinoid syndrome?**

While carcinoid tumors secrete bradykinin, histamine, prostaglandins, and kallikrein, the secretion of serotonin and/or 5-hydroxytryptophan are pathopneumonic of the syndrome. The most common location of these tumors is the appendix, ileum, and rectum, however, they can be found in bronchus, stomach, pancreas, duodenum and colon. Symptoms are related to the location of the tumor, with tumors in the small bowel and proximal colon more likely to produce the characteristic flushing, bronchoconstriction, gut hypermotility and hyperglycemia. The liver generally clears the mediators of this symptom complex, unless there are liver metastases.

O   **How are the symptoms of carcinoid syndrome treated?**

Octreotide (a somatostatin analog) blocks release of serotonin and mediators, as well as prevents the peripheral effects of mediators. A carcinoid crisis with severe hypotension and bronchoconstriction may require fluids and vasopressors, as well as octreotide.

O   **What is a pheochromocytoma?**

A pheochromoctyoma is a catecholamine-secreting tumor usually found in the adrenal medulla (90%) or paravertebral chromaffin tissue. They may secrete epinephrine, norepinephrine or other catecholamines. Ten percent are bilateral, and some may be familial or associated with a MEN (multiple endocrine neoplasia) syndrome or neurofibromatosis. Symptoms of hypertension, palpitations, headache, sweating, flushing, anxiety, tremor, and weight loss reflect excess catecholamines.

○ **How is pheochromocytoma managed intraoperatively?**

Intraoperative management depends on optimal preoperative preparation including: α-adrenergic receptor blockade (phenoxybenzamine or prazosin for 10-14 days), re-expansion of fluid volume and β-adrenergic receptor blockade for patients with persistent arrhythmias or tachycardia. Patient readiness is suggested with adequate blood pressure control to 165/90 mm Hg, orthostatic hypotension, resolution of ST-T changes on EKG and no more than one PVC every 5 minutes. All anesthetic agents have been used with success (isoflurane, sevoflurane, fentanyl, sufentanil, remifentanil and regional anesthesia). Invasive monitoring is essential, anticipating hypertension (treated with IV nitroprusside, phentolamine or magnesium) and transient arrhythmias (esmolol) on induction. After the tumor is isolated and the venous supply is secured, resuscitation with volume and direct-acting vasopressors (phenylephrine, dopamine, vasopressin or catecholamine infusions) may be required. Rarely, patients may remain hypertensive perioperatively. Dilutional anemia, hypotension and hypoglycemia should be anticipated following surgery.

○ **Why does epinephrine cause hyperglycemia?**

Epinephrine causes glycogenolysis in the liver and inhibits insulin release from the pancreas.

○ **What are preoperative considerations in diabetes mellitus (DM)?**

The type of DM, current treatment regimen, and complications from DM are the most important items to assess preoperatively; in addition, these patients may have related complications, such as atherosclerotic heart and peripheral vascular disease. The patient with type1 DM with an absolute deficiency of insulin will be prone to ketoacidosis if insulin is omitted, whereas the patient with type 2 DM will have insulin-resistance and may in fact have high levels of endogenous insulin; this second patient may be on oral agents, insulin, or both, and may be susceptible to nonketotic hyperosmolar coma. Classic complications from DM include the *triopathy* of nephropathy, neuropathy, and retinopathy.

The treatment regimen and degree of blood glucose control, as well as the prior considerations mentioned, will determine recommendations for medication management; preoperative instructions should include being NPO for surgery and treatment of potential hypoglycemia.

○ **What is features of the history and physical examination would suggest diabetic autonomic neuropathy?**

A clue about autonomic neuropathy may be a resting tachycardia, because parasympathetic neuropathy occurs before sympathetic neuropathy. Other cardiac effects of autonomic neuropathy include postural hypotension and silent ischemia. Gastroparesis may present as vomiting undigested food before breakfast, as well as having a "full stomach" despite strict observance of NPO guidelines. Other GI/GU manifestations include diarrhea, neurogenic bladder, and impotence. These autonomic symptoms have a parallel in the peripheral nervous system symptoms of pain and/or a characteristic stocking-glove pattern of numbness.

GI DISORDERS AND OBESITY

The Difficult Is That Which Can Be Done Immediately; The Impossible Is That Which Takes A Little Longer.
George Santayana

○ **Define obesity and morbid obesity.**

Obesity is body weight 20% greater than ideal weight. Morbid obesity is body weight more than two times ideal weight or greater than 100 pounds over ideal weight.

○ **Is an obese patient at greater perioperative anesthetic risk? Why?**

Yes, mostly due to cardiopulmonary morbidity.

1. Associated comorbidity; adult-onset diabetes mellitus, sleep apnea, DVT, pulmonary embolism, hypothyroidism, Cushing's disease, electrolyte abnormalities, obesity surgery or drug therapies.
2. Systemic physiologic changes; pulmonary (hypoxemia, impaired ventilatory response to CO_2), cardiac (hypertension, increased CO and blood volume, CAD, pulmonary hypertension, RVH, LVH, CHF, arrhythmia), GI (aspiration risk, cholelithiasis, fatty liver or cirrhosis), and unpredictable drug metabolism.
3. Technical challenges: difficult airway and ventilatory management, arterial and venous access, blood pressure monitoring, invasive monitoring and positioning.

○ **What is the effect of morbid obesity on preload, afterload and cardiac output?**

Cardiac output, blood volume (and therefore preload) and stroke volume increase in proportion to weight gain. Cardiac output increases 100 ml/min/kilogram of additional adipose tissue perfused. Systemic hypertension (increased afterload) occurs due to increases in CO and blood volume and the vascular changes inherent in the obese/diabetic patient.

○ **What is the incidence of hypertension and coronary artery disease in the obese patient?**

Systemic hypertension is 10 times more prevalent in morbidly obese patients; moderate in 50% and severe in 5 to 10% of these patients. The incidence of coronary artery disease is doubled compared to the non-obese population.

○ **What is the effect of obesity on cerebral, splanchnic and renal blood flow?**

Cerebral and renal blood flows are similar to non-obese patients, but splanchnic blood flow is increased.

○ **Are oxygen consumption, carbon dioxide production and basal metabolic rates changed in obesity?**

Total oxygen consumption and carbon dioxide production are increased because metabolic rate is proportional to body weight.

○ **Is a preoperative fasting period of eight hours for solids and milk prior to elective surgery sufficient for an obese patient?**

No. The obese patient is at risk of regurgitation and aspiration due to increased incidence of hiatal hernia, gastroesophageal reflux, gastroparesis, diabetes mellitus and the potential for difficult airway management. In addition, ninety percent of fasted morbidly obese patients have gastric volumes of greater than 25 ml and hyperacidic gastric fluid, greatly increasing their risk of acid aspiration pneumonitis.

O   **Describe hepatobiliary disease in the obese patient.**

Fatty infiltration of the liver is typical. Inflammatory, focal necrosis and cirrhotic changes may be present. Liver enzymes are generally elevated. Cholelithiasis is commonly associated with obesity.

O   **What are the medical complications of jejunoileal bypass?**

Hypokalemia, hypocalcemia, hypomagnesemia, anemia, renal stones, gout and liver abnormalities.

O   **How is the volume of distribution of drugs affected by obesity?**

Fat-soluble drugs have an increased volume of distribution, with the exception of fentanyl. Water-soluble drugs generally have a similar volume of distribution in obese and nonobese patients.

O   **How does obesity alter the pharmacokinetic profile of benzodiazepines and barbiturates?**

Benzodiazepines and barbiturates have an increased volume of distribution, more selective distribution to fat stores and decreased elimination half-life, resulting in lower serum drug concentrations and decreased clearance.

O   **What are the airway considerations for intubation of an obese patient?**

Obesity is a classical predictor of a difficult airway. Airway evaluation should include atlanto-occipital and temporo-mandibular range of motion, thyromental distance and visualization of the oral airway. Increased neck fat may limit cervical extension and a shortened distance between the mandible and sternal fat pads may impede laryngoscopy. Maintaining a tight mask fit and manual ventilation may be difficult.   The extra tissue within the oro-pharyngeal cavity may make laryngoscopy and intubation difficult.

O   **What precautions with the administration of premedication should be observed in the morbidly obese patient?**

Preoperative sedation and narcotics should not be given until the patient is in a safely monitored environment. The is particularly true if the patient has a history of obstructive sleep apnea, hypoxia, hypercapnia, pulmonary hypertension or an anticipated difficult airway. Due to the patient's increased risk of aspiration, H_2-receptor antagonists, metoclopramide and nonparticulate antacid prophylaxis would be prudent.

O   **Is the intramuscular route adequate for the obese patient?**

All drugs should be administered intravenously. Attempts to give intramuscular injections may result in a subcutaneous injection, which leads to unpredictable absorption and drug response.

O   **Which hemodynamic monitors would you choose for the obese patient?**

Non-invasive blood pressure monitoring may be difficult due to a discrepancy between cuff and upper arm size. A small cuff falsely elevates blood pressure readings and a large cuff gives falsely low readings. Intraarterial pressure measurements may be more accurate and permit arterial blood gas analysis for monitoring ventilatory status. Volume status and myocardial function may be followed with CVP or PAP monitoring. A 5-lead EKG should be used for detection of ischemia.

O   **What are the indications for use of a pulmonary artery catheter in an obese patient?**

Patients with evidence of significant cardiovascular disease (LV compromise, pulmonary hypertension and cor pulmonale), pulmonary dysfunction or hypoxia are indications for a PA catheter if the surgery is complex or will involve significant volume shifts.

O   **Are obese patient insulated and therefore at less risk of hypothermia?**

No. Cutaneous radiant heat loss depends on exposed body surface area and accounts for 90% of heat loss. Hypothyroidism and hypothalamic lesions may increase the risk of hypothermia.

O   **Would you perform general anesthesia without endotracheal intubation in an obese patient?**

Intubation is required for oxygenation, positive pressure ventilation and protection of the airway from aspiration.

O   **What alternative to an awake sedated fiber-optic intubation would be useful?**

The "awake look" with direct laryngoscopy is a useful practice. Topically anesthetize the mouth, pharynx, and supraglottic area with a local anesthetic solution and then gently introduce a standard laryngoscope and attempt to visualize the epiglottis and possibly arytenoids. If it is possible to see these structures, it is likely that intubation of the trachea following preoxygenation and rapid-sequence induction with cricoid pressure can be performed. However, muscle relaxation may lead to loss of pharyngeal tissue support, and lack of visualization can still be a problem even if the "awake look" is reasonable.

O   **If an obese patient is to be intubated, following induction of general anesthesia, what considerations are important?**

Cricoid pressure (Sellick's maneuver) should be applied in all cases. Adequate preoxygenation and denitrogenation of the patient using 3 minutes of spontaneous breathing with 100% oxygen should be performed. The availability of a second pair of experienced hands to facilitate two-man ventilation or adjust patient positioning is recommended. Availability of difficult airway devices is prudent.

O   **Is nitrous oxide a good choice in obese patients?**

Nitrous oxide is a logical choice for maintaining anesthesia unless high inspired oxygen concentrations are required to prevent hypoxia. N_2O is fat insoluble, rapid in onset and subject to limited metabolism. N_2O increases pulmonary vascular resistance and may exacerbate RV dysfunction in those patients with pulmonary hypertension.

O   **Do obese patients metabolize inhaled anesthetics differently from nonobese patients?**

Yes. The rate of biotransformation of methoxyflurane, enflurane and halothane is increased resulting in increased serum levels of fluoride ions, which may be potentially nephrotoxic. This is not seen with isoflurane and desflurane.

O   **Is the obese patient at increased risk for developing hepatitis following exposure to halothane?**

Yes. Risk factors associated with halothane hepatitis include obesity, female gender, familial predisposition and prior exposure.

O   **What are the inhalational anesthetic agents of choice in an obese patient?**

Isoflurane, sevoflurane and desflurane. The potential for inhalational anesthetic agents to cause end-organ injury is primarily dependent on the extent of their liver metabolism. All potentially decrease hepatic blood flow but are relatively safe if the mean arterial blood pressure and cardiac output are maintained. Isoflurane has the least detrimental effect on liver blood flow. A simultaneous decrease in the liver's metabolic demand tends to balance the oxygen supply-uptake ratio. Furthermore, these agents tend to be less fat soluble so residual anesthetic effects are minimized. Desflurane has the lowest fat solubility of the potent agents.

○   **What factors must be taken into consideration when calculating the dose of succinylcholine required for intubation in an obese patient?**

Pseudocholinesterase activity is increased requiring larger doses of succinylcholine (1.2-1.5 mg/kg). Dosing should be calculated on the basis of about 20 percent more than estimated lean body mass, rather than on actual body weight.

○   **What deleterious physiologic effects may result from supine positioning in the obese patient?**

Acute restrictive lung disease resulting in hypoxemia and hypercarbia; decreased FRC and time to desaturation following apnea, high peak inspiratory airway pressures causing hypoventilation or barotrauma; endobronchial intubation; and reduced preload to the heart (compression of the vena cava or high peak pressures) decreasing cardiac output and worsening ventilation-perfusion mismatch.

○   **Is regional anesthesia safe for the morbidly obese patient?**

Yes. Technical difficulties include layers of adipose tissue obscuring landmarks and necessitating the use of longer needles and positioning difficulties. For peripheral nerve blocks calculation of local anesthetic solution requirements should take into consideration estimated lean body mass. Weight will influence block height more so for epidural than spinal anesthesia. The potential for a difficult airway or aspiration risk is not circumvented. Cardiovascular and respiratory effects of high spinal may be detrimental to the patient. The patient must be able to tolerate the required surgical positioning. Laparoscopic surgery requires securing the airway due to further increasing elevated gastric pressure and the increased CO_2 load for which the patient may not be able to compensate.

○   **Does obesity effect block height during spinal anesthesia?**

Controversial. Many factors affect spinal anesthesia block height. The obese patient has decreased subarachnoid compliance, particularly when the patient is in the supine position. Using a hyperbaric spinal technique when the patient is given an injection while sitting and then placed supine may cause cephalad movement of the drug and an unpredictable increase in the height of the block. A reduction of drug dose 20 to 30% may be prudent. Few authors suggest weight is not related to block height during spinal anesthesia.

○   **What are the advantages of combined epidural-general anesthesia in the obese patient?**

Earlier ambulation, reduced risk of DVT, increase in postoperative pulmonary function and a possibly shorter hospital stay.

○   **What is the Pickwickian syndrome?**

Obesity-hypoventilation syndrome. Etiology is unclear. Symptoms include: decreased ventilatory response to CO_2 and O_2, sleep apnea, hypoxemia, hypercarbia, pulmonary hypertension, polycythemia and biventricular failure; evident in 5-10% of obese patients. The term originates from Charles Dickens' portrayal of Joe, the fat, somnolent, red-faced boy in the Posthumous Papers of the Pickwick Club, written in 1837. (Good cocktail info, but won't be on the boards.)

○   **What is the relationship between Pickwickian syndrome and body weight?**

Body weight is typically more than 130 kg and, in most cases, a very rapid increase in weight has occurred.

○   **Describe the classic triad of the obesity-hypoventilation syndrome.**

Obesity, alveolar hypoventilation and hypersomnolence.

○   **What is the pathophysiology of cor pulmonale in the Pickwickian syndrome?**

Right ventricular hypertrophy and failure results from chronic hypoxemia, hypercarbia, polycythemia and pulmonary hypertension.

○   **What are the commonest causes of small bowel obstruction?**

Adhesions account for approximately 60% of all small bowel obstructions followed by tumors (20%), hernias (10%) and Crohn's disease (5%). Other causes include intra-abdominal abscess from a ruptured appendix or diverticulum and intussusception.

○   **What is the primary anesthetic goal during induction for a patient with small bowel obstruction?**

Prevent regurgitation and subsequent aspiration of intestinal contents into the trachea and lungs.

○   **Why are patients with small bowel obstruction at high risk for aspiration?**

Risk factors for aspiration include: elderly, emergency surgery involving the upper abdomen, and obstruction to gastric and intestinal emptying resulting in large volumes (>0.4 ml/kg) of acidic (pH < 2.5) and nonacidic fluid containing bile, particulate and fecal material.

The small bowel is a secretory organ. Normally up to 9 liters of fluid can be secreted each day. When an obstruction occurs, fluid and air accumulate above the obstruction. In early obstruction, up to 1.5 liters of fluid can be sequestered in the gut. By the time a high- grade obstruction is established, up to 6 liters of fluid may be present.

○   **What measures can be taken to prevent aspiration?**

Preoperatively, the stomach should be emptied. This is usually achieved using a nasogastric tube for suctioning. Intubation of the trachea should be achieved either with the patient awake or with rapid sequence induction using cricoid pressure (Sellick's maneuver).

○   **Define body mass index (BMI). Is BMI gender specific?**

Body mass index is independent of gender and defined as the ratio of an individual's weight in kilograms to their height in square meters. BMI is a method of calculating ideal body weight.

Ideal body weight = BMI of 22-28

$$BMI = \frac{wt\ (kg)}{ht\ (m^2)}$$

○   **Define obesity and morbid obesity in terms of BMI.**

OBESITY = BMI OF 28-35
MORBID OBESITY = BMI > 35

○   **What changes in pulmonary volumes and function tests are associated with morbid obesity?**

The pulmonary function tests of obese patients show a restrictive pattern. Lung volumes are decreased including functional residual capacity (FRC), vital capacity, expiratory reserve volume and total lung capacity. Tidal volume and residual volume are normal. FEV_1 and maximum midexpiratory flow rate are normal or slightly decreased. Lung compliance is usually normal.

O   **In the obese patient, to what degree is the FRC decreased? How is this affected by anesthesia and patient positioning?**

FRC declines exponentially as BMI increases. This is further exacerbated by the supine and Trendelenburg position. In the anesthetized obese patient, FRC is decreased by 50% compared to 20% for the non-obese patient.

O   **Why is the morbidly obese patient at risk for hypoxemia following induction of anesthesia?**

Morbidly obesity is accompanied by hypoxemia due to V-Q mismatching. Changes in lung volumes results in closure of small airways and tidal volumes resting below closing volumes during normal breathing. FRC is greatly decreased, which is further exacerbated by anesthesia and the supine position. Total oxygen consumption is increased due to the large tissue mass. Consequently, following induction of anesthesia, with smaller oxygen stores and greater demands, the onset of hypoxemia can be rapid even in the setting of adequate preoxygenation. In addition, mechanical ventilation may be difficult due to decreased chest wall compliance and cephalad excursion of the diaphragm.

O   **What results are expected from arterial blood gas analysis of an individual with Pickwickian syndrome?**

Hypoxemia and hypercarbia.

O   **What is the pathophysiology of ischemia-reperfusion injury?**

Tissue hypoxia and acidosis are generally regarded as the major factors that mediate the pathological alterations associated with ischemia. But, it is the intrinsic ability of tissues to initiate and sustain an inflammatory response which may explain the vascular dysfunction and tissue injury produced by ischemia-reperfusion. Ischemia-reperfusion injury is initiated when the ischemic tissue is reperfused and production of reactive metabolites of oxygen and nitrogen causes accumulation of activated neutrophils. with neutrophil-endothelial adhesion, tissue damage results due to secretion of additional reactive oxygen species as well as proteolytic enzymes, In particular elastase. if the area of ischemic tissue is large, neutrophils also sequester in the lung, liver, splanchnic circulation and cardiovascular system resulting in the development of sirs (systemic inflammatory response syndrome) and mods (multiple organ dysfunction syndrome).

O   **What implications might ischemia-reperfusion injury have for the gastrointestinal tract?**

The cellular damage caused by splanchnic ischemia is less than that associated with ischemia and reperfusion injury. An example may be perinatal asphyxia and ischemia-reperfusion causing necrotizing enterocolitis or delayed primary function of a transplanted liver following reperfusion in the recipient.

O   **What is gastric tonometry?**

Gastric tonometry is a monitoring technique measuring carbon dioxide partial pressure in the gastrointestinal mucosa (stomach or intestine) as an indicator of tissue perfusion.

O   **What is the clinical significance of gastric tonometry?**

Early detection of splanchnic hypoperfusion and restoration of adequate splanchnic tissue perfusion may reduce the incidence of multiorgan failure. The difference between the arterial PCO_2 and the tonometry $PgCO_2$ is a reflection of stomach perfusion. In normally perfused mucosa, gastric mucosal $PgCO_2$ is close to $PaCO_2$. During hypoperfusion the calculated difference increases. If $PgCO_2$ minus $PaCO_2$ is greater than 20, perfusion is inadequate and fluids and/or inotropes should be considered.

O   **What are the signs of venous gas embolism during laparoscopy?**

Venous gas embolism is a rare but potentially lethal complication of laparoscopic surgery. Profound hypotension, hypoxemia, cyanosis, tachycardia or other dysrhythmias can occur. EKG changes may indicate right heart strain. A "millwheel" murmur may be auscultated with an esophageal or precordial stethoscope.

○   **Describe what happens to the end-tidal CO_2 during venous embolization of the insufflating gas.**

An initial increase in $ETCO_2$ due to pulmonary excretion of absorbed CO_2 is followed by a sudden decrease due to fall in cardiac output.

○   **By what route does CO_2 enter the bloodstream during laparoscopy?**

Gas embolism can occur through a tear in a vessel in the abdominal wall or peritoneum. The risk of embolic episodes decreases after completion of the pneumoperitoneum, because increased intra-abdominal pressure causes the injured vessel to collapse. Embolism resulting in sudden CV collapse can also occur due to inadvertent placement of the Veress needle directly into a vein or parenchymal organ.

○   **What is the immediate course of action should CO_2 embolism occur?**

Release of CO_2 pneumoperitoneum, ventilate with 100% O_2, check vital signs, and position the patient in steep head down and left lateral decubitus are recommended.

○   **What are the hemodynamic effects of pneumoperitoneum?**

As a result of increased intra-abdominal pressure during pneumoperitoneum, mean arterial blood pressure and systemic vascular resistance (afterload) are both increased while venous return (preload) is decreased.

○   **Are the cardiovascular effects of pneumoperitoneum clinically significant?**

At the typical insufflation pressures of 10-15 mm Hg, there is little effect on the cardiac output in healthy patients. However, in patients with limited cardiac reserve, the increase in afterload coupled with decreased preload may result in myocardial ischemia and decreased cardiac output.

○   **What are the principal respiratory complications of abdominal CO_2 insufflation for laparoscopy?**

Surgical exposure for laparoscopy requires the creation of a pneumoperitoneum. This is routinely achieved by intraperitoneal insufflation of CO_2. There are four principal respiratory complications that can result: subcutaneous emphysema, pneumothorax, endobronchial intubation and gas embolism. Pneumomediastinum and pneumopericardium can also occur.

○   **What are the causes of increased $PaCO_2$ during laparosopy?**

The list includes: absorption of CO_2 from the peritoneal cavity, V/Q mismatch (increased physiologic dead space), light/insufficient anesthesia (increased metabolism), depression of ventilation from anesthetics (spontaneously breathing patient) and accidental events such as endobronchial intubation, capnothorax, CO_2 emphysema or gas embolism.

○   **T/F: Endobronchial intubation does not occur during laparoscopic cholecystectomy because the patient is in reverse Trendelenburg (head up) position?**

False. The upward displacement of the diaphragm during pneumoperitoneum also causes cephalad displacement of the carina. Endobronchial intubation has been reported despite head up positioning of the patient.

○   **Describe the necessary action in the case of CO_2 pneumothorax in the absence of any cardiopulmonary compromise.**

Because CO_2 is highly diffusible, spontaneous resolution will occur within 30-60 minutes of exsufflation. In this scenario, thoracentesis may be avoided. Guidelines suggest to: stop N_2O, correct hypoxemia, apply PEEP and minimize intra-abdominal pressure. These guidelines do not hold true if pneumothorax is secondary to ruptured bullae in which case PEEP should not be applied and thoracentesis is mandatory.

O   **What is the mechanism for decreased cardiac output as a result of pneumoperitoneum?**

The mechanism is multifactorial including; decreased venous return (caval compression, pooling in lower extremities), increased venous resistance and increased systemic vascular resistance.

O   **How are myocardial filling pressures affected by abdominal insufflation and is this significant?**

Despite the decrease in venous return, there is a paradoxical increase in right atrial and pulmonary capillary wedge pressure presumably secondary to increased intrathoracic pressure as a result of pneumoperitoneum. Therefore, with regards to actual cardiac filling during pneumoperitoneum, CVP and PCWP may not be accurate measures.

O   **What are the principal concerns for the cardiac patient undergoing laparoscopic surgery?**

Hemodynamic alterations induced by laparoscopy are well documented and most pronounced in individuals with preexisting low cardiac output, low CVP and high SVR. Intraoperative risks imposed by these hemodynamic alterations should be carefully weighed against the postoperative benefits of laparoscopy particularly in patients with CHF, ischemic heart disease, cardiomyopathy, and/or significant valvular disease.

O   **What precautions can be taken to attenuate hemodynamic changes in the cardiac patient undergoing laparoscopy?**

Invasive monitoring (arterial catheter, pulmonary artery catheter, TEE) should be strongly considered. Hypovolemia should be corrected prior to surgery. Intravenous use of dobutamine, nitroglycerin or nicardipine may be used to treat low cardiac output states that are exacerbated by pneumoperitoneum. Slow insufflation of CO_2 and low intra-abdominal pressures (10 mm Hg) may attenuate some of the changes.

O   **What are the anesthetic contraindications for laparoscopy?**

Absolute anesthetic contraindications to laparoscopy have yet to be defined. Because of the physiologic alterations that occur, laparoscopy is undesirable in patients with elevated ICP, V-P or peritoneojugular shunts, severe cardiac disease and hypovolemia. Special care should be taken in patients with renal failure to avoid nephrotoxic drugs and optimize hemodynamics during pneumoperitoneum.

O   **Can laparoscopy be performed on individuals with V-P or peritoneojugular shunts?**

Yes. These shunts can be clamped prior to initiation of pneumoperitoneum.

O   **Which drugs will increase and decrease lower esophageal sphincter tone?**

>   Increase-
>   Protein meal
>   Coffee contains a protein that increases LES pressure
>   Bethanechol (Urecholine)
>   Metoclopramide (Reglan)
>   Antacids
>   alpha-adrenergic agents
>
>   Decrease-
>   Alcohol

Chocolate
Essence of peppermint
Smoking
Fatty foods
beta-adrenergic agents
Estrogen and progesterone
Caffeine decreases LES pressure
Calcium channel blockers
Diazepam
Barbiturates

○   **A patient with bile duct obstruction due to stones and cholangitis is scheduled for cholecystectomy. Are there any laboratory findings that would distinguish this cholestatic liver injury from that of viral hepatitis?**

Conjugated hyperbilirubinemia and a liver biopsy showing centrilobular cholestasis and neutrophils within edematous portal stroma.

○   **T/F: Dehydration and electrolyte disturbances in patients with chronic diarrhea suggests a secretory process, such as endocrine tumors or laxative abuse.**

True. Secretory diarrhea is caused by abnormal secretion or inhibition of absorption by the intestinal epithelium. Other mechanisms for diarrhea include: osmotic, inflammatory or conditions associated with deranged motility.

GENITOURINARY AND RENAL SURGERY

The Illiterate Of The 21ˢᵗ Century Will Not Be Those Who Cannot Read And Write, But Those Who Cannot Learn, Unlearn And Relearn.
Alvin Tofler

○ **What are the initial clinical effects of acute tubular necrosis on renal function?**

Loss of urinary concentrating ability caused by the breakdown of the energy requiring Na-K-ATPase pump in the thick ascending loop of Henle and a reduction in glomerular filtration rate (GFR) resulting from decreases in renal and glomerular blood flow and an abnormality in tubular integrity such as obstruction of tubular flow by cellular debris or backleak of ultrafiltrate.

○ **What level of spinal or epidural blockade is required to suppress the vasoconstrictor response to sympathetic stimulation that results in a reduction in renal blood flow and GFR?**

Neuraxial blockade from the level of T_4 to T_{10} is required, as sympathetic renal constrictor fibers are derived from T_4 to L_1 spinal cord segments through the celiac plexus. Sympathetic stimulation occurs secondary to surgical stress, general anesthesia, hypoxia, hypotension, pain, severe bleeding and strenuous exercise. Aortic cross-clamping below the renal arteries will increase renal vascular resistance despite adequate thoracic epidural blockade.

○ **What are the effects of airway pressure and PEEP on renal function?**

PEEP can decrease cardiac output and thus renal blood flow, glomerular filtration rate and urine output. Renin and aldosterone levels rise but not antidiuretic hormone. These effects are seen at 15 cm H_2O PEEP.

○ **What factors predispose to renal failure from myoglobinuria secondary to rhabdomyolysis?**

A low urine pH (<5.6) leads to myoglobin precipitation as ferrihematin in the proximal tubule. Hypovolemia, which causes a low tubular flow is another risk factor. Both of these contribute to renal failure by promoting tubular obstruction.

○ **What are the problems with renal function and sevoflurane?**

Sevoflurane is significantly metabolized by the liver and fluoride levels of 50 μM/L have been reported after prolonged exposure. There are no reports of impaired renal function after sevoflurane. Compound A is produced by interaction with CO_2 absorbent, and may be nephrotoxic at higher than clinically seen doses. Low fresh gas flows exacerbate Compound A production. FDA recommendations suggest Sevoflurane is safe for 2 MAC-hours at fresh gas flows 1-2 L/min. (MAC–hours is the product of concentration and time. For sevo = 2% x 2 hours = 1% x 4 hours = 2 MAC-hours). Longer exposures at high concentrations and low fresh gas flows have not been studied adequately. Compound A is not an issue above 2L/min of fresh gas flows.

○ **What are the effects of renal failure on the elimination of vecuronium, atracurium, cis-atracurium and mivacurium?**

The duration of neuromuscular blockade in renal failure is prolonged with vecuronium due to prolonged elimination half-life and lower plasma clearance. These effects are a consequence of a 30% elimination by the kidneys in healthy patients. Atracurium and cis-atracurium undergo pH dependent Hoffman elimination and are not dependent on renal excretion for termination of action. The duration of mivacurium can be prolonged

10-15 minutes in renal failure, which has been attributed to lwo plasma pseudocholinesterase levels in uremic patients or in those patients presenting after hemodialysis.

O   **A chronic renal failure patient requiring regular hemodialysis develops weakness and mild respiratory distress in the post anesthetic care unit. The patient has received vecuronium which has been reversed with neostigmine and atropine, in full and appropriate doses. What is the most likely explanation?**

The excretion of cholinesterase inhibitors (neostigmine, pyridostigmine and edrophonium) is delayed in patients with impaired renal function. This offsets the increased elimination half-life of vecuronium and makes recurarization an unlikely explanation. One should consider an interaction between antibiotics, diuretics or electrolyte disturbances with the muscle relaxant. In addition, mild hypothermia may be a contributory factor in the prolongation of action of any NMB due to slowed metabolic clearance.

O   **What are the problems with the use of sodium nitroprusside in renal impairment?**

Thiocyanate is a renally excreted metabolite of sodium nitroprusside, with a half life of 4-7 days, which is further prolonged in renal failure. Hypoxia, nausea, tinnitus, muscle spasm and psychosis can occur when levels exceed 10 mg/100ml. Hypothyroidism can result as thiocyanate inhibits iodide ion uptake by the thyroid gland. Oxyhemoglobin can oxidize thiocyanate to sulfate and cyanide, but it is too slow to be of clinical importance.

O   **What is TURP syndrome?**

Transurethral prostatic resection syndrome. Acute hyponatremia and cerebral edema resulting from excessive absorption of irrigating fluid causes restlessness, agitation, confusion, seizures and coma. Fluid overload may result in hypertension and bradycardia. Hypotension, widened QRS and ventricular ectopy, pulmonary edema, congestive heart failure and cardiac arrest may result. Hemolysis, septicemia, glycine toxicity with visual disturbances and air embolus can be associated.

O   **A patient is undergoing a TURP under spinal anesthesia and becomes disorientated and hypertensive one hour into the case. What is your next step?**

Ensure adequate oxygenation, ventilation and patency of the airway. Inform the surgeon of the change in the patient's mental status. Treatment consists of administering diuretics and fluid restriction, cautery of open venous sinuses, and rapid completion of the surgical resection. Retarding further fluid absorption by lowering the height of the irrigant is prudent. Hypertonic saline is rarely needed and carries the risk of further fluid overload and perhaps central pontine myelinolysis. NTG can be employed as a temporary measure to treat excessive preload.

O   **Where do "loop diuretics" act?**

Loop diuretics inhibit sodium and chloride reabsorption in the thick ascending limb of the loop of Henle.

O   **What are the potential side effects of thiazide diuretics?**

Hypokalemia (increased potassium secretion), metabolic alkalosis (increased hydrogen secretion), hyponatremia (impairment of renal diluting capacity), hyperkalemia, hyperuricemia, hyperglycemia and hyperlipidemia.

O   **What degree of nephron loss and fall in creatinine clearance is associated with uremia?**

The loss of 95% of functioning nephrons. The full manifestations of the uremia syndrome are seen only after the GFR decreases below 25 ml/min. Patients with clearances below 10 ml/min are dependent on dialysis for survival until successfully transplanted.

○   **What effect does renal failure have on the reversal agents for muscle relaxants?**

Fifty percent of neostigmine and 70% of pyridostigmine and edrophonium are excreted in the urine. Renal failure may prolong the duration of action of these drugs up to 100%.

○   **How does urinary sodium measurement reflect renal tubular function in the oliguric patient?**

Prerenal oliguria due to reduced renal perfusion is associated with a urinary sodium concentration < 20 mEq/L. A urine sodium > 40 mEq/l is indicative of intrinsic renal disease.

○   **Is succinylcholine a safe choice in the renal failure patient?**

If the patient has been dialyzed within 8 to 12 hours and the potassium concentration is normal, then succinylcholine is an appropriate choice. In most cases, renal failure patients are no more susceptible to an exaggerated hyperkalemic response induced by succinylcholine, than those with normal renal function. If the patient is hyperkalemic (the upper limit of normal to proceed with surgery is controversial but stated as 5.5meq/L)) use of a non-depolarizing muscle relaxants minimally dependent on the kidney for elimination would be appropriate (cis-atracurium, vecuronium, mivacurium). The concern is that the 0.5-1.0 meq/L increase temporarily seen after succinylcholine use might push an asymptomatic hyperkalemia into the range where cardiac conduction is affected.

○   **What percentage of the filtered sodium is reabsorbed by the renal tubules?**

Of the 25,000 mEq sodium filtered each day, 65% is reabsorbed in the proximal tubule, 25% is actively reabsorbed in the ascending loop of Henle and 9% by the distal tubule under aldosterone regulation. Only 1% of the filtered sodium is excreted in the urine.

○   **What is the mechanism of renal dysfunction following abdominal aortic aneurysm surgery?**

Acute tubular necrosis. Contributing factors include; intravascular volume depletion, embolization of atherosclerotic debris to the kidneys and iatrogenic surgical trauma to the renal arteries. Aortic cross-clamping reduces renal blood flow whether above the renal arteries (80 to 90%) or below (40%). Renal vasoconstriction and intrarenal redistribution of blood flow may account for the deterioration in renal function, but the pathophysiology is unclear. Mannitol, loop diuretics, renal vasodilators may be used clinically for renal protection, despite studies demonstrating little or no benefit.

○   **What factors determine renal blood flow (RBF)?**

The kidneys receive approximately 20% of the cardiac output or approximately 1 L/min of blood flow. The renal blood flow (RBF) is regulated by vascular smooth muscle tone. Anesthesia may decrease RBF by dropping cardiac output or mean arterial pressure (MAP). However, autoregulation works to preserve RBF by decreasing renal vascular resistance as MAP decreases. This occurs in normal and dennervated kidneys over a range of 60-160 mm Hg. Outside the autoregulatory limits, renal blood flow becomes pressure dependent. Glomerular filtration generally ceases when mean systemic arterial pressure is less than 40-50 mm Hg

In general, decreased RBF occurs with activation of the salt-retaining vasoconstrictor system that prevents hypovolemia and hypotension. This is triggered by exercise as well as by the insults of surgical stress, ischemia or sepsis via the effects of the sympathoadrenal system, the renin-angiotensin system, aldosterone and antidiuretic hormone.

On the other hand, increased RBF is favored by the salt-losing vasodilator systems which defend against systemic hypertension and hypervolemia through the effects of prostaglandins, kinins, and atrial natriuretic peptide.

○   **What effect does hypovolemia have on renin-angiotensin?**

While glomeruli connect the afferent and efferent renal arteries, modified smooth muscle cells (granular cells) lie between the juxtaposed vessels and produce renin. These cells are responsive to multiple stimuli, and secrete renin in response to actual hypovolemia (hemorrhage, diuresis, sodium loss or restriction) or effective hypovolemia (positive pressure ventilation, congestive heart failure, sepsis, or cirrhosis with ascites.)

○   **What effect does renin-angiotensin have on blood pressure?**

Renin cleaves angiotensinogen (liver) into the Angiotensin I. Angiotensin converting enzyme (ACE) in the lung and kidney cleaves Angiotensin I into the potent vasoconstrictor Angiotensin II. It takes about 20 minutes for the renin-angiotensin system to fully exert its effect.

Angiotensin II increases systemic blood pressure at the site of the arteriole. It has ten times the vasoconstrictor potency at the renal efferent arteriole as it does systemically. Thus moderate levels of Angiotensin II can maintain GFR even in the face of moderately decreased RBF. Angiotensin II further enhances systemic blood pressure by stimulating NaCl reabsorption by the proximal tubule, ADH secretion by the posterior pituitary, and aldosterone production by the adrenal cortex. Profound hypotension however, leads to renal decompensation. The kidney ceases its high-energy-consuming transport of sodium in the ischemic renal medulla and switches strategies to decrease GFR. High levels of Angiotensin II work towards this end by causing constriction of the glomerular mesangial cells, decreasing ultrafiltration. Angiotensin II also exerts negative feedback control by inhibiting further renin release, stimulating intrarenal prostaglandins, and stimulating ANP release.

○   **How is the release of ADH regulated?**

ADH, or vasopressin, is typically secreted when the serum osmolality exceeds the set-point of hypothalamic osmoreceptors, typically between 280 and 290 mOsm/kg. Psychiatric stress can also stimulate its secretion. Hypovolemia, detected by decreased left atrial and pulmonary vein stretch-receptors, or hypotension signaled from aortic and carotid baroreceptors are more potent and overriding triggers. Surgical stress is also a profound stimulus and typically lasts two to three days after the surgical procedure. A syndrome of inappropriate ADH secretion (SIADH) can occur in a number of processes, commonly including head trauma or neurosurgery and neoplasms, particularly bronchogenic carcinoma. In contrast, patients in septic shock have inappropriately low ADH levels although the pathologic mechanism is unknown.

○   **How do the different vasodilators used for induced hypotension differ in their effects on renal blood flow?**

The selective DA_1-dopaminergic agonist fenoldopam is capable of providing deliberate hypotension, without any significant decrease in renal blood flow. Nitroglycerin decreases renal blood flow less than sodium nitroprusside which is associated with renin-angiotensin and sympathetic stimulation. Trimethaphan abolishes autoregulation and causes the greatest decrease in renal blood flow.

○   **How is GFR calculated?**

In the absence of the polysaccharide inulin, that is filtered but neither secreted nor absorbed, creatinine clearance will reflect GFR and is calculated as:

Creatinine Clearance = ([Creatinine]Urine / [Creatinine]Plasma) X Urine Flow Rate

An alternate formula that can provide an estimate when only a single plaasma creatinine value is known:

Male Creatinine Clearance = [(140 - age] x lean body weight] / (72 X [Creatinine]Plasma)

The product of this equation needs to be multiplied by 0.85 to accurately estimate female GFR.

○   **Can GFR be accurately determined in a hypovolemic patient?**

No. Serum creatinine levels are subject to volume status and can be diluted by perioperative administration of IV fluids. Creatinine clearance has several limitations varying with muscle mass, physical activity, protein intake, and catabolism, and can be falsely elevated by ketoacidosis, barbiturates and cephalosporin antibiotics as a result of laboratory assay interference.

O   **Why is a normal serum creatinine still consistent with impaired renal function, especially in the elderly?**

Serum creatinine concentrations are dependent on dietary protein intake and muscle tissue turnover. Elderly people have less muscle mass and thus lower serum creatinines. Creatinine is freely filtered at the glomerulus with minimal secretion in the distal tubule and no reabsorption. Because of the wide ranges of normal for serum creatinine, a 50% increase may still be within the normal range yet represent a significant reduction in glomerular filtration rate which will not be recognized unless a baseline value is known or a formal creatinine clearance study is performed (24 hour urine collection with serum and urine measurements needed).

O   **What is the fractional excretion of sodium?**

FENa is defined by (Urinary Na/ Plasma Na) divided by (Urinary Cr/ Plasma Cr) x 100%. A prenal picture is suggested by a ratio < 1% and intrinsic renal disease by a ratio > 3%. Diuretic therapy can overcome the kidneys ability to retain sodium, thus a high urine Na does not necessarily reflect loss of tubular function. However, low Urine Na in the setting of diuretics indicates an intense prerenal state.

O   **How does urine specific gravity and osmolality help determine renal tubular function?**

A high specific gravity (>1.030) or an osmolality (>1050 mOsm/kg) means that there is unimpaired tubular function. Urine specific gravity (1.010) or osmolality (290 mOsm/kg) that is the same as plasma is suggestive of renal disease. A dilute urine (50-100 mOsm/kg) may still indicate renal disease as the urine dilution mechanism fails after the concentrating ability.

O   **What are the hormonal causes of oliguria?**

Normal urine output does not rule out renal failure just as oliguria may be due to a number of factors independent of GFR. Urine output depends upon tubular excretion of solute and water, which is determined hormonally by levels of circulating renin, ADH, aldosterone, and catecholamines. Surgical stress is a profound stimulus for the release of ADH, typically persisting for two to three days after the surgical procedure. Surgical stress also leads to the elaboration of high levels of angiotensin II, which causes increased NaCl resorption at the proximal tubule, elaboration of aldosterone and contraction of the glomeruli mesangial cells with a physiologic decrease in GFR.

O   **What are the differential diagnosis and laboratory abnormalities associated with perioperative oliguria?**

Perioperative oliguria can be broken down into three categories: prerenal, intrinsic renal, and post-renal.

Prerenal oliguria is the clinical result of poor renal perfusion. It can be caused by hypovolemia, low cardiac output states, aortic or renal artery clamping, thromboembolic phenomena, hemorrhage or transfusion reaction. Lab values include FENa<1, U_{Na} <25, BUN/Cr Ratio> 20:1, Urine osmolality >500.

Intrinsic renal oliguria results from a variety of injuries – either ischemic, toxic, or immune mediated. It can be caused by shock states; exposure to antibiotics, chemotherapeutics, contrast dyes, free hemoglobin or myoglobin, or cellular debris; or acute interstitial nephritis such as hypersensitivity reactions; or acute glomerulonephritis. U_{Na}>40, FENa>1, Urinary osmolality <350.

Post-renal oliguria can occur with mechanical obstruction of the urinary tract, and resolves with alleviation of the obstruction. Calculi, tumors, blood clots, edema or surgical ligation can be causative. Postrenal oliguria in the absence of a foley catheter can also occur due to voiding dysfunction. Voiding dysfunction can result from disruption of sacral parasympathetic motor innervation of the bladder from residual spinal or epidural block. It can also be caused by high dose intravenous or neuraxial morphine due to its anticholinergic effect. Any other residual anticholinergic (antagonizing bladder parasympathetics) or α-adrenergic (agonizing bladder sympathetics) drug can have the same effect.

O   How is postoperative oliguria treated?

Immediate post-operative oliguria is most often prerenal or postrenal in nature. Correcting prerenal oliguria involves medically achieving cardiovascular homeostasis by addressing issues of hypovolemia, abnormal cardiac rate, dysrhythmia, hypocontractility and decreased systemic vascular resistance. Normal vital signs coupled to a urinalysis consistent with prerenal oliguria may suggest renal thromboembolism, a surgical issue.

Postrenal oliguria is usually treated with a foley catheter or catheter irrigation. Ultrasound for bladder scan can be a valuable diagnostic tool for this condition, though it may confound the diagnosis by showing an empty bladder after a bladder perforation.

Intrinsic renal failure is treated conservatively by maintainance of adequate renal perfusion pressure and stimulation of diuresis with furosemide, mannitol, or low-dose dopamine infusion. More aggressive treatment includes dialysis. The attempts to pharmacologically prevent intrinsic renal failure have not been met with success. However, the negative effects of specific toxic exposures can be diminished. For example the use of homocysteine and aggressive hydration along with nonionic contrast dyes provides some benefit in high risk situations. Calcium channel blockers have been found to ameliorate the effects of cyclosporine, cisplatin and contrast dye as long as hypotension is avoided. Minimizing ATN in the setting of hemolysis or rhabdomyolysis can be attempted with aggressive fluid management and urine alkalinization. A low urine pH (<5.6) leads to myoglobin precipitation as ferrihematin in the proximal tubule, and hypovolemia causes a low tubular flow and sludging. If oliguric ATN cannot be avoided by these measures, however, there has been much interest generated recently in using ANP to promote dialysis-free survival.

O   What are some of the laboratory or electrolyte effects that may accompany acute renal failure?

The major problem arising from acute renal failure is the inability to maintain the dynamic balance between dietary intake of essential substances and production of waste products. This results in:
- a decrease in serum sodium and calcium.
- a daily rise in serum potassium of 0.3 to 3 mEq/L except when there is concomitant potassium loss from diarrhea or vomiting.
- metabolic acidosis.
- a progressive rise in serum urea, creatinine, uric acid, magnesium, sulfate, phosphate, some amino and organic acids and polypeptides.
- a decrease in serum proteins particularly albumin.
- elevation of total lipids, cholesterol, phosphorous, and neutral fats.
- hyperglycemia, which may or may not be insulin resistant.

O   What are some of the metabolic and systemic effects that may accompany acute renal failure?

The kidney functions both as an endocrine and an excretory organ. Thus disorders of renin-angiotensin and aldosterone secretion occur, contributing to the hypertension that develops in patients with severe renal disease. Heart failure and abnormalities in liver function and blood coagulation may also occur. Infection is common and difficult to treat because the altered excretion of antibiotics leads to rapid development of toxic levels of these drugs.

O   What are some of the laboratory or electrolyte effects that accompany chronic renal failure?

Metabolic acidosis, hyperkalemia, hypocalcemia, hypermagnesemia and hyperphosphatemia are seen. Reduced erythropoietin production results in a chronic anemia. Coagulopathies are common and may accompany platelet dysfunction.

○ **What are some of the systemic effects that accompany chronic renal failure?**

There is altered hydration status with unpredictable intravascular fluid volume. Systemic hypertension, congestive heart failure, and attenuated sympathetic nervous system activity are often seen. Chronic anemia results in increased cardiac output, and shifts the oxyhemoglobin dissociation curve to the right. Pruritis occurs, the intensity of which may be reduced by erythropoietin. In addition, there is increased susceptibility to infection, as there is decreased activity of phagocytes. Most chronic renal failure patients succumb to sepsis.

○ **How is magnesium excreted?**

Because circulating Mg is partially protein-bound, only 70-80% is filtered across the glomerulus. In general, only 3% of the filtered magnesium escapes reabsorption and is excreted, though this can increase or decrease depending on magnesium status. Mg is unique in that most of it (50-60%) is reabsorbed in the thick ascending loop of Henle or distal convoluted tubule rather than in the proximal convoluted tubule (20-30%). It is also unique that alterations in Mg excretion are dependent upon changes in loop transport. Most of Mg transport is passive, diffusing with NaCl down an electrical gradient. Mg wasting can therefore be induced with a loop diuretic. Mg transport in the thick loop is influenced by serum levels of calcium and Mg which bind a receptor of the thick ascending limb cells and inhibit K transport on the luminal side. This in turn will decrease NaCl absorption thereby increasing Mg excretion. In the distal convoluted tubule, active transport may involve a Na / Mg exchanger.

○ **The nephrologist cautions you against using morphine intraoperatively for a patient with chronic renal failure. What are the issues that need to be considered? What are your alternate choices for analgesia?**

Morphine is a prototypical example of an opioid with active metabolites that are dependant on renal clearance mechanisms for elimination. Morphine is principally metabolized by conjugation in the liver and is eliminated via renal excretion of water soluble glucuronides (morphine 6 glucuronide, morphine 3 glucuronide). The kidney also plays a role in the conjugation of morphine, accounting for nearly 40% of its metabolism. Morphine 6 glucuronide is a mu agonist with greater potency than morphine. Patients with renal failure can develop very high levels of morphine 6 glucuronide and life threatening respiratory depression. Like morphine, meperidine is metabolized in the liver to several metabolites that are eventually excreted by the kidney. Normeperidine, the chief metabolite has analgesic and CNS excitatory effects including seizures at high levels. In contrast to morphine and meperidine, the clinical pharmacology of the fentanyl congeners is not grossly altered by kidney failure, and their large volume of distribution (Vd) minimizes any effect that decreased plasma protein binding may potentially play. Sufentanil pharmacokinetics are not altered in any consistent fashion by renal disease, although greater variability exists in its clearance and elimination half-life. No delay in recovery after alfentanil administration should be expected in patients with renal failure. Neither the pharmacokinetics nor the pharmacodynamics of remifentanil is altered by impaired renal function.

○ **One of your colleagues suggests that you use the same induction dose of sodium thiopental in patients with renal failure as you would in healthy patients, as the termination of clinical effect is due to redistribution and not metabolism or excretion. Your clinical experience does not support this. Why?**

Sodium thiopental is 75-85% protein bound to albumin and due to low plasma protein levels in renal failure one would expect greater free drug available to cross the blood brain barrier. Sodium thiopental also has weakly acidic properties with a pKa in the physiological range, making greater unionized levels available in the typically acidemic chronic renal failure patient. These changes may increase free drug availability from 15% in healthy patients to 28% in renal failure patients.

○ **What level of regional anesthesia is required for Extracorporeal Shock Wave Lithotripsy?**

A T_6 sensory level assures adequate anesthesia, as renal innervation is derived from T_{10}-L_2.

○   **What concerns are there following a regional technique for Extracorporeal Shock Wave Lithotripsy?**

The patient may initially become severely hypotensive due to vasodilation from the regional technique, compounded transiently by the warm water of the bath. On the other hand, hydrostatic pressure from the water bath on the legs and abdomen causes a redistribution of venous blood centrally, as well as a hydrostatically mediated increase in SVR. As a result, arterial blood pressure is likely to stabilize. The sudden increase in central venous volume, however, can precipitate congestive heart failure in patients with marginal cardiac reserve. When the patient leaves the bath the compressive effects of the bath are lost and the blood pressure again falls. If an epidural technique with loss-of-resistance to air is used and a large volume of air injected, this air can provide an interface for energy absorption which can result in epidural tissue damage. Foam tape used to secure epidural catheters should be clear of the blast path as this tape can absorb up to 80% of the shock wave energy and result in a failed lithotripsy.

○   **What is the importance of the EKG during Extracorporeal Shock Wave Lithotripsy?**

There is a risk of cardiac dysrhythmias due to the discharge of shock waves independent of the cardiac cycle. To minimize this problem the EKG is coupled to the lithotripsy so that the shockwaves are triggered by the R wave of the EKG. Therefore it is important that a good reliable EKG signal is obtained preferably with waterproof EKG electrodes. Shock wave induced cardiac arrhythmias occur in 10-14% of patients undergoing lithotripsy despite the fact that shock waves are synchronized with the patient's ECG and are delivered in the refractory period of the cardiac cycle. These arrhythmias are believed to be due to mechanical stresses on the conduction system exerted by the shock waves and can manifest as PACs, PVCs, Afib or SVT. EKG artifact during ESWL is also common.

○   **What are the absolute contraindications to Extra Corporeal Shock Wave Lithotripsy?**

Pregnancy, untreated bleeding disorders, and abdominal pacemakers are the only absolute contraindications to extra corporeal shock wave lithotripsy. Orthopedic instrumentation and abdominal aortic aneurysms are acceptable as long as they are not in the blast path.

○   **What determines the absorption of irrigating solution in transurethral resection of the prostrate?**

The following principles govern the amount of irrigating solution: (1) The height of the container of irrigating solution above the surgical table determines the hydrostatic pressure driving fluid into prostatic veins and sinuses. (2) The duration of surgical time for resection is proportional to the quantity of fluid that is absorbed. On average 10-30 mL of fluid is absorbed per minute of resection time, with as much as 6 to 8 L absorbed in some cases lasting up to 2 hours. Whether patients suffer complications as a result of absorption of irrigating fluid depends on the amount and type of fluid absorbed.

○   **What is the cause of transient blindness after transurethral resection of the prostate?**

Systemic absorption of glycine.

Glycine is a non essential amino acid which has a distribution similar to γ-aminobutyric acid, one of the inhibitory neurotransmitters. It has been suggested that glycine also is a major inhibitory transmitter acting in the spinal cord, brain stem, and retina. In addition, absorption of glycine may result in CNS toxicity as a result of its oxidative biotransformation to ammonia. Blood ammonia levels as high as 500uM have been detected. Deterioration of CNS function is said to occur when ammonia levels exceed 150 uM. In a prospective study examining glycine metabolism , blood ammonia levels were increased postoperatively in 12 of 26 patients in whom 1.5 % glycine levels were also measured. Of interest, glycine and ammonia levels did not correlate; in fact the opposite relationship was prevalent. Furthermore, high ammonia levels were not necessarily associated with CNS symptoms of toxicity.

○   **What are some of the bleeding complications associated with a TURP?**

A hypertrophied prostate is highly vascular and operative bleeding could be significant (2-5 ml/min of resection time, 20-50 ml/g of prostate.) Abnormal bleeding after TURP occurs in less than 1 percent of cases. The coagulopathy is deemed by some to be due to systemic fibrinolysis caused by prostatic release of plasminogen activator, which converts plasminogen into plasmin. Others believe that the bleeding diathesis is secondary to DIC triggered by the systemic absorption of resected prostate tissue, which is thromboplastin rich. If primary fibrinolysis is suspected, an intravenous bolus and infusion of aminocaproic acid may be an effective antidote.

O   **What level of spinal anesthesia is desirable for a TURP?**

An anesthetic level to T_{10} is necessary. A spinal anesthetic provides adequate anesthesia for the patient and good relaxation of the pelvic floor and the perineum for the surgeon. The signs and symptoms of water intoxication and fluid overload can be recognized early in an awake patient. An anesthetic level above T_{10}, however, may prevent the recognition of a bladder perforation.

O   **What symptoms may be associated with bladder perforation during TURP?**

Bladder perforation during TURP is a relatively common complication (1.1%) and may result in the urologist noting a diminished return of irrigating fluid. Most bladder perforations are extraperitoneal and occur during difficult resections with the cutting loop, knife electrode or resectascope tip, although others can occur from bladder overdistension with irrigation fluid. An extraperitoneal perforation typically results in pain in the periumbilical, inguinal, or suprapubic region. An intraperitoneal perforation may cause back pain or refer pain to the upper abdomen, the precordium or the shoulder. Other signs and symptoms may include pallor, sweating, abdominal rigidity, nausea and vomiting. The differential diagnosis for such symptomatology is broad and can range from myocardial ischemia or infarction to abdominal aneurysmal leak or rupture to tension pneumothorax. Epidural hematoma might be suspected with severe back pain and a working spinal block. Less critical considerations could range from acute appendicitis or cholecystitis to gastritis or peptic ulcers.

O   **What are the complications of lithotripsy?**

The complications of lithotripsy vary depending upon the technique. Any of the techniques can cause renal parenchymal damage and bleeding with subsequent postoperative urine outflow obstruction. Bacteremia and septicemia can also ensue.

Laser lithotripsy raises specific concerns for ureter mucosal damage or perforation with the rather sharp wire over which the laser is transmitted. Eye damage can occur from stray laser energy.

Percutaneous lithotripsy can result in perforation of bowel or great vessels. Patients are subject to all the risks of a prone patient, including loss of airway, blindness, neuropathy and positioning induced ischemia to the nose, breasts or genitalia. As the surgical site is near the diaphragm, pneumothorax is a possibility.

ESWL can induce cardiac dysrhythmia (10-14%), fatal pulmonary hemorrhage, hypotension, bony fracture and flank ecchymosis or hematoma. It can trigger congestive heart failure and can induce epidural nerve damage after epidural placement with loss of resistance to air. It can cause orthopedic implant or pacemaker destruction and inappropriate AICD firing. It could even cause fetal demise or AAA rupture in the poorly selected patient.

O   **What are the potential complications of intraperitoneal insufflation of CO_2 for laparoscopy?**

The main respiratory complications of intraperitoneal insufflation include endobronchial intubation, a 30-50% decrease in pulmonary compliance, and pneumothorax.

Cardiovascular risks include those of gas embolism, pneumomediastinum or pneumopericardium, increased vagal tone and dysrhythmia, and hypercarbia. There is a simultaneous decrease in venous return, increased vascular resistance of intraabdominal organs, increased systemic vascular resistance and resultant decreased cardiac output.

O   What are the particular complications of laparoscopy associated with urogenital surgery?

While unintentional extraperitoneal insufflation can always occur in laparoscopic cases, genitourinary surgery often intentionally demands such extravasation of gases. This carries additional risk of CO_2 subcutaneous emphysema. The large retroperitoneal area has facile communication with the thorax and can extend via the subcutaneous tissue to the head and neck. Postoperative pharyngeal swelling from submucous CO_2 can lead to airway compromise. The large surface area exposed can lead to marked acidosis. Postoperative oliguria may be caused by increased perirenal pressure from the insufflated gas.

O   What is a safe insufflation pressure for laparoscopy?

There is no truly safe pressure limit for laparoscopy. However, keeping pressures at or below 10-15 mm Hg is usually well tolerated, though tolerated less well in the obese, sicker ASA II or III patients.

O   What are the causes of renal failure after cardiopulmonary bypass (CPB)?

CPB induces hypotension and nonpulsatile flow which promotes renal vasoconstriction and decreased RBF. Surgery and CPB cause the release of norepinephrine, as well as activation of angiotensin with a renin release that persists well after CPB. Pump mediated platelet activation and elaboration of thromboxane as well as tissue release of endothelin may both add to renal vasoconstriction. Aortic cross-clamping may release aortic atheroemboli that circulate to the kidney.

Patients undergoing mitral valve replacement studies have shown that patients whose postoperative left atrial pressure decreases by 7 mm Hg compared to preoperative levels have a decrease in both sodium excretion and urine flow rate. This coincides with decreased circulating levels of ANP. While ARF after CPB occurs in less than 2% of patients, the mortality associated with it remains between 60-90%.

CARDIAC SURGERY

It Is Not The Brains That Matter Most, But That Which Guides Them - The Character, The Heart,
Generous Qualities, Progressive Ideas.
Fyodor Dostoyevsky

○   **What is the most common site of aortic aneurysm?**

The abdominal aorta. About 75% of all arteriosclerotic aneurysms are confined to the abdominal aorta, usually below the renal arteries. The other 25% are in the thoracic aorta, most commonly the arch over the descending portion.

○   **What are the most common sites of aortic dissection?**

Over 85% arise in one of two locations: 1) The ascending aorta within several centimeters of the aortic valve, and 2) The descending thoracic aorta distal to the origin of the subclavian artery at the site of the ligamentum arteriosum.

○   **Which hereditary disorders are associated with aortic dissection?**

Marfan's syndrome and Ehlers-Danlos syndrome.

○   **What is the most common presenting symptom of aortic dissection?**

Severe pain located in the anterior chest (ascending and arch dissections) and midscapular in the back for descending. This symptom is found in more than 90% of patients, typically abrupt and severe in onset, described as tearing in nature.

○   **What is the best imaging study for diagnosis of aortic dissection?**

MRI for hemodynamically stable patients (sensitivity 98.3% and specificity 97.8%) and transesophageal echocardiography for unstable patients, which can be performed in 15 minutes. Aortography is the gold standard, but used selectively due to its higher complication rate.

○   **Describe the medical management of aortic dissection.**

Acute medical management of all dissections generally involves medical therapy, even if definitive treatment is urgent surgery. The principles of medical management include:
- oxygenation
- monitoring (EKG, intra-arterial blood pressure, CVP, PAP, urine output, SpO_2)
- control of systolic blood pressure to 105 to 120 mm Hg (vasodilators)
- decreasing ejection velocity and heart rate (beta-blockers)
- transfusion as needed
- pain control

○   **What are the most commonly used drugs for the treatment of aortic dissection?**

Nitroglycerin, nitroprusside (vasodilators); beta-blockers and labetalol (decrease heart rate and contractility). Nitroglycerin is a relatively weak agent. Nitroprusside is generally very effective. Use of this agent alone, however, can result in increased shear forces associated with increased heart rate, thus, it is generally wise to use a beta blocker when administering nitroprusside. When nitroprusside is ineffective or contraindicated, labetalol is also an effective agent. This drug, a combination alpha-blocker and non-selective beta blocker, depresses shear forces as well as systolic blood pressure. Trimethaphan is a second-line agent for refractory hypertension, but the side effects of tachyphylaxis (develops within the first 24 hours), severe hypotension, somnolence, sympathoplegia and pupillary dilation renders this a seldom-used drug. More recently, some have advocated the use of nicardipine (Cardene), and effective vasodilator that works via calcium channel blockade.

○   **What are the most common side effects of nitroprusside?**

Reflex tachycardia in clinical doses. For overdose/toxicity, nausea, restlessness, somnolence, hypotension and cyanide toxicity. This generally develops after at least 48 hours of continuous use.

○   **You suspect severe LV systolic dysfunction in a patient newly admitted to the ICU. A pulmonary artery catheter is inserted, however, your pressure transducer is malfunctioning and your cardiac output machine is broken. What laboratory test will confirm your suspicions?**

Mixed venous oxygen saturation will determine whether the cardiac output and oxygen delivery is matched to oxygen demand. The normal SvO_2 is 75%, with a 5-10% decrease considered significant and usually preceding hemodynamic changes.

○   **What is the law of Laplace?**

The Laplace equation states: wall tension = P x R/ 2h

P = intraventricular pressure (dynes/cm^2)
R = inner radius (cm)
h = wall thickness

A simplified equation that describes the factors governing wall stress in the left ventricular chamber. According to Laplace, wall stress equals the pressure within a chamber multiplied by the radius of the chamber, divided by twice the chamber's wall thickness. When the heart dilates or fills to high pressures, wall tension increases, the LV must work harder and myocardial oxygen demand increases.

○   **A sustained ventricular tachycardia is well controlled with lidocaine 2 mg/min in a 55-year old man following a non-Q wave MI. He has a known history of ischemic cardiomyopathy. Day 3 of his admission, his speech becomes slurred, he is lethargic and when he is aroused he becomes very agitated. What should you do?**

The patient has classic findings of lidocaine-induced CNS toxicity, and you should strongly consider stopping this drug. Elderly patients and patients with heart failure or hepatic insufficiency are especially at risk due to the hepatic metabolism of lidocaine.

○   **What are the acute hemodynamic effects of furosemide administration?**

Pulmonary venous pressure falls. Furosemide causes mainly venodilation and reduces preload within 15 minutes of intravenous bolus. Diuresis starts 30 minutes after administration and peaks at 1 to 2.5 hours.

○   **A 72-year old woman admitted to the ICU with pulmonary edema is much improved after overnight diuresis, with a negative fluid balance of 4 liters. She suddenly develops polymorphic ventricular tachycardia requiring cardioversion. Her regular medications include furosemide 80 mg po bid. What is the likely etiology?**

Acute ischemia or infarction and electrolyte abnormalities, especially hypokalemia and hypomagnesemia may induce torsades de pointes in CHF patients after vigorous diuresis – especially in patients on chronic diuretics.

○   **A 65-year old man with known severe hypertension, CHF and COPD is intubated for acute pulmonary edema and suspected pneumonia. BP is 190/110 mm Hg, oxygen saturation is 94% on 60% oxygen. You successfully lower his blood pressure to 140/80 mm Hg with intravenous sodium**

nitroprusside, however, the patient develops chest pressure and his oxygen saturation decreases to 86%. What happened?

Three vascular effects of nitroprusside are the likely culprits, one pulmonary, and two cardiac. Nonselective dilation of the pulmonary arteriolar bed can worsen ventilation-perfusion mismatch, especially in patients with COPD or pneumonia, and cause desaturation. This desaturation may make coronary oxygen delivery insufficient and cause myocardial ischemia, leading to chest pain. "Coronary steal" (reduced perfusion to coronary arteries with fixed obstruction in the setting of arteriolar dilation by nitroprusside of arteries feeding non ischemic areas) may lead to ischemia and chest pain, with the decreased function of the heart causing some degree of pulmonary congestion and increasing V/Q mismatch. Finally, a decrease in coronary artery perfusion pressure related to a lowered aortic diastolic pressure may be the culprit. The presenting diastolic BP of 110mm Hg may have been necessary to perfuse the myocardium. Chest pain and arterial oxygen desaturation follow as described above.

O   **A 70-year-old man with systolic heart failure is refractory to appropriately administered escalating doses of furosemide. Suggest an option to treat his diuretic resistance.**

Loop diuretics is the only class of diuretics effective as single agents in moderate to severe CHF. Often, adding a second agent with a different site of action in the nephron, - e.g. a thiazide diuretic that prevents fluid reabsorption at a site distal to the loop of Henle - will enhance diuresis.

O   **Describe the typical findings for cardiac output, arterial-mixed venous oxygen difference and systemic vascular resistance in systolic congestive heart failure.**

Cardiac output is low, arterial-mixed venous oxygen difference is increased and systemic vascular resistance is increased.

O   **A 27-year-old man with past history of receiving chemotherapy for a hematologic malignancy presents with worsening dyspnea on exertion for several months. Exam reveals jugular venous distension (JVD) and rales throughout both lung fields. X-ray of the chest demonstrates cardiomegaly. Echocardiogram shows four chambers dilation with severely reduced LV function. What chemotherapeutic agent might the patient have received?**

Doxorubicin, which can present with cardiomyopathy, even years after its initial administration.

O   **Give several reasons why dobutamine is a superior inotropic drug versus dopamine for the treatment of congestive heart failure.**

Dobutamine acts as a vasodilator (SVR and PVR reduction) improving left and right ventricular systolic function, whereas dopamine, even at intermediate infusion rates, may cause peripheral vasoconstriction. Dobutamine is a direct agonist which causes less tachycardia at low doses and a greater increase in coronary blood flow, thereby, increasing cardiac output with less increase in myocardial oxygen demand.

O   **You place a pulmonary artery catheter in a severely malnourished alcoholic patient with peripheral edema and cardiomegaly. Findings include: elevated cardiac output, decreased arterial-mixed venous oxygen difference and systemic vascular resistance. What diagnosis should you consider?**

These are classic hemodynamic findings in beriberi heart disease (thiamine deficiency) and alcoholic cardiomyopathy in a patient with end-stage liver disease.

O   **What are the two most common causes of post-cardiopulmonary bypass bleeding, excluding surgical causes?**

Residual heparin, platelet dysfunction/thrombocytopenia.

O   **Name four beta-agonist inotropic drugs.**

Dopamine, dobutamine, norepinephrine and epinephrine.

○   **Name three vasodilator drugs used in cardiac surgery.**

Nitroprusside, nicardipine, and nitroglycerin.

○   **How do you treat hypertension during cardiopulmonary bypass (CPB)?**

Nitroprusside, isoflurane administered by calibrated vaporizer in the oxygenator gas inlet line and phentolamine in pediatric CPB. Hypertension is caused by high systemic vascular resistance or excessive perfusion flow and is treated with vasodilators.

○   **What is a type II reaction to protamine?**

Idiosyncratic anaphylactic or anaphylactoid reaction, presumably due to prior sensitization or patients with fish allergy.

○   **If a patient experiences a possible type II reaction to protamine coming off CPB and becomes severely hypotensive, what should you do?**

Stop protamine, give 100% oxygen, discontinue anesthetic agents, aggressively address intravascular volume expansion and selectively give a pulmonary vasodilator into the right side of the heart, and a vasoconstrictor/inotrope into the left (e.g. epinephrine). For refractory hypotension, re-institute cardiopulmonary bypass.

○   **What hemodynamic information is available from cardiac catheterization data?**

Cardiac output, cardiac index, right-sided pressures; atrium, ventricle and pulmonary artery, pulmonary capillary wedge pressure, and calculations of different types of vascular resistance (total pulmonary vascular resistance, systemic vascular resistance). Calculation of valve orifice area and detection and measurement of intra and extracardiac shunts is also reported. Cardiac output is usually 5 L/min (CI = 2.5 L/min/m^2). Total pulmonary resistance (PA pressure – LA pressure)/CO = 1.4 Woods units or 205 +/- 50 dynes.sec.cm. Systemic vascular resistance (MAP – CVP)/CO = 1130 +/- 18 dynes.sec.cm.

○   **What is the best assessment technique to measure LV preload?**

LVEDV (left ventricular end-diastolic volume), has traditionally been measured with a pulmonary artery catheter as LVEDP, assuming that LVEDP is equal to LA pressure, which is equal to wedge pressure. Other monitors measure stroke volume, maximum acceleration (contractility) and left ventricular ejection time (LVET) as a measure of preload status.

○   **T/F: The number of beta $_1$ receptors per unit area of the sarcolemma is fixed.**

False. Beta $_1$ receptors can increase and decrease in various disease states. These changes are called *upregulation* or *downregulation* of receptor density. In addition, the receptors can be desensitized or "internalized" by chemical changes making them unavailable for signal transmission.

○   **What factors contribute to *myocardial oxygen supply and demand*?**

The myocardium accounts for 11% of the total body oxygen consumption, but the coronary circulation receives only 4% of the cardiac output. *Myocardial oxygen supply* (arterial oxygen content, coronary blood flow = coronary artery diameter x coronary perfusion pressure) and *myocardial oxygen demand* (heart rate, wall tension, contractility) determine myocardial oxygen balance. Myocardial ischemia occurs when there is an imbalance between supply and demand, and it is usually predominantly subendocardial.

○   **T/F: Sinus tachycardia is associated with an increased thromboembolic risk.**

False. Sinus tachycardia is an increase in the normal heart rate to > 100 bpm. It usually respresents a normal physiological response to exercise or high adrenergic states, and rarely represents the presence of organic heart disease. Persistent sinus tachycardia may suggest an underlying cause such as infection, hyperthyroidism, anemia, and hypercarbia for many causes. As the synchrony between the atria and ventricle is maintained, there is seldom any hemodynamic changes, unless at very fast rates there is decreased LV filling.

○   **What is the relationship between cardiac output (CO) and mixed venous oxygen content (CVO_2) in the Fick equation?**

Cardiac Output (L/min) = VO_2 (oxygen consumption)/CaO_2 – CVO_2, where CaO_2 is the arterial oxygen content and CVO_2 is the mixed venous oxygen content. (This assumes no intracardiac shunt is present)

○   **What are the determinants of myocardial oxygen supply?**

The product of arterial oxygen content and the coronary blood flow.

○   **What are the variables affecting left ventricular filling in normal subjects?**

Age is the major independent factor affecting LV filling in normal subjects. Other variables include: gender, heart rate, systolic and diastolic blood pressure, aortic root and left atrial dimensions, left ventricular mass index, and left ventricular shortening fraction.

○   **Is there any morbidity associated with a junctional rhythm?**

Hypotension. Junctional rhythms may take the form of a tachycardia or an escape rhythm during significant bradycardia or high-grade atrioventricular block. The morbidity is usually related to the underlying cause. Junctional tachycardia is often a symptom of digitalis toxicity, recent cardiac surgery for valve replacement or acute MI. Junctional bradycardia is symptomatic of increased vagal tone or the presence of sinus node disease (sick sinus syndrome or complete heart block).

○   **A patient presents in septic shock, CVP < 8 mm Hg, mean arterial pressure < 60 mm Hg, SVO_2 = 70%. Would you fluid resuscitate this patient or start pressors?**

Pressors are drugs that make the blood pressure go up. There are five components of blood pressure: preload, contractility, afterload, rate and rhythm.   Resuscitation should start with oxygenation SpO_2 > 95%, pH > 7.3 and < 7.5, crystalloid or colloid infusion to CVP 8-12 mm Hg. Drugs causing profound alpha constriction should be avoided if systolic pressure > 90 mmHg as renal blood flow increases to that point, and then decreases. If the SVO_2 is < 70%, transfuse with packed RBC to a Hct > 30% and then start inotropes to maintain the SVO_2 > 70%.

○   **What is the effect of pressors on preload?**

End-diastolic pressure (LVEDV) is used as a clinical index of preload. In the normal heart, RV preload is determined by venous return which is dependent on venous tone, blood volume, heart rate, gravity and the changes in pleural pressure generated during ventilation. LV preload is dependent on RV preload, atrial contraction, ventricular compliance, and pulmonary vascular resistance. Pressors can increase or decrease preload depending on their relative effects on vascular resistance, heart rate and cardiac output.

○   **What is the definition of coronary artery dominance?**

Dominance is defined by the source of the posterior descending artery (PDA), which is usually 70% right (right coronary artery), 20% balanced and 10% left (left circumflex artery).

❍   **What are the sources of noncoronary collateral flow (NCCF)?**

NCCF to the heart is supplied from noncoronary routes such as mediastinal, pericardial and bronchial collateral channels, through pericardial reflections surrounding pulmonary and systemic veins as well as from the vasa vasorum along major blood vessels. The NCCF functions as supplemental feeding arteries during myocardial ischemia. Abnormal sources include: a left superior pulmonary vein that drains into the coronary sinus and right heart, patient ductus arteriosus or a systemic to pulmonary artery shunt, anomalous systemic venous drainage into the left heart, and aortic regurgitation.

❍   **During cardiopulmonary bypass how does the perfusionist maintain constant venous return?**

The reservoir. With membrane oxygenators the reservoir is the first component of the extracorporeal circuit which receives venous drainage as well as the cardiotomy drainage. Blood then passes to the arterial pump. The reservoir serves as a capacitance chamber which buffers the fluctuations between venous return and arterial outflow. This protects the patient from the risk of systemic air embolism if venous drainage is reduced and the system is effectively pumped dry. The reservoir also serves as an air trap and allows administration of blood, fluids or drugs to the circuit.

❍   **List several causes of hypotension during CPB.**

Most incidents on bypass present as hypotension and most are attributable to human error. An incidence of 0.4 to 1% associated with permanent neurologic injury or death rate of 1 in 1000 to 1 in 1500 has been reported. Hypotension related to the CPB is especially common on initiation of bypass, but may be caused by: anything limiting pump flow (low venous return, electrical failure, gas embolism, clotting, line separation, blood leaks, mechanical failure, and failure of the oxygenator), aortic dissection, low peripheral resistance (transfusion-related complications, anaphylactic or anaphylactoid reactions, hematocrit < 18-20%, drug effects especially anesthetic or vasodilators). Again, the determinants of BP – preload, contractility (in this case roller pump function) and afterload need to be investigated.

❍   **What are the hemodynamic changes associated with mitral regurgitation?**

Mitral regurgitation produces volume overloading of the left ventricle. Anatomic structures integral to competency of the mitral valve include: posterior LA wall, anterior and posterior valve leaflets, chordae tendinae and papillary muscles and their attachments to the LV wall. Acute MR (non-compliant LA) results in increased left atrial pressure and decreased cardiac output which can cause pulmonary edema, pulmonary hypertension and RV failure. Compensatory changes lead to worsening of the MR as a result of tachycardia and increase systemic vascular resistance. Chronic MR (compliant LA) is compensated by LV hypertrophy and dilation and LA dilation, so pressures remain low in the LA and there is little effect to the pulmonary vasculature and RV until late in the progress of the disease.

❍   **Describe the physiologic effects of nitric oxide on cardiac function.**

NO relaxes arteriolar smooth muscle and inhibits platelet aggregation. Nitroglycerine generates NO which causes coronary artery vasodilation. In the heart, NO inhibits L-type Ca^{2+} channels but stimulates sarcoplasmic reticulum (SR) Ca^{2+} release, leading to variable effects on myocardial contractility.

❍   **T/F: The classic signs of traumatic cardiac tamponade include distended neck veins and muffled heart sounds?**

False. The classic signs of cardiac tamponade are usually absent. If the blood in the pericardial sac is clotted, needle pericardiocentesis will also be negative.

❍   **During cardiopulmonary bypass with a temperature of 28^0C and a hematocrit of 24%, the temperature corrected $PaCO_2$ is 50 mmHg and uncorrected $PaCO_2$ is 60 mmHg. What is the appropriate management?**

Increase the fresh gas flow in the oxygenator. In a bubble and membrane oxygenator, CO_2 transfer is proportional to total gas flow. The higher the total gas flow the lower the CO_2. At higher flows it may be necessary to add CO_2 to prevent hypocarbia.

O   **What are the contraindications to intraaortic balloon pump (IABP)?**

Relatively few. Contraindications include: aortic aneurysm, aortic dissection, severe aortic insufficiency, severe peripheral vascular disease and irreversible brain damage.

O   **What are the main determinants of myocardial oxygen consumption (MVO2)?**

Ventricular wall tension, preload (LVEDV), afterload (systemic vascular resistance), contractility (dP/dT) and heart rate.

O   **During cardiopulmonary bypass the activation of fibrinolysis results in postoperative bleeding complications. What are the treatment strategies to miminize blood loss?**

During CPB, activation of fibrinolysis results in an increased activation of plasminogen and the reduction of plasmin inhibitors. CPB also initiates elastase release which may be an indicator of postoperative inflammatory reaction and could correlate with a reduction in AT III.

The use of lysine analogs (epsilon aminocaproic acid or tranexamic acid) in cardiac surgical patients results in less chest tube drainage but significant decreases in transfusion requirements have not been consistently documented. Aprotinin inhibits thrombin activation, fibrinolysis and has a protecting effect on thrombocytes. Aprotinin has been demonstrated to be highly effective in reducing bleeding and transfusion requirements in high risk patients undergoing repeat median sternotomy or in patients who are taking aspirin. Results from multicenter studies of aprotinin show there is no greater risk of early graft thrombosis, MI, or renal failure in aprotinin treated patients. The incidence of stroke may be lower in aprotinin treated patients.

O   **What are the key features of coronary blood flow?**

Flow is tightly coupled to oxygen demand. When oxygen consumption increases (normally 8-10 O_2 min/100g), there is an increase in coronary blood flow that is nearly proportionate to the increase in MVO_2. The myocardium has the highest A-VO_2 gradient of a vital organ (10-13 ml/100 ml). Autoregulation occurs between 60 and 200 mm Hg perfusion pressure. Mediators for autoregulation of coronary blood flow include adenosine and nitric oxide. Sympathetic activation results in coronary vasodilation and increased coronary flow due to increased metabolic activity (increased heart rate and contractility) despite direct vasoconstrictor effects mediated by α_1-adrenoceptors. Flow in the left coronary artery is pulsatile in nature. Flow is lower during systole with isovolumetric contraction and ejection than during diastole therefore, the endocardium is more susceptible to ischemia especially at lower perfusion pressure. Tachycardia limits flow in diastole, which is significant in patient with coronary artery disease with limited reserve.

Coronary blood flow is proportional to coronary perfusion pressure divided by coronary vascular resistance. Coronary perfusion pressure is determined primarily by the aortic diastolic pressure and coronary vascular resistance is determined by external compressive forces as well as metabolic, endothelial and neural factors which regulate intrinsic coronary tone via auto-regulation.

O   **What is the incidence and risk factors for adverse neurologic outcome following CABG surgery?**

The overall incidence is reported as 6.1%. Adverse cerebral outcomes included: focal injury; stupor or coma; or seizures, memory deficit or deterioration in intellectual function. Risk factors include: age, proximal aortic atherosclerosis and history of neurological disease. The landmark study by Newman et all demonstrated the incidence of cognitive decline was 53% at discharge, 36 % at six weeks, 24% at six months, and rising to 42 % at 5 years. Possible mechanisms include: progression of concomitant disease, stress of major OR or specific events during CABG surgery (atheroemboli, microemboli, cerebral hypoperfusion and systemic inflammatory response).

○   **What factors increase SVO$_2$ (mixed venous oxygen saturation)?**

SVO$_2$ varies directly with cardiac output, hemoglobin and arterial saturation and inversely with oxygen consumption. The normal SVO2 is 75%. When the SVO$_2$ is less than 30%, tissue oxygen balance is compromised and anaerobic metabolism ensues.

○   **What conditions result in inadequate tissue oxygenation?**

Hypoxic hypoxia (inadequate PO$_2$ in arterial blood), anemic hypoxia (decrease in hemoglobin or conditions where Hg is ineffective in binding oxygen ie: carbon monoxide poisoning), circulatory hypoxia (inadequate cardiac output) and histotoxic hypoxia (cyanide poisoning).

○   **What is the indication for venodilators (or lasix and rotating tourniquets) in the treatment of congestive heart failure?**

To reduce preload in patients presenting with dyspnea due to high filling pressures causing pulmonary congestion.

○   **What is the mean arterial pressure (MAP)?**

MAP is calculated from the systolic and diastolic pressures as: diastolic pressure + 1/3 (systolic-diastolic pressure). Most practitioners agree that the MAP should be maintained between 60 mm Hg and 70 mm Hg to ensure adequate perfusion of vital organs. Another formula is (systolic + 2 x diastolic)/3

○   **Albert Nobel stabilized nitroglycerin for dynamite and some postulate that he died of nitroglycin toxicity. What are the adverse effects of nitroglycerin (NTG)?**

Headache, hypotension, methemoglobinemia and hypoxemia due to V/Q mismatch.

○   **What is the mechanism of NTG in the treatment of myocardial ischemia?**

1. Venous dilation: a. reduces preload which decreases intra-myocardial wall tension and intraventricular work, b. reduces left ventricular filling pressure which decreases myocardial oxygen demand and ischemia, c. increases cardiac output in CHF with no or little decrement change in normal hearts

2. Arterial dilation: a. dilates large coronary arteries, b. antagonizes vasospasm, c. increases coronary collateral blood flow, d. decreases systemic vascular resistance.

○   **What is the differential diagnosis of hypotension (specific to cardiac surgery) following CABG?**

Preload: bleeding

Rhythm: the incidence of atrial fibrillation or flutter is 20-30%, especially on day 2 or 3 postop

Left or right ventricular dysfunction and low cardiac output: inadequate protection of the myocardium during aortic cross-clamping, pulmonary edema, acute left ventricular distension or other trauma, uncorrected valvular lesion or valvular incompetence, reduced coronary blood flow due to graft occlusion, pericardial tamponade with cardiac compression or intracardiac shunting.

Low serum levels of thyroid hormone

Systemic vascular resistance low: normothermic perfusion or longer pump times, rewarming after hypothermic CABG, sepsis, vasodilator therapy.

○   **What is the conventional TEE view for detection of intraoperative myocardial ischemia?**

The transgastric short-axis view at mid-papillary level is most commonly employed for ischemia detection. A satisfactory alternate is the four-chamber view, switching intermittently to the long-axis.

○   **What are the physiologic effects of IABP counterpulsation therapy?**

The tip of the IABP lies in the descending aorta just below the origin of the left subclavian artery. Inflation and deflation of the balloon are synchronized to the patient's cardiac cycle. Inflation at the onset of diastole augments diastolic pressure and increases coronary perfusion pressure as well as improves the relationship between myocardial oxygen supply and demand. Deflation occurs just prior to the onset of systole with improvement in cardiac output, ejection fraction, wall tension and a decrease in heart rate, PCWP and systemic vascular resistance.

○   **What are the factors that affect left-to-right shunt in patients with VSD?**

Four types of VSDs: membraneous, muscular, outflow tract and endocardial cushion type. The larger the defect the more pressure is transmitted to the right ventricle. When the VSD is more than 50% of the area of the aortic root the RV and LV pressures will equalize. The determining factor at this point for the amount of left-to-right shunting becomes the relative systemic and pulmonary vascular resistances. Muscular ventricular septal defects become smaller during systole allowing less shunting. Symptoms with VSD usually start with a QP:QS ratio of 2.5:1 or more. A combination of ASD and VSD will increase to left-to-right shunting at the ventricular level. Aortic stenosis, aortic insufficiency, mitral stenosis and pulmonary stenosis will also influence the shunt flow.

○   **Which clinical situations may be associated with heparin resistance from acquired antithrombin deficiency?**

Heparin binds to plasma proteins including platelet factor 4, fibrinogen, factor VIII and histidine-rich glycoproteins. Many of the heparin-binding proteins are acute phase reactants, so the phenomenon of heparin resistance due to altered clearance is often encountered in acutely ill patients, those with malignancy and during peri- or postpartum periods. Drug-induced causes include aprotonin and nitroglycerine (controversial). Its association with low antithrombin levels is also a point of heated discussion in the literature and includes: infective endocarditis, intraaortic balloon counterpulsation, oral contraceptives, shock, low grade intravascular coagulation, prior heparin or streptokinase therapy, presence of clot within the circulation, neonatal respiratory distress syndrome, and increased platelets or factor VIII levels.

○   **Describe the TEE findings of mitral regurgitation associated with myocardial infarction and sudden hemodynamic collapse.**

Rupture of the posteromedial papillary muscle (accounting for 90% of papillary muscle ruptures), a wide gap in mitral coaptation, eccentric significant mitral regurgitation swirling in the left atrium, with a large flow convergence.

○   **A patient with HOCM (hypertrophic cardiomyopathy) presents in acute heart failure and is treated with diuresis, nitrates and inotropic agents. What would you predict would be the outcome of this therapy?**

The patient's condition becomes more critical. The correct management is volume administration, slowing the heart and increasing afterload. The key pathophysiology of HOCM is a hypertrophied interventricular septum which can lead to "functional" outflow tract obstruction if the ventricle is empty or hypercontractile. An associated anomaly called systolic anterior motion (of the anterior mitral leaflet) or "SAM" contributes to the obstruction when the anterior leaflet bulges into the outflow tract resulting in mitral regurgitation. Both outflow tract obstruction and mitral regurgitation are exacerbated by inotropic therapy and hypovolemia.

○   **What are the limitations of the ACT clotting test in monitoring high-dose heparin anticoagulation?**

The ACT is less precise than the PTT, and lacks high correlation with the PTT or with heparin antifactor Xa levels. The ACT is influenced by a number of variables including the platelet count, platelet function, lupus anticoagulants, factor deficiencies, ambient temperature, hypothermia and hemodilution. As the various methods are not standardized, results from different methods are not interchangeable. Aprotinin will prolong celite-based ACTs but generally not kaolin-based ACT, unless very high initial bolus doses of aprotinin are administered.

○   **How do you determine if an unexpected PTT prolongation is due to heparin contamination?**

Measure the PTT before and after heparinase treatment. Heparinase degrades unfractionated heparin, most importantly the pentasaccharide sequence which is the antithrombin binding site required for heparin anticoagulation. The resulting small fragments lack anticoagulant activity.

○   **Describe the maneuvers a nurse anesthetist should perform in the event of a massive air embolism on CPB.**

Position the patient in steep Trendelenburg with bilateral compression of the carotid arteries, wait until the surgeon and perfusionist have stopped the pump and isolated the patient from the circuit, performed retrograde perfusion through an exit wound in the aorta, removed the aortic cannula, purged the arterial circuit of air and placed the aortic cannula in the SVC. The perfusate temperature is decreased to 20 degrees Celcius and once all of the air is expelled from the aorta, the aortic cannula is placed in the ascending aorta and the CPB restarted at high flow rates. The coronary arteries are massaged and all 4 heart chambers vented. The MAP is increased to 65 mm Hg, the FiO_2 is set at 100% and the $PaCO_2$ in maintained in the low 30s. The nurse anesthetist should administer steroids and mannitol. Discontinue bypass with the systolic pressure > 100 mm Hg and low filling pressures. Contact the Hyperbaric Facility.

○   **What are the EKG signs of right ventricular infarction?**

A routine 12 lead EKG may not be very helpful. Inferior ischemic changes accompanied by ST depression in lead V1, V2 or V3 or ST elevation in lead III greater than lead II may be suggestive. A more common method of assessing RV infarction is the 15 lead EKG with elevated ST segments of 1 mm or more in at least one of the leads V4R, V5R or V6R. Presence of Q or inverted T waves is not considered an indicator of ischemia or infarction.

○   **What are the clinical findings frequently associated with a right ventricular infarct?**

Second or third degree AV block requiring inotropic, chronotropic or pacemaker support, elevated jugular venous pressure and an inability to tolerate preload reduction (especially nitroglycerine or morphine administration).

○   **Why is it so critically important to avoid atrial arrhythmias in a patient with aortic stenosis?**

Narrowing of the aortic orifice from 2.5 or 3.5 cm^2 to about 1 cm^2 leads to concentric left ventricular hypertrophy and a reduction in left ventricular compliance. Left ventricular filling during diastole depends on adequate preload as well as atrial contraction which contributes less than 20% of filling in the normal heart, but may contribute twice this amount in aortic stenosis. As the aortic valve area diminishes below 1 cm^2 to 0.5 cm^2, the left ventricle will begin to dilate and the patient may develop atrial fibrillation and symptoms of pulmonary congestion or syncope with exertion.

○   **Describe the pathophysiology of aortic regurgitation.**

Volume overload of the left ventricle, with dilatation and eccentric hypertrophy. The left ventricle generates a very large stroke volume, aided by peripheral dilatation, to make up for the regurgitant backwards flow through the aortic valve during diastole. The heart rate is usually elevated as this reduces the proportion of time spent in diastole. With severe, compensated AR the regurgitant flow may exceed 20 L/min, giving a total cardiac output of 25 L/min.

○ **What are the anesthetic considerations for mitral regurgitation?**

Cardiac output is optimized when the heart is full and reasonably fast, with the blood pressure maintained at low-normal with afterload reduction. Bradycardia should be avoided as it is associated with an increase in ventricular size leading to valvular dilatation and an increase in the regurgitant fraction. Contractility of the left ventricle is difficult to determine without a PAC or TEE so one should avoid myocardial depression acknowledging that these patients will often require inotropic support during general anesthesia.

○ **What are the indications for transvenous pacemaker insertion?**

Bradycardia, tachyarrhythmias, and other conduction system disturbances. The purpose of temporary transvenous pacemaker insertion is to provide standby pacing in the event of sudden complete heart block, to increase heart rate during periods of symptomatic bradycardia and to control sustained supraventricular or ventricular tachycardia with overdrive pacing.

○ **Describe triggering and timing of inflation and deflation of the IABP.**

The most common method of triggering the IABP is from the R wave of the patient's EKG. Inflation starts in the middle of the T wave at the beginning of diastole which is noted on the dichrotic notch on the arterial waveform and deflation is set to occur prior to the ending of the QRS complex, immediately prior to the arterial upstroke. The arterial waveform may be used if synchronization with the EKG mode is difficult, as in tachyarrhythmias or poor EKG signals.

○ **What markers are used for the laboratory diagnosis of myocardial infarction?**

None is completely sensitive and specific for myocardial infarction and timing is important, as well as correlation with the patient's symptoms and EKG findings. Creatine kinase (total: mostly found in skeletal muscle) and creatine kinase-MB fraction (15 to 40% of isoenzyme CK in cardiac muscle is MB, with < 2% in skeletal muscle) are routinely monitored. CK-MB rises in serum within 2 to 8 hours of onset of infarction, peaks for 12 hours and then falls over the next 1 to 3 days. The cardiac index is the ratio of CK to CK-MB and is a sensitive indicator of myocardial injury. CK-MG isoforms 1 and 2 can also be measured electrophoretically, but this is labor intensive, with false positive test results in patients with congestive heart failure. Troponins I and T are highly specific for myocardial injury. They begin to increase following MI within 3 to 12 hours, and remain elevated 5 to 9 days for troponin I and up to 2 weeks for troponin T. Measuring the rise in myoglobin may help in determing the size of the myocardial infarction. LDH begins to rise 12 to 24 hours after the event, peaks in 2 to 3 days and gradually dissipates in 5 go 14 days. With myocardial injury isoenzyme 1 is greater in concentration than iso-2, which is inverse to the normal relationship.

○ **Discuss the EKG diagnosis of myocardial ischemia.**

EKG findings depend on the duration (acute versus evolving/chronic), extent (transmural versus subendocardial) and localization (anterior versus inferior-posterior) of ischemia or infarction. EKG abnormalities (ST segmenet, T or Q waves or left bundle branch block) may indicate myocardial ischemia within 90 minutes of onset of symptoms, with serial EKGs more diagnostic than a single tracing. Transmural ischemia is seen with ST elevation and sometimes tall positive T waves; the overlying leads of an area of subendocardial ischemia show ST segment depression and ST elevation in lead aVR. Severe ischemia or MI can occur with slight or even absent ST-T changes.

O   **A patient scheduled for vascular surgery has evidence of myocardium at risk for ischemia on preoperative diagnostic imaging studies. How can you decrease the risk of perioperative ischemia and atrial fibrillation?**

Prophylactic beta-blockade at least 7 days in advance of moderate-to-high risk surgery, titrating the patient's heart rate to 60 to 70 beats per minutes. Postoperatively narcotics and additional beta-blockers should be given to reach a target heart rate of 80 beats per minute. This is a class 1 recommendation from the American College of Cardiology/American Heart Association guidelines.

O   **What is the treatment of pericardial tamponade?**

In this condition, blood or fluid collects within the pericardium preventing the ventricles from adequately filling. Treatment is pericardiocentesis in symptomatic patients, keeping the patient "oxygenated, fast, full and tight." Potential causes include bacterial or viral infections, dissecting thoracic aortic aneurysm, heart surgery, blunt or stab injury to the heart, lung cancer, acute MI, renal failure, hypothyroidism, systemic lupus erythematosus or radiation therapy to the chest.

O   **What is the risk of pulmonary artery rupture using a PA catheter?**

Estimated at 0.2% of patients, associated with a 50% mortality rate. Rupture of the pulmonary artery usually occurs if the PA catheter balloon is overinflated while in the wedged position.

O   **Does echocardiography have a role in the diagnosis of pulmonary embolism?**

Echocardiography can be helpful in the diagnosis of pulmonary embolism, although the gold standard is still pulmonary angiography. TEE findings may include: evidence of acute right ventricular pressure overload with right ventricular dilation and hypokinesis, pulmonary hypertension and the paradoxical motion of the interventricular septum due to a shift by a dilated right ventricle or direct identification of thrombotic masses in the pulmonary arteries or floating intracavitary thrombi. Results of TEE are highly dependent on the expertise of the echocardiographer.

O   **Immediately following aortic crossclamp you notice ST depressions. What hemodynamic factors have led to this myocardial ischemia?**

Sudden dramatic increase in afterload prevents ventricular emptying, produces a sudden increase in preload, wall tension, and subendocardial myocardial oxygen demand.

O   **What differentiates LV versus RV increased function?**

The LV is a pressure pump that increases strength of contraction while the RV is thinner walled and responds more to volume.

EYES, EARS, NOSE, THROAT SURGERY

It Is The Tragedy Of The World That No One Knows What He Doesn't Know – And The Less A Man Knows, The More Sure He Is He Knows Everything.
Joyce Cary

○ **What are the causes of recurrent laryngeal nerve (RLN) injury?**

Stretching of the nerve (retraction or positioning injury), direct surgical trauma, ischemia or misadventure during endotracheal intubation.

○ **How is the diagnosis of RLN injury made?**

The patient may complain of hoarseness or a weak voice. Direct or indirect laryngoscopy reveals the ipsilateral vocal cord in a paramedian position due to the unopposed action of the cricothyroid muscle on the same side, resulting in an incompetent glotttis. The RLN innervates all the intrinsic muscles of the larynx except for the cricothyroid and inferior pharyngeal constrictors. Bilateral injury results in closure of the glottis following extubation, creating a true asphyxial emergency.

○ **What special anesthetic considerations are necessary for patient safety during laser surgery?**

Unintentional injury during a laser procedure may include direct laser exposure in non-target areas and indirect injury due to ignition of the drapes or endotracheal tube resulting in burns. Preventive measures include wearing appropriate protective eyewear, using roughened surfaces on metal surgical equipment, moistening combustible materials, maintaining deep anesthesia or using muscle relaxants to prevent unintentional movement, limiting FiO_2, consider nasotracheal intubation and/or using a laser-safe tube. All personnel must complete a laser safety module and be prepared to extinguish a flame.

○ **What measures can be taken to reduce the risk of laser-generated airway fires?**

- Use of a specially designed metal, wrapped or laser-proof endotracheal tube
- Inflation of the endotracheal tube cuff with saline or water. The fluid acts as a heat sink and allows more energy to be absorbed before perforation and if penetrated the escaping liquid helps extinguish any fire
- Avoid nitrous oxide which supports combustion
- Reduction in inspired oxygen concentration to less than 30% (helium or air)
- Choice of ventilation techniques not requiring an endotracheal tube such as jet ventilation
- Nasotracheal intubation
- Reduction of heat by limiting laser exposure (short, frequent bursts)
- Moistening exposed flammable surfaces

○ **What are the major risk factors for airway fires?**

The requirements are fuel (combustible material), oxygen and heat (flame). The fuel is usually supplied as a polymer endotracheal tube, oxygen from the anesthesia machine, and heat by either a laser or electrocautery device.

○ **Describe the emergency management of an airway fire.**

The acceptable management of an airway fire includes: discontinue ventilation, turn off the oxygen supply, remove the endotracheal tube from the airway, extinguish any residual flames in the airway with sterile water or saline and remove any smoldering residue from the patient's airway. Re-establish the airway and ventilate with air until it is certain that nothing remains burning and then switch to 100% oxygen. Bronchoscopy should be performed immediately while ventilating with a jet ventilator or using the smallest endotracheal tube possible. Re-intubate if tracheal/airway damage and ensuing edema is suspected. Steroids should be given and airway gases humidified. A chest x-ray should be performed and the patient observed in the ICU. If the airway burn is significant, tracheostomy and mechanical ventilation may be necessary.

〇   **What are the causes of inspiratory stridor in infants?**

Upper airway obstruction including obstruction from enlarged tonsils and/or adenoids, midface hypoplasia, laryngomalacia or other congenital laryngeal anomalies and infectious processes such as croup. All of these abnormalities occur above the thoracic inlet.

〇   **What are the anesthetic implications of the use of intraocular sulfur hexafluoride (SF_6)?**

SF_6 is injected into the posterior chamber of the eye to facilitate retinal re-attachment. In patients with an intact globe, SF_6 can absorb nitrous oxide resulting in bubble enlargement and an increase in intraocular pressure. If used, NO_2 should be replaced with 100% oxygen 15 minutes before the injection procedure. In addition NO_2 should be avoided in any subsequent general anesthetic administered within 10 days.

〇   **What are the anesthetic implications in the management of bleeding during middle ear surgery?**

Successful surgery in the middle ear requires a bloodless operative field. Infiltration of the surrounding tissues with epinephrine-containing solutions provides some hemostasis, but often intraoperative hypotension must be induced. Care should be taken to choose appropriate patients for this technique, as hypotension may induce ischemia of perfusable organs and tissues. A recent article has advocated the use of propofol versus isoflurane for this technique because propofol helps to maintain middle ear blood flow autoregulation. Elevation of the head of the OR table to reduce CVP and improve venous drainage of the head and neck may be helpful, but can predispose the patient to venous air embolism.

〇   **What is the most feared complication of infection in the retropharyngeal space?**

Descending necrotizing mediastinitis, with mortality rates approaching 50%.

〇   **What fascial space(s) is involved in Ludwig's angina?**

The submandibular space, with secondary involvement of the submental space.

〇   **What is Ludwig's angina?**

It is a cellulitis of the floor of the mouth caused by bacterial infection of the sublingular and/or submandibular tissues. It can rapidly lead to stridor and eventually asphyxia and death due to acute airway obstruction. Antibiotic therapy is usually ineffective due to mixed bacterial flora and poor penetration into the space.

〇   **How is the airway secured in a patient with Ludwig's Angina?**

Awake intubation or cricothyroidotomy under local anesthesia is preferred. The patient should not be anesthetized prior to securing the airway.

〇   **What is the most common origin of infection in patients with Ludwig's angina?**

Dental abscesses.

〇   **What are the most common local findings in patients with Ludwig's angina?**

Swelling of the floor of the mouth and tongue, fever, and suprahyoid firmness without fluctuation.

○   **What is the most common cause of death in Ludwig's angina?**

Acute airway obstruction (75%).

○   **What two means of maintaining the airway are recommended in Ludwig's angina?**

Tracheostomy or cricothyroidotomy, with tracheostomy preferred.

○   **What are the most important organisms in Ludwig's angina?**

Aerobic streptococcus, staphylococcus, bacteroides, and peptostreptococcus.

○   **What is the antibiotic of choice for Ludwig's angina?**

Penicillin, although clindamycin or ampicillin/sulbactam should be considered with the recent rise in beta-lactamase producing organisms.

○   **What are the most common presenting signs of anterolateral pharyngeal space infections?**

Trismus, fever, chills, swelling at the angle of the mandible and medial bulging of the pharyngeal wall.

○   **What are the most common findings on lateral neck x-rays in patients with retropharyngeal abscess?**

Prevertebral soft tissue widening, air-fluid levels, loss of cervical lordosis and cervical osteomyelitis.

○   **What are the consequences of N_2O administration in middle ear surgery?**

Inhaling a high concentration of nitrous oxide can result in increasing pressure in a noncompliant cavity such as the middle ear. Normally the pressure in the middle ear is passively vented via the Eustachian tube but surgical trauma, edema or underlying disease may obstruct the Eustachian tube and prevent decompression.

○   **Is nitrous oxide contraindicated in middle ear surgery?**

Middle ear pressure rises with N_2O administration and with its removal negative pressure may develop as the N_2O is rapidly reabsorbed if the middle ear does not communicate with the atmosphere. Rupture of the tympanic membrane, nausea, vomiting and development of serious otitis have been documented. It is generally recommended that the N_2O be discontinued 10-30 minutes before closure of the middle ear.

○   **What are the limits of epinephrine injection when given for hemostasis?**

Classically, epinephrine administration during anesthesia is limited to *2.1* mcg/kg with halothane, 10.9 mcg/kg with enflurane and *6.7* mcg/kg with isoflurane. Children seem to be able to tolerate higher doses than adults. Volatile anesthetics sensitize the myocardium to the atrial and ventricular arrhythmogenic effects of epinephrine.

○   **Are non-depolarizing muscle relaxants contraindicated in surgery where facial nerve preservation is a concern?**

To identify the facial nerve at least 10-20% of the muscle twitch response must be preserved. Realistically, the use of non-depolarizing muscle relaxants may be implicated as contributory if the patient demonstrates facial nerve dysfunction postoperatively. Despite monitoring, the surgical risk of facial nerve paralysis is 0.6-3.0%.

O   **A patient develops ventricular ectopy during right radical neck dissection. Does this operation raise specific concerns of arrhythmia?**

Prolonged Q-T interval resulting in a lower threshold for ventricular arrhythmia is commonly associated with right but not left radical neck dissection. This presumably results from trauma to the right stellate ganglion and cervical autonomic nervous system during dissection. Torsades de pointes is a possible arrhythmia.

O   **What is the risk of hemorrhage and mortality after elective tonsillar and adenoid surgery?**

Postoperative hemorrhage occurs at a rate of 0.06-0.9% in various studies. Mortality has been reported at 1:10,000 in the 1960's; with more recent studies, mortality has been estimated to be 1:14,000, unadjusted for age.

O   **When is bleeding after adenotonsillectomy likely to occur?**

Three fourths of bleeds after adenotonsillectomy occur within the first six hours after surgery. The remaining 25% occur in the remaining 24 hours. Occasionally bleeding occurs as late as 5-10 days after surgery and is usually associated with infection.

O   **A 5-year-old presents 10 hours after tonsillectomy vomiting frank blood. He is tachypneic, hypotensive and anxious. Can he under go mask induction before an IV is established?**

No. An IV or IV's should be started and intravascular volume replaced prior to induction and a rapid sequence planned. If no IV can be started, and emergent induction is required to control bleeding, IM ketamine would be a better choice, with the most rapid control of the airway possible to prevent aspiration. Transfusion of blood should be dictated by following serial hematocrits. The end point of fluid replacement should be return of blood pressure and heart rate toward normal.

O   **Beyond fluid replacement how should the child be prepared for surgery?**

The child should be typed and cross-matched as indicated by hematocrit. Coagulation studies should be obtained. The child should be treated as a full stomach.

O   **How should a child with post-tonsillectomy bleed be induced?**

Awake intubation is not practically feasible in an anxious frightened child. Options include either rapid sequence induction or mask induction with cricoid pressure. Regardless of the method chosen, two suction catheters, duplicate laryngoscopes and endotracheal tubes are prepared and a physician experienced in emergent cricothyroidotomy should be present. If hemorrhage is brisk, laryngoscopy and intubation may be performed with the head turned to the lateral position.

O   **A 4-year-old child presents to the emergency department. The child was well six hours earlier but has since developed a fever and dyspnea. The child is leaning forward, drooling and complaining of a sore throat. How should this child be managed?**

The diagnosis of acute epiglottitis must be considered until ruled out. The child should be kept calm and transported immediately to the operating room. In the presence of an anesthesia provider and otolaryngologist fiberoptic pharyngoscopy or indirect laryngoscopy is performed to either confirm or eliminate the diagnosis. A lateral radiograph of the neck may be helpful, if the clinical condition permits.

O   **How does one induce anesthesia in a child with epiglottitis?**

On a nurse or parent's lap the child is pre-oxygenated. Ventilation is not assisted during inhalational induction. An IV is established only after the patient is deeply anesthetized with the subsequent administration of 0.01-0.02 mg/Kg IV atropine. Muscle relaxants should be avoided. Gentle laryngoscopy should be performed by the individual who is most experienced The endotracheal tube should be at least one size (0.5 mm) smaller than would normally be used and preloaded with a stylet.

○ **Should a rapid sequence induction be performed in a child with epiglottitis?**

No. Laryngoscopy should be performed under deep general anesthesia without muscle relaxants to minimize the possibility of complete loss of the airway. Complications from aspiration have been rare.

○ **Five minutes after intubating a child with epiglottitis frothy secretions are suctioned from the endotracheal tube, why?**

Patients with epiglottitis are known to develop negative pressure pulmonary edema as a complication. This is due to generation of high negative inspiratory pressures against an obstructed laryngeal inlet. It occurs only after relief of airway obstruction which facilitates increased venous return and thus extravasation of fluid from damaged alveolar capillaries.

○ **How is negative pressure pulmonary edema treated?**

It usually requires supportive care and is generally self-limited; it may be improved with PEEP/CPAP.

○ **How long should an epiglottitis patient remain intubated?**

Inflammation resolves in 24 to 72 hours. Some practitioners recommend revisualization of the epiglottis prior to extubation. Others believe this is unnecessary and that leak around the endotracheal tube can be used safely as a guide to readiness for extubation.

○ **At what age does laryngotracheobronchitis (croup) occur?**

It occurs at ages 6 months to 6 years and typically lasts less than 5 days. This is in contrast to children with epiglottitis, a disease that typically occurs in older children ages 2 to 6, but may occur into adulthood.

○ **How does the presentation of laryngotracheobronchitis (croup) differ from that of epiglottitis?**

The onset of croup is usually insidious. The child presents with low-grade fever, inspiratory stridor and a "brassy" or "barking" cough. Subglottic narrowing of the airway produces the characteristic "steeple sign" in lateral cervical spine x-rays. Respiratory distress may develop slowly or acutely.

○ **What is the treatment for croup?**

Treatment begins with humidified oxygen. If tachypnea and cyanosis are present aerosolized racemic epinephrine may be helpful. The use of corticosteroids is controversial. If symptoms persist for more than 7 days, or the child is less than 4 months of age, laryngoscopy should be considered to rule out other causes.

○ **Is a recent upper respiratory infection a contraindication to myringotomy and tube insertion?**

Typically this procedure is accomplished using mask inhalation anesthesia. The children often have accompanying upper respiratory infections (URI's) and it is the drainage of middle ear fluid that eradicates this problem. No significant difference in post-operative morbidity has been observed in children asymptomatic and those with uncomplicated URI's who undergo myringotomy and tube placement and do not require endotracheal intubation.

○ **How often do neonates with cleft lip and palate have associated anomalies?**

Associated congenital anomalies occur thirty times more frequently. Ten to twenty-five percent have anomalies of other organs.

O   **When should a child with cleft lip or palate have it repaired?**

The lip is usually repaired at 3 months of age provided there are no associated anomalies. Many surgeons have adopted "Musgrave's" rule of ten to determine appropriate timing of lip closure. (Hemoglobin >10 gm, > 10 weeks of age, weight ≥10 kg and WBC < 10,000). The palate can be closed up to 4 years of age, but speech development is optimized if repair is before 18 months of age.

O   **A child presents with wheezing and is using accessory muscles to breathe. The child appears otherwise well. Examination shows hyperlucency in the right upper lobe. What is your presumptive diagnosis?**

Aspiration of a foreign body should be strongly suspected. It is the most common cause of wheezing refractory to medical treatment in children. Death by asphyxiation due to aspiration is the leading cause of death in children < 1year old, followed by motor vehicle accidents. Children present with wheezing, coughing and gagging. Cyanosis, hemoptysis, intercostal muscle retractions, and use of the accessory respiratory muscles may be observed. Most foreign bodies are radiolucent but a chest x-ray may demonstrate atelectasis or obstructive emphysema.

O   **How is anesthesia induced in a child who has aspirated a foreign body?**

An inhalational induction is the safest method. Avoid assisting ventilation since this may drive the foreign body further into the airway causing complete obstruction or contribute to air trapping distal to the object. Rectally administered medication may be used to assist with induction in the uncooperative patient.

O   **How is the diagnosis of sleep apnea syndrome confirmed?**

Sleep apnea syndrome is confirmed by the presence of one of the following findings during graphic recording of respiration in natural sleep:
Complete cessation of airflow at the mouth or nose
Oxygen desaturation to $SpO_2 \le 80\%$
Obstruction for 10 seconds or more with no air movement and paradoxical movement of the chest and abdomen

O   **What causes sleep apnea?**

Both anatomic and neurologic causes are responsible for the pathogenesis of sleep apnea. Obstructive sleep apnea (OSA) is caused by narrowing of the upper airways during sleep. In most patients, snoring predates the development of obstructive events by years. A critical subatmospheric pressure is generated during inspiration that overcomes the ability of the airway muscles to maintain airway patency. Obesity also tends to decrease the size of the upper airways. Central sleep apnea is due to the loss of central stimulatory drive to the ventilatory muscles. Sleep apnea can be due to both mechanisms, although mixed apneas are usually classified as variants of OSA.

O   **What is the innervation of the larynx?**

The superior laryngeal branch of the vagus nerve supplies sensation above the vocal cords and function of the cricothyroid muscle (tension of the vocal cords) and a portion of the transverse arytenoid muscle. The recurrent laryngeal nerve provides innervation to all remaining intrinsic laryngeal muscles and sensation below the vocal cords.

O   **What sequelae result from superior laryngeal nerve injury?**

Superior laryngeal nerve injury would cause loss of sensation above the vocal cords and decreased ability to shorten and adduct the true vocal cords. This results in decreased vocalization ability and a reduction in upper airway protective reflexes.

O   **What are the consequences of bilateral denervation of the carotid bodies in bilateral neck dissection?**

Bilateral carotid body denervation is associated with increased resting $PaCO_2$ and the loss of the normal respiratory and blood pressure responses to acute hypoxia. Hypertension is also common and should be aggressively treated. Serious respiratory depression may occur after opioid administration.

O   **Is atlantoaxial instability more likely in the pediatric population?**

Yes, the pediatric patient has several predisposing factors including a disproportionally large head, immature cervical musculature, ligamentous laxity and wedge shaped cervical vertebrae. This makes children especially prone to C_1-C_2 subluxation. Extreme rotation and extension should be avoided. Other co-morbidities or syndromes that increase the chances of atlantoaxial instability include rheumatoid arthritis, ankylosing spondylitis, and Down's Syndrome.

O   **What is the differential diagnosis of partial airway obstruction in children?**

Extrinsic pathology: hypertrophied tonsils/adenoids, infection, cystic hygroma, vascular abnormalities, and neoplasm.
Intrinsic pathology: epiglottitis, croup, subglottic stenosis, vocal cord paralysis, laryngeal stricture anomalies (webs, cysts, etc.).

O   **What complications should one be aware of in surgery for head and neck cancer?**

Open neck veins allow entrainment of air into the venous system. This potentially devastating complication can be reduced if not eliminated by placing the patient in a slight head down position. Tumors involving the major vessels in the neck can require sacrifice of one or both internal jugular veins resulting in decreased cerebral perfusion pressure and cerebral edema. Cardiac arrhythmia is also a concern. Occasionally a carotid artery may need to be ligated if infiltrated with tumor.

O   **A patient develops worsening hoarseness after tonsillectomy. How should you respond?**

Hoarseness is a common problem following extubation. Usually hoarseness resolves within 5 to 7 days. Hoarseness that worsens or persists for > 7 days requires evaluation by an otolaryngologist to rule out vocal cord injury.

O   **What is the incidence of laryngeal injury after short-term intubation?**

The overall incidence is 6.2 percent. The most common complication is hematoma of the vocal cords (4.5%). Mucosal laceration occurs in approximately 1 in 1000 intubations. Perforation of the trachea is a rare complication usually occurring with the use of a stylet and forceful passage. Subcutaneous emphysema should prompt investigation.

O   **What are the risks of intranasal cocaine?**

Cocaine may cause ventricular fibrillation, cardiac arrest, respiratory depression, agitation, hypertension and tachycardia. It is contraindicated for use in patients on monoamine oxidase inhibitors. It should be used with caution in patients with hypertension or CAD.

O   **What are the risks of general anesthesia in a patient with peritonsillar abscess?**

Difficulty in intubation should be expected due to distorted anatomy, edema and trismus. Accidental rupture of the abscess with spillage of pus into an unprotected airway is a risk. If possible the abscess should be drained by needle aspiration under local anesthesia prior to induction of general anesthesia.

O   **Name three anesthetic techniques for microlaryngoscopy.**

1. 95% of operations can be done with a small 5.0 mm I.D. endotracheal tube placed near the posterior commissure. Only 5% of microsurgical laryngeal procedures involve the lower third of the vocal cords.
2. Jet ventilation through the laryngoscope. This technique is contraindicated in children.
3. Apneic oxygenation technique with intermittent ventilation.

O   **What is the difference between a unilateral and bilateral mandibular fracture?**

A unilateral mandibular fracture is stable; a bilateral fracture is unstable. With a bilateral mandibular fracture the posterior fragment may be distracted posteroinferiorly by the muscles of the floor of the mouth leading to obstruction of the pharynx by the base of the tongue.

O   **How does a Le Fort I fracture complicate anesthetic management?**

A Le Fort I fracture is a horizontal fracture through the maxilla which results only in a mobile palate and it presents little problem to the nurse anesthetist. Patients may be intubated either orally or nasally providing intranasal damage has been ruled out.

O   **What are the anesthetic concerns with a Le Fort II fracture?**

A Le Fort II fracture involves the nose and, therefore, nasal intubation is relatively contraindicated. Because the force necessary to create this fracture is substantial, one must be suspicious of an occult fracture at the base of the skull.

O   **What is the most likely cause of bradycardia seen during eye surgery?**

Always suspect the oculocardiac reflex – a trigeminal vagal reflex. Never forget possible hypoxia though.

O   **Describe the afferent limb of the oculocardiac reflex.**

Transmission occurs via the trigeminal nerve, through the ciliary ganglion to the ophthalmic division of the trigeminal nerve and there from the gasserian ganglion to the sensory nucleus of the 4th ventricle.

O   **Describe the efferent limb of the oculocardiac reflex.**

The vagus nerve carries output from the sensory nucleus of the 4th ventricle.

O   **Stimulation of the oculocardiac reflex causes what cardiovascular perturbations?**

Bradycardia, nodal rhythm, premature ventricular contractions, ventricular fibrillation or asystole.

O   **What is the most important therapy for bradycardia due to the oculocardiac reflex?**

Stop the stimulus!

O   **After you stop the stimulus how do you treat persistent bradycardia and prevent further episodes?**

Give atropine (or other anti-cholinergic), ventilate and oxygenate, and deepen the level of anesthesia.

THORACIC SURGERY

A Wise Man Is He Who Knows How Much Is Enough.
Chinese Proverb

O   Does cessation of smoking reduce perioperative pulmonary risk?

Yes. Cessation for 48 hours decreases the level of carboxyhemoglobin and 4 to 6 weeks decreases postoperative complications. The most beneficial effect occurs after 2-3 months with an improvement in closing volume, increase in maximum voluntary ventilation and reduction in sputum.

O   What preoperative pulmonary tests are needed in patients for thoracic surgery?

Arterial blood gas, spirometry, and chest x-ray. A bronchoscopy, flow-volume loops and computed tomography (CT) of the chest may be indicated. Occasionally, split lung function studies are appropriate if first line tests suggest resection may leave a patient ventilator-dependent.

O   Are there any contraindications to lung resection?

A predicted residual FEV_1 of less than 800 ml in a 70-kg patient.

O   Which thoracic surgeries may need one lung ventilation?

When the procedure requires immobility or collapse of a lung for ease of dissection or surgical access (repair of thoracic aortic aneurysm, lung resection ranging from pneumonectomy to segmental resection, thoracoscopy, esophageal surgery, single lung transplantation, anterior approach to the thoracic spine and bronchoalveolar lavage). Patient-related factors include: isolation of infection or bleeding to one lung, separate ventilation of each lung or severe hypoxemia due to unilateral lung disease.

O   Does a mediastinoscopy require one lung ventilation?

No

O   What are the complications with a mediastinoscopy?

Most common is hemorrhage because of the proximity of major blood vessels and the vascularity of certain tumors.

Second most common is a pneumothorax, usually right-sided. Recurrent nerve damage is the third most common complication and is permanent in 50% of cases. Autonomic reflexes can be stimulated due to manipulation of the trachea or the aortic arch. Obstruction of the innominate artery may occur which will result in decreased cerebral blood flow. Less common complications may include tracheal collapse, tension pneumomediastinum, mediastinitis, hemithorax, and chylothorax.

O   Which vesssels are more likely to be injured during a mediastinoscopy?

SVC, pulmonary artery and azygous vein are the most commonly injured. The right radial arterial line will indicate compression of the innominate artery by the mediastinoscope but it is rarely injured.

O   What are the absolute indications for double-lumen tubes or one-lung ventilation?

Patient-related:

Protection of a healthy lung from a contaminated lung due to infection or massive hemoptysis
Separate ventilation of each lung (bronchopleural fistula, tracheobronchial disruption, cyst or bulla)
Severe hypoxemia due to unilateral lung disease

Procedure-related:
Surgical opening of major airways, disruption of bronchial system or unilateral cyst or bullae
Repair of thoracic aortic aneurysm
Esophageal surgery
Bronchoalveolar lavage of one lung
Anterior approach to the thoracic spine

○   **What are the relative indications for double-lumen tubes or one-lung ventilation?**

Surgical exposure requiring the collapse of one lung (thoracoscopy, pleural surgery, lobectomy, pneumonectomy, bullectomy, lung volume reduction, surgeries on the descending thoracic aorta, thoracic spine, esophagus, or for pulmonary endarterectomy).

○   **What methods are used for lung separation?**

Endobronchial intubation with a double-lumen tube or a single-lumen tube or use of an endobronchial blocker deployed through a single lumen tube to occlude one of the mainstem bronchi.

○   **Which method is available for children?**

Endobronchial intubation or an endobronchial blocker. There is no double-lumen tube small enough for a child less than about 10 years of age.

○   **What are the advantages of double-lumen tubes?**

Ability to ventilate or collapse either lung sequentially, access to both lungs for endotracheal suction or application of CPAP.

○   **What are the disadvantages of double-lumen tubes?**

Misplacement, laryngeal trauma, bronchial trauma from low volume, high pressure cuff, tracheal cuff easily torn on teeth, difficult to insert if the larynx is not easily visualized, need to change to single lumen if post-operative ventilation is required.

○   **How do you check placement of a double-lumen tube?**

Advance the double-lumen through the larynx under direct visualization (tip anterior and then rotated to the left after passing through the cords), with blind advancement until the resistance of the carina is felt, then pull back slightly and inflate the tracheal cuff. Confirm tracheal placement with auscultation of bilateral breath sounds and the presence of CO_2 on capnography.

Placement of the double-lumen tube should be confirmed after the patient is turned to the lateral position. Inflate the (left) bronchial cuff, clamp the tracheal lumen and check for unilateral left-sided breath sounds.

The tube should be advanced if you still hear air entry on the right-side.

Right and no left-sided air entry indicates that the tube is in the right bronchus.

Unclamp the tracheal lumen and clamp the bronchial lumen. Check for unilateral right breath sounds.

A diminution of breath sounds may be heard if the bronchial cuff is partially occluding the distal trachea; the tube needs to be advanced.

As each lumen is clamped (tracheal and bronchial) the vent should be opened to determine if there is a leak present. Direct visualization of the carina and blue edge of the bronchial balloon in the left mainstem bronchus with a fiberoptic bronchoscope placed in the tracheal lumen should confirm clinical findings. The best test for proper placement is fiberoptic visualization (carina below tracheal lumen, blue bronchial balloon top visualized in the main stem.) This should be followed by appropriate one-lung ventilation observed with the chest open.

O   **What size fiberoptic bronchoscope should be used when placing a standard single lumen endotracheal tube?**

The standard adult FO will pass through an ETT 7.0 mm or greater, but because of decreased cross-sectional area available for ventilation, a pediatric FO should be used for ETT< 8.0 mm.

O   **What uses can be made of the suction port on a fiberoptic bronchoscope?**

Oxygen insufflation and limited suctioning depending on size. Oxygen insufflation can be effective at clearing secretions.

O   **How can jet ventilation be accomplished through a fiberoptic bronchoscope?**

The Luer lock connection of a hand-held jet ventilation device attaches to the biopsy port of a FOB (fiberoptic bronchoscope). The tip of the FOB must be in the trachea and the glottis must be open to avoid barotrauma. Driving pressure, inspiratory time and ventilatory rate are dictated by the operator. Using a driving pressure of 50 psi results in a tracheal pressure of 6-8 mm Hg, FiO_2 of 88-93%, and PaO_2 of 340-478 mm Hg.

O   **What percentage of double-lumen tubes are placed incorrectly and not detected by auscultation?**

About 30%. Less common for non-disposable tubes (Robertshaw) and more common for disposable tubes (Mallinckrodt). This is why confirmation of placement with a fiberoptic bronchoscope, especially after turning to the lateral position, is mandatory.

O   **How can one-lung ventilation be accomplished in a patient with a tracheotomy or stoma?**

A shorter DLT (Sheridan), an endobronchial blocker, or endobronchial intubation may be used. Unless laryngectomy has been performed it may be possible to intubate with the usual equipment via the larynx.

O   **For one-lung ventilation is a right or left-sided tube more commonly used and why?**

A left-sided tube. The distance between the right upper lobe bronchus and the right mainstem bronchus is 2.1 cm in females and 2.3 cm in males. The distance between the left upper lobe bronchus and the left mainstem bronchus is 5 cm in females and 5.3 cm in males. Therefore, it is easier to obstruct the right upper lobe with the bronchial cuff. For this reason right-sided double lumen tubes are NEVER used in current, routine thoracic anesthetic practice.

O   **What kinds of complications can occur with a DLT?**

Injury to the larynx, trachea or bronchus, malpositioning with failure to collapse the lung or failure to ventilate.

O   **What are the positioning complications of a left-sided DLT?**

A left-sided DLT down the right-side can result in obstruction of the right upper lobe and unexpected ventilation of the contralateral lung. If the tube is not advanced far enough into the left bronchial lumen, the cuff may still be in the trachea resulting in normal ventilation deflated but partial to complete tracheal obstruction when the cuff is inflated. A right-sided tube commonly obstructs the right upper lobe. It is less likely for a left-sided tube to obstruct the left upper lobe unless advanced way too far when impingement of the tracheal lumen on the carina can result in failure to ventilate the right side, in addition to left upper lobe collapse.

○   **What serious complications could occur with malpositioning?**

Complete obstruction of the trachea with the inability to ventilate. Inadvertent ventilation of the intended lung for isolation resulting in barotrauma and cardiac arrest if pneumothorax or bullae are present. Blood and purulent secretions may be disseminated to the contralateral lung.

○   **What F_iO_2 is recommended with one lung ventilation?**

100% for the highest safety margin, but this should be limited to the shortest period possible and weaned as tolerated, accepting $SaO_2 > 90\%$ or lower in patients who have received chemotherapeutic agents (especially bleomycin). The presence of nitrogen in inspired air splints open alveoli and decreases atelectasis.

○   **What complications can be associated with a high inspired oxygen concentration?**

Oxygen toxicity, especially in patients with a history of bleomycin therapy (ARDS and pulmonary fibrosis) and absorption atelectasis.

○   **What tidal volume should be used for one-lung ventilation?**

There is no specific tidal volume, but aim to keep peak inspiratory pressures between 30 to 40 mm Hg, minimizing the risk of barotrauma. Pneumothorax of the dependent lung may be life threatening. In theory, a tidal volume < 8 ml/kg results in decreased FRC and more atelectasis in the ventilated lung. TV >15 ml/kg may increase airway pressure and pulmonary vascular resistance, which may divert blood flow to the non-ventilated lung, and result in more shunting. However, the increased use of pressure control ventilation may improve safety by avoiding inadvertent high tidal volumes and pressures being applied to one lung on initiation of OLV. Also the use of smaller tidal volumes during video-assisted thoracoscopic surgery has proven safe and effective.

○   **What is the ideal respiratory rate?**

As low as is required to avoid air trapping.

Permissive hypercapnia is well tolerated during general anesthesia in most patients. The major risk is for those patients with right ventricular dysfunction who will not tolerate the pulmonary hypertension associated with high $PaCO_2$ and acidosis (pH < 7.10).

○   **What are the deleterious effects of hypocapnia?**

In one lung ventilation hypocapnia will increase pulmonary vascular resistance in the dependent lung, inhibit hypoxic pulmonary vasoconstriction in the nondependent lung (secondary to a vasodilator effect), increase shunt, decrease PaO_2 and reduce tissue extraction of oxygen by shifting the oxyhemoglobin curve to the left.

○   **What should the peak inspiratory pressure be after lobectomy, pneumonectomy, or lung transplant? Why?**

Ideally, the PIP should not exceed 30 mm Hg, to prevent possible damage to the bronchial stump or new suture line. For such patients, volume targeted pressure-controlled ventilatory modes are typically used to limit the potential for barotrauma. Permissive hypercapnia is tolerated if required.

○   **How do you test for integrity of the suture line on the bronchial stump?**

Prior to closing the chest the surgeon will check for air bubbles as you apply a "PEEP maneuver" of 35- 40 mm Hg to the surgical lung, with the bronchial stump submersed in saline.

○   **What complications can occur with one lung ventilation, despite correct tube placement?**

Hypoxemia, hypercapnia, increasing airway pressure, air trapping, pneumothorax, arrhythmias and hypotension.

O   Is the decrease in PaO$_2$ caused by right or left one-lung ventilation equivalent?

Theoretically, collapse of the right lung involves more lung segments than the left resulting inor a greater decrease in PaO$_2$. In practice, the collapsed lung may well be diseased and have minimal contribution to ventilation and oxygenation. Patients with normal lungs requiring OLV for surgical access often develop more hypoxia.

O   What factors contribute to a decrease in arterial oxygenation during one-lung ventilation with surgery performed in the lateral decubitus position?

Increased V/Q mismatch in the ventilated dependent lung accounts for a third of the 35-40% shunt that occurs during one-lung anesthesia. The major cause of hypoxemia is the pulmonary arteriovenous shunting of deoxygenated blood through the non-ventilated lung. Hypoxic pulmonary vasoconstriction in the non-ventilated lung is the most important variable determining PaO$_2$. Other contributory factors: gravity, application of PEEP, use of very small tidal volumes, atelectasis, secretions and increased interstitial fluid in the dependent lung.

O   Once the treatable causes of hypoxemia are ruled out what are your options?

Add oxygen insufflation or continuous positive pressure airway pressure (CPAP 5 cm H$_2$O) to the non-ventilated lung first after sustained positive pressure reinflates alveoli. Increase CPAP until further lung expansion will compromise surgical exposure. Then positive end expiratory pressure (PEEP 5 cm H$_2$O) to the ventilated lung is applied. Incrementally increase the CPAP and PEEP in alternate lungs until the optimal balance is achieved, permitting maximum PaO$_2$. Intermittent inflation of the collapsed lung, high frequency jet ventilation to the collapsed lung and differential lung ventilation are other options. Finally, returning to two lung-ventilation, even temporarily, may be necessary. For pneumonectomy, the surgeon can clamp the pulmonary artery to the nondependent lung, eliminating shunt from this source.

Treatable causes include: inadequate FiO$_2$, tidal volume, respiratory rate; improper positioning of the ETT; obstruction (secretions, kinking).

O   How does CPAP work?

CPAP = continuous positive airway pressure delivered throughout the respiratory cycle during spontaneous breathing. It maintains the patency of the non-ventilated alveoli, allowing some oxygen uptake in these alveoli. It works best if a tidal volume is delivered to the collapsed lung to create slight expansion before applying CPAP, otherwise it takes 45 minutes for full effect. This must be balanced with encroachment of the lung into the surgical field. It is unacceptable for video-assisted thoracoscopic surgery as it obstructs the surgical field.

O   How does PEEP work?

PEEP = positive end-expiratory pressure applied during mechanical ventilation where the airway pressure at end-expiration remains above ambient pressure. It increases lung volume at end expiration, increasing FRC resulting in lower pulmonary vascular resistance, improving V/Q mismatch, limiting atelectasis and thereby improving PaO$_2$. If the FRC is adequate and the PaO$_2$> 80 mmHg, PEEP may have a negative effect due to redistribution of blood flow from the ventilated lung to the non-ventilated lung and reduction of cardiac output.

O   What are the causes of increasing peak airway pressures during OLV?

Problems are isolated to the anesthetic machine, double-lumen endotracheal tube or patient (lungs or chest wall). Switching to manual ventilation will exclude ventilator dysfunction.

Endotracheal tube factors:
Kinked or occluded (secretions, debris, cuff herniation)
Malposition (too far with tracheal lumen against the carina, pulled back with both lumens in the trachea and the bronchial cuff occluding the trachea)
Loss of lung isolation with soiling into the dependent lung

Patient factors (affecting the dependent hemithorax or lung):
Tension pneumothorax
Bronchospasm
Overinflation of the lung
Pulmonary edema
ARDS
Positioning, i.e., Trendelenburg
Chest wall - if the chest is closed; chest wall rigidity due to narcotics, surgeon leaning on the chest wall or light anesthesia/paralysis

❍ What factors would contribute to arrhythmias and hypotension?

The most important causes are hypoxemia, hypercapnia and myocardial ischemia. Also likely is pericardial manipulation, especially with a left thoracotomy and pulling of the great vessels. Always check tube position and evaluate for air trapping and pneumothorax.

❍ What is hypoxic pulmonary vasoconstriction (HPV)?

This is an important local physiologic response of the lung to areas of alveolar hypoxia (and to a much lesser extent mixed venous desaturation) resulting in pulmonary vasoconstriction. The mechanism involves either a direct effect of hypoxia on the pulmonary vasculature or mediated by the release of leukotrienes. An increase in pulmonary vascular resistance will divert blood to more oxygenated alveoli, thereby reducing V/Q mismatch and preventing hypoxemia.

❍ Does HPV work with one-lung ventilation?

Yes. HPV in the non-ventilated lung shifts blood flow to the ventilated lung. HPV is typically preserved when using less than 1 MAC of volatile agents.

❍ What physiologic effect does HPV have on OLV?

Improvement in oxygenation due to decrease in V/Q mismatch.

❍ What other factors will effect blood flow to either lung?

Surgical stimulation, vascular clamping, the application of PEEP, preexisting lung disease and gravity.

❍ What effects are seen when there is surgical stimulation of lung tissue?

Stroking or compressing the lung causes the release of prostaglandin and endothelium-derived relaxing factor resulting in vasodilatation and increased blood flow to the manipulated lung which is normally the non-ventilated lung, increasing V/Q mismatch.

❍ Will pre-existing lung disease affect the shunt fraction with one-lung ventilation?

If the non-ventilated lung has a reduction in blood flow due to preexisting disease this will create less of a shunt when one-lung ventilation is instituted. However, if the lung to be ventilated has a decrease in flow secondary to pre-existing disease then there will be an increased shunt as more blood flow and higher PA pressures overcome HPV that may exist in certain locations of the ventilated lung.

○ **How much shunt is created when one-lung ventilation is instituted in a healthy lung?**

If HPV is intact, the shunt is usually 25-30%.

○ **What PaO$_2$ does this give the patient if breathing 100% oxygen?**

150-210 mm Hg.

○ **What is a normal shunt fraction?**

5-10%.

○ **What effect does the lateral decubitus position have with two-lung ventilation?**

Increase V/Q mismatch, relatively good ventilation but poor perfusion to the non-dependent lung, poor ventilation with good perfusion to the dependent lung. West's zones of the lung are rotated 90° from upright, air moves up and blood moves down secondary to gravity. The fractional blood flow is 40% to the non-dependent lung and 60% to the dependent lung. The shunt fraction is normal.

○ **Is there a difference with right or left lateral decubitus positioning?**

Yes. If the left lung is nondependent (right lateral decubitus position) it gets 35% of the blood flow. When the right lung is nondependent (left lateral decubitus position) it gets 45% of the blood flow.

○ **What effect does lateral decubitus positioning have on one-lung ventilation?**

An obligatory shunt is still created because the non-ventilated lung still receives blood flow but this is less pronounced due to the aid of gravity pushing more blood to the dependent ventilated lung. Fractional blood flow is 22.5% to the nondependent lung and 77.5% to the dependent lung. The resulting shunt fraction is 27.5%. This causes a significant decrease in PaO$_2$ which may continue to decrease for 45 minutes.

○ **What other factors will affect blood flow to the nondependent lung?**

Gravity (vertical gradient), surgical interference (lung stroking or compression), preexisting lung disease (of either the nondependent or dependent lung), pneumothorax (dependent lung), vascular clamping of the opposite pulmonary artery or airway positive pressure.

○ **What must you take into consideration when using inhalation agents with these patients?**

Inhaled anesthetic agents are dose dependent vascular dilators which inhibit HPV above 0.5 MAC, thereby, increasing blood flow to the non-ventilated lung.

○ **Would nitrous oxide be a good choice?**

No. 100 % FiO$_2$ is the best choice. With nitrous oxide, there is the chance of air expansion in air-filled spaces (bulla, air trapping, pneumothorax). Nitrous oxide increases pulmonary vascular resistance and depresses HPV (reported in dog model at MAC equivalent > 0.5). Nitrous oxide also limits the FiO$_2$.

○ **What about narcotics and intravenous anesthetics?**

They have no effect on HPV and oxygenation is well preserved. Many patients rely on hypoxic pulmonary drive, so with long acting narcotics there is a propensity for respiratory depression in these patients. Avoid drugs which cause histamine release.

O   **Which drugs are known to cause histamine release?**

Morphine, meperidine, atracurium, d-tubocurarine, mivacurium, atracurium, and doxacurium.

O   **How would you treat bronchospasm?**

Identify and correct the underlying cause. If bronchoconstriction is the diagnosis: administer 100% O_2, lengthen expiration time, deepen the level of anesthesia (inhaled anesthetics), aerosolized albuterol treatment or injected down the ETT, subcutaneous terbutaline, IV epinephrine (infused to effect, not CPR doses), IV aminophylline (probably useless in acute attacks) and steroids. Other mild bronchodilators include magnesium sulfate and atropine.

O   **What effect has inhaled nitric oxide been shown to have on pulmonary vasculature?**

Nitric oxide is an endothelium-derived vasodilator that is administered as an inhaled gas. NO decreases pulmonary artery pressure in patients with reactive pulmonary vasoconstriction. This may improve PaO_2 in patients with preexisting pulmonary hypertension and ARDS (without improving mortality), and reduce right ventricular afterload improving right ventricular failure, without causing systemic hypotension.

O   **Are there any special considerations when extubating patients with a DLT or endobronchial blocker in place?**

Stimulation of the carina may cause laryngospasm or bronchospasm. Hemorrhage or bronchopleural fistulae can occur due to the suturing of an endobronchial tube or blocker to the bronchial wall.

O   **Is there any indication for leaving a DLT in place?**

If the patient requires postoperative ventilation, the double-lumen ETT is usually removed and replaced with a conventional single lumen ETT. Indications for leaving the DLT in place would be: history of difficult intubation, risk of inducing hypoxemia or requirement for PEEP, differential ventilation of the lungs, and residual bronchopleural fistula or possibility of cross contamination of the lungs.

O   **What if the patient needs postoperative ventilation?**

If the patient has a DLT it is best to change it to a single lumen ETT. If the patient has been given a large amount of fluid and the airway is edematous or the patient was a difficult intubation and there is a potential for losing the airway, the DLT should be changed over a tube exchange catheter (Sheriden or Cook). The risks of leaving the DLT in place include tracheal or bronchial trauma, increased airway resistance and difficulty clearing secretions.

O   **When is rigid bronchoscopy indicated?**

For foreign bodies, massive hemoptysis, vascular tumors, for small children, endobronchial resection and mediastinal tumors causing compression of the airway.

O   **How is ventilation accomplished with a rigid bronchoscope?**

Apneic oxygenation, apnea and intermittent ventilation when the eye piece is closed, or jet ventilation.

O   **What are the anesthetist's concerns with anterior mediastinal masses?**

A potentially catastrophic situation following induction of anesthesia secondary to airway obstruction (due to positioning or paralysis) and/or compression of the SVC (superior vena cava syndrome), pulmonary vessels or heart (reduced venous return from compression or positive-pressure ventilation) resulting in hypotension.

○ **How can the airway be assessed preoperatively in a patient with a mediastinal mass?**

Ask the patient if they are able to breathe without difficulty when supine (or if there is difficulty with any particular position), review the chest x-ray and CT scan of the chest (tracheal deviation, compression or obstruction distal to the carina) and evaluate the flow-volume loops in the upright and supine positions (airway obstruction). Lack of any symptoms at all - including cough or hemoptysis - in an adult usually indicates that airway obstruction will not occur. In a child, lack of symptoms is NOT an indication that the airway will not obstruct due to the more compliant cartilaginous versus bony nature of the supportive rib cage.

○ **How can cardiac involvement be assessed preoperatively?**

CT evaluation of the mass and involvement of surrounding structures, echocardiogram upright and supine (cardiac function, direct myocardial invasion, pericardial fluid), EKG and observing the effect of a Valsalva maneuver on the pressure tracing from an arterial line placed prior to induction (mass impeding venous return causing hypotension).

○ **What are your anesthetic options in a patient with a symptomatic anterior mediastinal mass found on preoperative evaluation?**

Local anesthesia for cervical or scalene node biopsy, preoperative radiation or chemotherapy for mass reduction and/or for symptomatic patients prior to general anesthesia. Prophylactic cannulation of the femoral vessels with cardiopulmonary bypass on standby. A rigid bronchoscope should be immediately available to lift the mass off of the airway, and multiple individuals to re-position the patient (often prone) to move the mass off of critical structures.

○ **What options are available for general anesthesia?**

Awake fiberoptic intubation with an armored ETT passed distal to the potential obstruction, 100% oxygen, volume loading, IV access in lower extremities, determine the ability to ventilate prior to paralysis, standby rigid bronchoscope, standby cardiopulmonary bypass. Consider strongly an inhalation or slow ketamine induction and spontaneous respirations, if awake fiberoptic with placement distal to the obstruction is not possible.

○ **What is the primary disease associated with thymectomy?**

Abnormalities of the thymus gland (anterior mediastinal mass) associated with myasthenia gravis (MG).

○ **What are the perioperative considerations for patients with myasthenia gravis?**

Clinical presentation: ocular, bulbar or skeletal muscle involvement (aspiration risk and respiratory insufficiency requiring postoperative ventilation).

Associated syndromes: anterior mediastinal mass, autoimmune diseases (hypothyroidism, diabetes mellitus, rheumatoid arthritis and collagen vascular disease), arrhythmia and cardiomyopathy.

Drug therapy: immunosuppressants (steroids, azathioprine, cyclophosphamide), anticholinesterases (myasthenic versus cholinergic crises leading to weakness), plasmapheresis.

Drug interactions or side effects: altered response to muscle relaxants, adrenal insufficiency with chronic steroid use, medications which exacerbate myasthenic symptoms.

○ **What are the effects of neuromuscular blocking drugs in myasthenic patients?**

Sensitive to nondepolarizing muscle relaxants (start with one-tenth of the usual dose of short or intermediate acting MR or preferably, avoid all muscle relaxants) and theoretically resistant to depolarizing muscle relaxants, even if the patient is in remission. Resistance to depolarizing relaxants has not been shown to be clinically relevant.

○   **What is myasthenic syndrome?**

Eaton-Lambert syndrome, often seen in patients with small cell carcinoma of the lung. Predominantly men presenting with proximal limb weakness (legs > arms) which improves with exercise. Muscle pain is common. Reflexes are absent or decreased. Patients are sensitive to depolarizing and nondepolarizing muscle relaxants. Therapeutic response is poor with anticholinesterase drugs.

○   **What are the choices for pain control after thoracic surgery?**

IV narcotics, patient-controlled analgesia, thoracic epidural with narcotics and/or local anesthetics, intrathecal narcotics (single dose), and paravertebral intercostal nerve blocks.

○   **What nerve damage can occur during thoracic surgery?**

Intercostal nerve damage is the most common. Branches of the brachial plexus, recurrent laryngeal nerve and the phrenic nerve may be injured. The brachial plexus is easily damaged during lung transplantation with the "clam shell" incision and retraction.

○   **What nerve damage can occur during thoracic aortic surgery?**

The left recurrent laryngeal nerve courses around the aorta, and injury may lead to vocal cord paralysis. The left vagus nerve lies in the esophagoaortic groove but due to bilateral innervation, injury would be clinically asymptomatic. Phrenic nerve injury is also possible either from direct surgical trauma or from ice in the pericardium (incidence 1.7-11%). The left phrenic nerve courses along the posterior pericardium before dividing and penetrating the diaphragm lateral to the left border of the heart.

○   **How do you diagnose auto-PEEP?**

Observe the end-expiratory pressure on the airway pressure gauge (some ventilators have an expiratory hold feature for this purpose). If this value is greater than the external PEEP you set, the difference is the auto-PEEP.

○   **What is the cause and treatment of auto-PEEP?**

Breath stacking seen when the inspiratory phase begins before the expiratory phase is completed during mechanical ventilation due to a fast respiratory rate or short expiratory time and in patients who have difficulty in exhaling gas during spontaneous ventilation because of airway obstruction.

Treatment consists of adjusting ventilator settings allowing for full exhalation and bronchodilator therapy. If this is not sufficient, interrupt ventilation periodically to allow complete exhalation.

○   **How can you predict the postoperative FEV$_1$?**

The ratio of the number of lung segments resected to the total number can be used to calculate the expected decline in FEV$_1$ following lung resection. This may overestimate the decline. A radioisotope perfusion scan will delineate the contribution of the diseased lung to overall ventilation/perfusion.

○   **Can the choice of anesthetic technique influence postoperative lung function?**

Patients undergoing upper abdominal and thoracic procedures under general anesthesia exhibit a reduction in lung volumes (VC and FRC) which may take 7 to 14 days to normalize. Complete reversal of neuromuscular blockade, minimal residual sedation or narcosis, effective thoracic epidural analgesia and incentive spirometry is the ideal plan to minimize postoperative pulmonary complications. The ability to cough effectively and clear secretions is crucial.

○   **What additional information is useful when interpreting an FEV$_1$/FVC ratio of 60%?**

Response to bronchodilators and apparent effort.

O   **Which diagnosis is provided by flow-volume loops but not spirometry?**

Flow-volume loops aid in the anatomic localization of airway obstruction and indicates if the obstructive component is variable or fixed.

The ratio of FEF_{50} or mid-VC ratio (forced expiratory flow at 50% of FVC) and FIF_{50} (forced inspiratory flow at 50% FVC) determines the nature of the obstruction:

FEF_{50}/FIF_{50} = no change in fixed airway obstruction
FEF_{50}/FIF_{50} > 1, variable extrathoracic obstruction
FEF_{50}/FIF_{50} < 1, variable intrathoracic obstruction

O   **Which pulmonary function tests have been related to increased perioperative pulmonary complications following abdominal or thoracic surgery?**

	Abdominal	Thoracic
FVC	< 70% predicted	< 70% predicted or < 1.7L
FEV_1	< 70% predicted	< 2L (pneumonectomy)
		< 1 L (lobectomy)
		< 0.8 L (segmentectomy)
FEV_1/FVC	< 65%	< 35%
MVV	< 50% predicted	< 50% predicted or 28 L/min
RV		< 50% predicted
DLCO		< 50%
VO_2		< 15 ml/kg/min

The best indicator is probably maximum breathing capacity (MVV, maximum ventilatory volume). In a patient scheduled for pneumonectomy: FEV_1 > 2 L, FEV_1/FVC > 50% MVV > 50% and RV/TLC < 50%, then one liter of FEV_1 will remain in the residual postoperative lung.

O   **How do you assess adequacy of ventilation when using jet ventilation?**

Jet ventilation at low frequencies for microlaryngoscopy requires an oxygen supply at 30 to 50 psi, inspiratory time of 1.5 seconds, passive free egress of gas over an expiratory time of 6 seconds resulting in a ventilator rate of 6 or 7 breaths/min. Movement of the chest wall is assessed to determine adequacy of tidal volume, with arterial blood gases needed to measure CO_2. Pulse oximetry is used to monitor oxygenation.

High-frequency jet ventilation delivers a *small tidal volume breath* from an O_2 source of 5 to 50 psi at a rate of 60 to 100 per minute through a small-bore cannula with an interposed cycling mechanism allowing high frequencies of 10 to 15 Hz. CO_2 clearance is determined by arterial blood gas measurements.

O   **What are the causes of bronchopleural fistula?**

Rupture of a lung abscess, bronchus (typically traumatic), bullae, cyst or parenchymal tissue (barotrauma) into the pleural space. Bronchial erosion by carcinoma or chronic inflammation or breakdown of a bronchial suture line following pulmonary resection also creates a communication between the airways or lung parenchyma and the pleural space.

O   **What are the nurse anesthetist's considerations for bronchopleural fistula?**

Achieving adequate ventilation (awake intubation to secure airway), avoiding a pneumothorax (chest tube insertion) and preventing contamination of the healthy lung (using a double-lumen tube). This is one of the best clinical indications for using high-frequency ventilation, which allows a reduction in peak airway pressures, and a reduction of gas flow across the fistula, and is particularly good when applied via a double lumen tube to the side with the fistula while applying normal ventilation to the unaffected side.

○   **What thoracic aortic surgery typically requires deep hypothermic circulatory arrest (DHCA)?**

Aneurysms or dissections involving the aortic arch or ascending aortic lesions where distal application of the cross clamp would be needed. Bleeding from arterial sites after congenital heart surgery may also require DHCA for repair. The safe limit of DHCA with interruption of cerebral blood flow is 45 to 60 minutes.

○   **How is cerebral protection achieved during DHCA?**

Cooling on cardiopulmonary (femoral-femoral) bypass, surface cooling with the head packed in ice, EEG monitoring to maintain isoelectric tracing with thiopental and retrograde (internal jugular vein) or anterograde (innominate artery) selective cerebral perfusion with cold oxygenated blood (may extend the safe time of DHCA to 90 minutes). Mannitol, furosemide and steroids are given to limit cerebral edema and ischemic injury following reperfusion.

○   **What is the major determinant of cerebral dysfunction following DHCA?**

Circulatory arrest time, age.

○   **What techniques are used for spinal cord protection during thoracoabdominal aortic surgery?**

Hypothermia (34 degrees C), distal aortic perfusion with extracorporeal support, CSF drainage (for up to 72 hours postoperatively), and possibly drug therapies (many have been tried including: barbiturates, corticosteroids, calcium channel blockers, dextrophan, magnesium, naloxone and intrathecal papaverine).

○   **How is distal aortic perfusion achieved?**

Left heart bypass (LHB) with outflow typically from the left atrium and inflow typically into the left femoral artery. Oxygenation is via the lungs.

○   **What are the major complications associated with LHB?**

Right ventricular dysfunction and hypoxemia. Distal perfusion with extracorporeal support has been shown to reduce the incidence of paraplegia (risk of 10 to 20% for simple thoracoabdominal repair), but is probably not beneficial if the cross-clamp time is less than 20 to 30 minutes.

○   **What heart chambers are usually injured following blunt cardiac trauma?**

The right ventricle is most commonly injured followed by the ventricular septum, the LV and the right atrium. Valve injury and injury of the coronary arteries are also reported.

○   **What are the major complications associated with cardiac trauma?**

Exsanguination typically occurs in the field. For survivors, compensated cardiac tamponade may be revealed on induction of anesthesia. Sternotomy or pericardiotomy can result in exsanguination; cardiopulmonary bypass should be on standby. Femoral cannulation should be planned if there is radiological or echocardiographical evidence of intracardiac or aortic injury. Myocardial infarction can result from coronary artery injury and a ventricular septal defect from septal injury.

○   **Which types of lasers are used during airway surgery and how do techniques differ for proximal and distal airway surgery ?**

A YAG solid state laser (Yttrium Aluminum Garnet emitting near infrared invisible light at 1064 nm) is typically used for debulking, coagulating and removing obstructing tumors in the airway. Proximal airway laser surgery requires a rigid bronchoscope with intravenous anesthesia and jet ventilation; a flexible bronchoscope passed through a large (> 8.0) ETT may be used for distal airway surgery.

O **What potential complications occur during laser surgery?**

Bleeding, pneumothorax and airway fire.

O **What precautions should be taken to avoid airway fire?**

Avoid $FiO_2 > 30\%$ (ideally minimize FiO_2) and have a calibrated oxygen analyzer in line. Secure ETT in a proximal position as only PVC ETTs are available in these sizes and they are flammable. Keep the laser tip as far as possible from the flammable flexible bronchoscope tip. Limit laser firing to short bursts. Ensure good communication between anesthesia and surgeon should higher FiO_2 be needed between laser bursts.

O **How do you treat an airway fire?**

Turn off oxygen and gases
Remove the source of the fire (i.e. laser, ETT, bronchoscope).
Extinguish residual fire with sterile water.
Reintubate to assess the airway for damage (consider bronchoalveolar lavage and steroids).
Obtain CXR and monitor for pulmonary dysfunction.

O **How is the thoracic duct injured and what are the possible sequelae?**

Thoracic duct injury may occur during attempted insertion of left internal jugular or subclavian intravenous catheters (it enters the left SC vein just prior to IJ insertion), although sequelae are rare if injury is limited to needle puncture. Avulsion or rupture causing chylothorax can occur with hyperextension injury at the time of spinal trauma, during surgical mobilization or injury to the aortic arch, the esophagus, or the left subclavian artery or rarely spontaneously during coughing or vomiting. Chylothoraces are reported to have a high mortality but this may be due to the fact that 50% of chylothoraces are associated with tumor infiltration.

O **What steps are taken in diagnosing an intraoperative pneumothorax in an intubated and ventilated patient?**

Initial signs of reduced SpO_2 or hypercarbia will most likely be due to reduced lung compliance, i.e. reduced tidal volume on pressure controlled ventilation or increased airway pressure with a volume controlled ventilatory mode. Arterial desaturation will then occur with hemodynamic instability (tachycardia, hypotension) being a late sign. Tension pneumothorax is far more likely during IPPV and nitrous oxide administration, and may be suspected from observing bulging hemidiaphragms. A CXR provides a definitive diagnosis. Needle and tube thoracostomy will be accompanied by a distinctive hiss with relief of the tension pneumothorax.

O **What sequelae of thoracic lymphoma are important to the nurse anesthetist?**

Thoracic lymphoma primarily involves anterior mediastinal lymph nodes, possibly producing a mass effect on the trachea or bronchi, superior vena cava and heart chambers (typically right atrium as it is anterior and compressible). It can also lead to a pericardial effusion that may present with tamponade physiology.

O **Describe important features of the design of thoracostomy tube drainage systems.**

Underwater seal
Drainage chambers for up to 2000 mls fluid
Ability to apply suction up to -40 cm H_2O
Parallel chambers to allow grading of an airleak

By contrast underwater seal post-pneumonectomy involves a balanced system that prevents volume and pressure changes in the thoracic cavity with subsequent mediastinal shift and hemodynamic compromise. There is no option to inadvertently apply suction to these systems

O   **What are the major considerations for providing safe anesthesia for lung volume reduction surgery in patients with severe bullous emphysema ?**

The patient needs to have minimal sedation but good analgesia at the end of the case. This involves the use of thoracic epidural analgesia with local anesthetics and as little epidural opiate as required. Minimal, short acting opiates may be used at induction and the volatile agent must be totally cleared prior to extubation. Using TIVA or propofol toward the end of the case to allow time for excretion of the volatile agent is effective. The patient may be difficult to ventilate and selective ventilation of bullae will result in ineffective gas exchange and distension of the bullae with potential hemodynamic effects similar to a tension pneumothorax. The treatment for overdistension is to temporarily disconnect the ventilator to allow deflation. Pressure controlled ventilation with a low respiratory rate (6-10 breaths/min) is mandatory and permissive hypercapnia is tolerated. Postoperative intensive care is required, with early mobilization and continuous epidural analgesia for at least 72 hours.

NEUROSURGERY

The Ultimate Measure Of A Man Is Not Where He Stands In Moments Of Comfort And Convenience, But Where He Stands At Times Of Challenge And Controversy.
Dr. Martin Luther King, Jr.

○ **What are the main components of an SSEP (somatosensory evoked potential) signal?**

Amplitude and latency. Amplitude is the size of the recorded wave and latency is the time lag between sensory nerve stimulation and when the signal is received.

○ **What medications decrease SSEP amplitude and/or prolong latency?**

Volatile anesthetics and propofol. Nitrous oxide causes a decrease in SSEP amplitude without a change in latency when used alone or when added to a narcotic based anesthetic. In general, opioids cause a dose-dependent increase in latency and decrease in amplitude of SSEPs. Opioids can be used in patients requiring intraoperative SSEP monitoring but large bolus administration should be avoided during the critical times of surgery.

○ **How will the administration of muscle relaxants affect the SSEP signal?**

The signal would be improved due to elimination of the background "noise".

○ **A patient is positioned prone for Harrington rod instrumentation and during surgery the SSEP signals decrease in both lower extremities. Excluding medications, what could be the cause of these findings?**

- Cold irrigation of the spinal cord
- An electrode dislodged from the skin or disconnected from the computer resulting in loss of signal
- Spinal cord stretch or pressure causing ischemia
- Pedicle screw placement with impingement on the spinal cord or nerve root
- Improper limb positioning causing nerve compression
- Hypotension
- Hypothermia

○ **Describe proper SSEP electrode placement?**

SSEP signals are intended to evaluate sensory nerve signal conduction. A signal is produced in the periphery and recorded at the brain. In order to ensure a signal is propagating down a nerve there are intermediate sites of signal recording in the periphery. For upper extremity SSEPs the signals are normally produced at the wrist over the ulnar nerve, sensed in the brachial plexus at Erb's point, and then finally sensed in the brain by scalp electrodes. Lower extremity signals are produced at the posterior tibial nerve at the ankle and sensed in the popliteal fossa, as well as the brain.

○ **What parts of the spinal cord do SSEP and MEP signals interrogate?**

SSEP signals interrogate the posterior columns, while MEP signals interrogate the anterior horn. Therefore, SSEP signals will not detect anterior cord ischemia and cannot detect the onset of motor paralysis (unless caused by whole cord ischemia).

○ **How will the administration of muscle relaxants affect the MEP signal?**

271

In contrast to SSEPs, it will eliminate them. On the other hand, the same anesthetic agents that decrease SSEP signals will also decrease MEP signals to an even greater degree.

○   **Why is MEP monitoring performed during AAA repair?**

To determine if cross clamping of the aorta reduces blood flow through the artery of Adamkiewicz sufficiently to cause ischemia of the anterior spinal cord resulting in paralysis.

○   **What is the neurological prognosis of victims with traumatic spinal cord injury?**

Cervical spinal cord injuries are more common than thoracic, thoracolumbar or lumbar injuries. Approximately one-third of patients with an upper cervical spinal cord injury die at the scene. Of those that make it to the hospital most are neurologically intact. At least 5% of spine injury patients experience onset of neurologic symptoms, or worsening of preexisting symptoms, after arrival to the hospital.

○   **What level of cervical spine injury results in dependence on mechanical ventilation?**

C_4 or higher.

○   **What is the correct technique to intubate a trauma patient with suspected cervical spine injury using direct laryngoscopy?**

The cervical collar generally must be removed, cricoid pressure applied and neck movement minimized with bimanual stabilization performed by an assistant. Care must be taken to avoid neck traction as it may worsen neurologic damage.

○   **How do you prevent cerebral vasospasm?**

Anticipate and treat it before it happens. The only medication shown to be beneficial in the prevention of cerebral vasospasm is nimodipine. Calcium channel blockers and magnesium have not been shown to improve outcome.

○   **A 55 year old patient with subarachnoid hemorrhage undergoes clipping of a cerebral aneurysm and is treated in the neurointensive care unit for cerebral vasospasm. What therapy has been shown to improve outcome?**

Triple H therapy (hypertension, hemodilution, and hypervolemia) is the mainstay of therapy.

○   **How does thiopental affect the brain?**

Thiopental decreases cerebral blood flow by vasoconstriction and causes a decrease in the functional cerebral metabolic rate ($CmRO_2$).

○   **What causes a decrease in the basal $CmRO_2$?**

Only hypothermia decreases the basal $CmRO_2$ of the brain.

○   **Which anesthetic agents decrease brain $CmRO_2$?**

Propofol, etomidate, thiopental, volatile anesthetics and to a lesser extent benzodiazepines, lidocaine and nitrous oxide decrease brain $CmRO_2$. Opioids do not decrease $CmRO_2$.

○   **Can you reliably use a standard pulse oximeter probe in the MRI scanner?**

No. Ordinary wiring from the pulse oximetry probe can act as an antenna and attract enough radiofrequency energy to distort the MRI images or cause patient burns. The MRI magnetic field also causes pulse oximetry reading artifact.

O   **What are the implications of spinal anesthesia in a patient with pseudotumor cerebri?**

Spinal anesthesia poses no additional risk for this patient given the lack of a CNS lesion and mass effect in the presence of elevated ICP. This patient is actually at a lower risk for post dural puncture headache and in fact, drainage of CSF is therapeutic to reduce headache pain associated with benign intracranial hypertension.

O   **Describe intracranial compliance in terms of the volume-pressure relationship.**

The cranial cavity is a fixed space. Initially, increases in intracranial volume are well compensated for with minimal increases in pressure. However, when the capacity to compensate for volume expansion is exhausted even a small further increase in volume will dramatically increase pressure. Intracranial compliance ($\Delta V/\Delta P$) has been exhausted when intraventricular injection of 1 ml saline results in a 4 mm Hg increase in ICP.

O   **Describe the clinical manifestations of subarachnoid hemorrhage (SAH)?**

Headache, loss of consciousness, pulmonary edema, and decreased ventricular wall motion. The pulmonary and cardiac manifestations are thought to be secondary to norepinephrine release.

O   **Which EEG rhythm waves correspond to the various depths of anesthesia?**

Theta waves are seen during moderately deep anesthesia and delta waves during deep anesthesia. Alpha waves are predominant in the resting awake adult. Beta waves are seen during mental activity and possibly light anesthesia.

O   **What causes EEG burst suppression intraoperatively?**

High dose propofol, isoflurane (2 MAC), barbiturates, etomidate, severe hypoxia, and profound hypothermia (< 15-20 degrees Celsius).

O   **During carotid endarterectomy surgery carotid clamping results in an ipsilateral slowing of the EEG amplitude signal. What does this mean and how can it be treated?**

EEG evidence of cerebral ischemia. Pharmacologically elevating the blood pressure may shunt blood from the contralateral side of the brain to the affected side. If this does not rectify the problem then the surgeon can place a carotid bypass shunt.

O   **In general, how do vasoactive drugs affect cerebral blood flow?**

Vasodilators and vasoconstrictors both tend to increase CBF. Vasodilators produce the same effect in the brain, as in the periphery. Increased cerebral vessel diameter allows for more cerebral blood flow. In contrast, vasoconstrictors only constrict vessels in the periphery, producing an increased driving pressure through the same diameter cerebral vessels, which results in increased cerebral blood flow.

O   **Cerebral autoregulation is effective over what range of mean arterial pressures (MAP)?**

MAP 50-150 mm Hg.

O   **Explain how hyperventilation can actually improve blood flow to the diseased area of brain in a patient with a gliobastoma tumor?**

The key is that in general cerebral autoregulation is not preserved in diseased areas of brain. Hyperventilation leading to a decrease in $PaCO_2$ will cause cerebral vasoconstriction in normal vessels and preferential shunting of blood flow toward the diseased area of brain. This is the "reverse steal phenomenon".

O   **Name the three components of intracranial volume.**

Brain (1400 ml, 85%), Blood (150 ml, 10%), and CSF (75-100 ml, 5%)

O   **How does mannitol influence intracranial pressure?**

Intracranial volume is reduced by the increased osmolality caused by mannitol in the blood pulling water out of the brain compartment. Mannitol is also a weak vasodilator and causes a transient increase in cerebral blood volume. The overall affect of mannitol is to decrease ICP.

O   **What effect does $PaCO_2$ have on intracranial pressure?**

$PaCO_2$ causes cerebral vasodilation and increases cerebral blood flow 2-4% per mm Hg increase in $PaCO_2$ within the range of 20 and 80 mm Hg. The increased CBF leads to increased intracranial blood volume resulting in an increase in ICP.

O   **Describe the arterial blood supply to the spinal cord.**

A single anterior spinal artery supplies blood to the anterior two-thirds of the spinal cord. Paired posterior spinal arteries supply blood to the posterior one-third of the spinal cord.

O   **How is spinal cord blood flow determined?**

Spinal cord blood flow = MAP minus CVP (or ICP, if ICP is greater than CVP). Autoregulation is intact and drug effects on spinal cord blood flow mimic those changes seen in cerebral blood flow. Mass effect (or stretch) can decrease spinal cord blood flow just as it does cerebral blood flow.

O   **In an elderly patient undergoing elective abdominal aortic aneurysm repair what techniques can be employed to minimize the potential for anterior spinal artery syndrome?**

The goal is to minimize the potential for spinal cord ischemia by maximizing blood flow to the spinal cord and decreasing metabolic rate. Spinal cord blood flow is determined by MAP minus ICP, therefore a lumbar drain would allow for lowering ICP and improving blood flow. Moderate hypothermia is advantageous as it decreases metabolic rate. Hyperglycemia can worsen ischemia-induced neurologic injury so monitoring and tight control of serum glucose is essential.

O   **A patient is positioned at a 45 degree incline for sitting craniotomy. Monitoring includes an arterial line with the transducer placed at wrist level (20 cm below the earlobe) and central line with the catheter tip at the SVC/RA junction. The surgeon has just opened the dura. BP 110/50 mm Hg, CVP 10 mm Hg. What is this patient's cerebral perfusion pressure (CPP)?**

CPP = MAP minus CVP, or ICP whichever is greater. In this problem CVP is greater since ICP is zero with the dura open.

MAP is calculated by ((2*DBP) + SBP)/3, or 210/3, therefore MAP = 70 mm Hg. However, the MAP at the earlobe is used for CPP calculation. The transducer is 20 cm H_2O lower than the earlobe. 1 cm H_2O = 0.74 mm Hg. Therefore three quarters of 20 is 15 and the MAP at the ear is 15 mm Hg less than 70, or 55 mm Hg. The calculation then is MAP 55 mm Hg – CVP 10 mm Hg equals 45 mm Hg. The CPP is 45 mm Hg.

O   **What are the possible side effects of nitroprusside used to induce deliberate hypotension?**

Sodium nitroprusside is a nonselective potent vasodilator. It results in both systemic (hypotension) and pulmonary vasodilation (loss of hypoxic pulmonary vasoconstriction, shunting, hypoxemia). Nitroprusside is metabolized by a liver-based enzyme, rhodonase, to thiocyanate which is renally excreted. Prolonged infusions in patients with liver or renal impairment may predispose the patient to cyanide toxicity and hypoxemia. Rebound hypertension is possible with discontinuation of a sodium nitroprusside infusion.

❍   How does induced deliberate hypotension affect ICP?

All vasodilators cause an increase in intracranial blood volume and hence increase ICP.

❍   What pulmonary findings should be anticipated in a patient scheduled for scoliosis surgery?

Commonly in severe scoliosis there is decreased oxygenation secondary to ventilation-perfusion mismatching (with a normal $PaCO_2$). The pulmonary function tests reveal a restrictive pattern with normal FEV_1/FVC ratio and decreased TLC, FRC, IC, ERV and VC. Impaired respiratory muscle function results in an inspiratory force 70% of normal. Scoliosis patients may develop increased pulmonary resistance leading to pulmonary hypertension and right ventricular hypertrophy or dysfunction.

❍   How are neurogenic motor evoked potentials (NMEPs) produced?

The signal is generated at the spinal cord by direct electrode contact and then sensed at the popliteal fossa or posterior tibial nerve. Spinal cord stimulation must occur in a dry field or the current will be dissipated away from the motor neurons of the spinal cord. These signals are relatively resistant to suppression by anesthetic agents and are not eliminated (may actually be improved) if muscle relaxants are given.

❍   What postoperative complications might you expect after resection of a fourth ventricle tumor?

Brainstem swelling may cause central apnea (compression of the respiratory center) or difficulties swallowing (9th cranial nerve nucleus). Of note, fixed and dilated pupils would not be seen with brainstem swelling. The nucleus of the 3rd cranial nerve lies above the tentorium cerebelli and supratentorial pressure is required to cause uncal herniation compressing pupilloconstrictor fibers of the occulomotor nerve producing a fixed and dilated pupil.

❍   How is the diagnosis of cerebral vasospasm made?

Clinical signs and symptoms of cerebral ischemia to the areas supplied by the constricted cerebral artery raise the possibility of cerebral vasospasm. The diagnosis can be confirmed by transcranial doppler, contrast CT, MRA or cerebral angiography.

❍   What is cerebral metabolic uncoupling and how is it produced?

Normally CBF increases to areas of increased metabolic rate and decreases to areas of decreased metabolic rate. Volatile anesthetics decrease $CMRO_2$ and at the same time cause vasodilation and an increase in CBF. This uncoupling phenomenon produces luxury perfusion, or increased perfusion to brain that actually requires less nutrient deliver, because of decreased neuronal activity.

❍   What are the methods for detection of venous air embolism during a sitting craniotomy?

Precordial doppler is the most common method employed and is as sensitive as TEE. A pulmonary artery catheter can be used to detect pulmonary embolism if there is evidence of right heart failure. End tidal nitrogen is relatively insensitive. Even less sensitive is a decrease in end tidal CO_2. Presence of PACs is slightly more sensitive than $ETCO_2$ change. Least sensitive is a decrease in pulse oximetry.

❍   What factors have been implicated in the development of delayed ischemic deficits from cerebral vasospasm following subarachnoid hemorrhage?

Blood in the basilar cistern, hypovolemia and hyponatremia.

○   **70 year old man does not regain consciousness after a 4 hour resection of a large meningioma. What could be the cause of delayed emergence?**

The possibilities are pharmacologic, endocrine/metabolic or structural causes. Common pharmacologic causes include residual effect of volatile agents, opioids, benzodiazepines, or muscle relaxants. Metabolic causes include hypothermia, hypocapnea (which raises the pH and decreases ionized calcium), hypoxia, hyponatremia, acidosis and hypoglycemia. Unrecognized hypothyroidism might also be a culprit. Structural causes are related to the surgical site with bleeding or swelling leading to elevated ICP or a post-ictal state following seizures.

○   **What are the cardiovascular effects of a cervical spinal cord injury?**

Spinal shock due to loss of sympathetic tone leading to vasodilation, relative hypovolemia and hypotension. Unfortunately, because the cardiac accelerator fibers (T_1-T_4) are located below the level of injury the normal tachycardic response to hypovolemia will be absent. The patient will not likely be able to compensate for the lowered SVR and will require pressor support.

○   **What are the EKG findings of SAH?**

The EKG changes originate from the centrally mediated norepinephrine surge associated with SAH and range from ST segment changes and T wave abnormalities to prolonged QT intervals, presence of U waves and P wave abnormalities.

○   **How do propofol and isoflurane differ in their effect on CBF and $CMRO_2$?**

Propofol and isoflurane decrease cerebral metabolic rate. Isoflurane increases cerebral blood flow which results in an uncoupling of CBF and $CMRO_2$. In contrast, propofol causes cerebral vasoconstriction and a decrease in CBF to the areas of decreased metabolic demand. The decrease in metabolic rate is more pronounced than the decrease in blood flow.

○   **What is EEG burst suppression?**

An EEG pattern of deep sedation where periods of electrical silence are interrupted by brief episodes of activity.

○   **What is the treatment for patients in acute neurogenic shock?**

Lack of sympathetic tone produces relative hypovolemia and hypotension. Fluids are the first line of therapy followed by a vasoconstrictor such as norepinephrine. Lesions above the cardiac accelerator fibers (T_1-T_4) may be associated with bradycardia which can be treated with atropine, dopamine, isoproterenol or epinephrine.

○   **Should anxiolytics be given preoperatively to a patient with a brain tumor?**

This decision can only be made on an individual patient basis. In patients with documented or suspected elevation in ICP it is prudent to avoid sedatives. Hypoventilation leading to elevated $PaCO_2$ and increased CBF can worsen elevated ICP. In addition, preoperative sedation may preclude immediate postoperative neurological assessment.

○   **Can you intubate a patient in the MRI scanner?**

Only if you use a MRI compatible laryngoscope blade and handle.

○ **Intracranial bleeding can occur from what vessels during the transphenoidal approach to pituitary tumor resection?**

The transphenoidal approach has many advantages (lower morbidity and mortality, lower incidence of diabetes insipidus, no need for brain retraction) but does not allow the same degree of peri-pituitary structural visualization as the transcranial approach. Significant bleeding can occur from the cavernous sinuses or carotid arteries.

○ **When does cerebral vasospasm usually occur relative to the onset of SAH?**

It usually occurs 4 days to 2 weeks after the initial bleed.

○ **At what CBF does cerebral ischemia become apparent on the EEG?**

20 ml/100g/minute. Normal global CBF is 50 ml/100g/minute. Neuronal damage is thought to occur at CBF below 10 ml/100g/minute.

○ **How does systemic hypertension effect cerebral autoregulation?**

Chronic uncontrolled hypertension will shift the upper and lower limits of the cerebral autoregulation curve to the right (to higher pressures). This phenomenon can be reversed by adequate blood pressure control but it will take at least a few months to shift the cerebral autoregulation limits back towards normal.

○ **What are the different ways that ICP can be measured?**

A bolt (extra dural pressure monitor), an intraventricular catheter (usually lateral ventricular placement), and a camino (ICP measured with placement in the ventricle or brain matter).

○ **Transient neurologic syndrome (TNS) following spinal anesthetia is most common using which local anesthetic agent?**

Lidocaine. Contributing factors include: a dose greater than 75 mg, concentration exceeding 2%, lithotomy positioning and epinephrine added to the solution. The dose of lidocaine has not been definitively proven to correlate with an increased incidence of TNS.

○ **Immediately prior to induction of anesthesia a patient scheduled for resection of a brain tumor begins seizing. How should this be managed?**

ABCs and stop the seizure activity (thiopental or benzodiazepine) with subsequent EEG monitoring to evaluate for continuing seizure activity. Seizures result in increased metabolic demand on the brain and increased CBF. The additional volume of blood within the cranial vault may further increase ICP.

○ **What is the Cushing's triad?**

Elevated ICP, hypertension and bradycardia.

○ **Which volatile anesthetic provides the best cerebral protection?**

Isoflurane has classically been the answer but no advantage has been established over the newer volatile anesthetics, sevoflurane and desflurane.

○ **The surgeon reports that the patient's brain is tight. What are the treatment choices?**

Hyperventilation to a $PaCO_2$ of 25-30 mm Hg, elevate the patient's head, administer thiopental (cerebral vasoconstrictor and decreases $CMRO_2$), make sure there is no obstruction to cranial venous outflow (check head position), and reduce ICP by opening the CSF drain, if this is an option.

ORTHOPEDIC SURGERY

Sticks And Stones May Break My Bones, But Words Will Make Me Go In A Corner And Cry By Myself For Hours.
Eric Idle

○   **What are the boundaries of the epidural space?**

The epidural space is bounded anteriorly by the posterior longitudinal ligament, laterally by the periosteum of the vertebral pedicles and the intervertebral foramina and posteriorly by the ligamentum flavum and the anterior surface of the lamina. Superiorly the space extends to the foramen magnum, where dura is fused to the base of the skull. Caudally, it ends at the sacral hiatus.

○   **What anatomic structures are encountered during correct placement of an epidural needle, using the midline approach?**

As the epidural needle enters the midline of the back between the spinous processes, it passes through the skin and subcutaneous tissue, followed by the supraspinous ligament, the interspinous ligament, the ligamentum flavum and finally, the epidural space.

○   **Injection of lidocaine for which regional nerve block will result in the highest blood concentration of this local anesthetic?**

Intercostal nerve block. The rate of systemic vascular absorption of local anesthetics is proportionate to the vascularity of the site of injection.

○   **A 44 year-old construction worker is about to undergo an open reduction and internal fixation of a fracture of the distal left radius. Brachial plexus anesthesia is provided via an axillary approach, using 40cc of a 1.5% lidocaine solution with epinephrine 1:200,000. The patient's hand and fingers are numb to pin prick. Upon incision over the distal radius however, the patient reports pain. Which peripheral nerve requires supplemental anesthesia?**

The musculocutaneous nerve.

○   **What are the important landmarks for peripheral nerve block for an amputation of the leg below the knee?**

Femoral nerve: Anterior superior iliac spine, pubic tubercle, and lateral to the femoral artery.

Sciatic nerve: Classic approach of Labat (posterior approach): posterior superior iliac spine, greater trochanter of the femur, and the sacral hiatus;
Anterior approach: Anterior superior iliac spine, pubic tubercle, greater and lesser trochanter of the femur.

○   **What are the sequential systemic effects of a lidocaine overdose when an excessive total dose has been delivered with a single injection brachial plexus block?**

Toxic effects (CNS and cardiac) in increasing order of severity are light-headedness, tinnitus, numbness of the tongue and perioral tissues, a metallic taste, confusion, auditory and visual hallucinations, and eye movements not unlike nystagmus; muscle twitching, and unconsciousness; tonic-clonic seizures, coma, and respiratory arrest; hypertension, tachycardia, hypotension, decreased contractility and cardiac output; sinus bradycardia, ventricular dysrhythmias, and circulatory arrest.

○   **The function of which nerve is frequently spared after placement of an interscalene brachial plexus block?**

As blockade of the inferior trunk of the brachial plexus is often incomplete with the interscalene approach, function of the ulnar nerve (C_8-T_1) is frequently spared. These nerves can join the sheath below the level where the block is placed.

○ **What clinical findings would you expect to find with a pulmonary embolism following deflation of a pneumatic tourniquet placed on the thigh? What is the mechanism?**

Sudden, unexplained hypotension, hypoxemia and/or bronchospasm (wheeze, increase in peak airway pressures, decrease in SpO_2). A decrease in end-tidal CO_2 from increased dead-space ventilation is suggestive, but not specific. Should invasive monitoring be in place, an elevation of the central venous pressure and pulmonary artery pressure may be observed from mechanical obstruction of the right ventricle, pulmonary hypertension, acute ischemia from coronary embolization, or combinations thereof.

Significant pulmonary embolism is rare, but has been reported with pneumatic tourniquet inflation (pre-existing clot) and deflation (decreased fibrinolysis or release of plasminogen activators secondary to the inflated tourniquet or the metabolic conditions distal to it). Patients at risk for upper leg and pelvic DVT include: advanced age, bed rest, prior DVT or pulmonary embolism, morbid obesity, venous insufficiency, oral contraceptive use among young female patients and malignancy. The risk of embolism from immobilization increases with time. Embolization of fat, marrow or air may occur from high-volume, and pressurized cement use, especially in the femoral canal.

○ **What are the significant anatomical landmarks for a median nerve block at the elbow?**

The median nerve can be blocked at its location just medial to the brachial artery on a line connecting the medial and lateral epicondyles of the humerus (intercondylar line) at a depth of about 5 cm.

○ **What are the significant anatomical landmarks for a radial nerve block at the elbow?**

Lateral epicondyle of humerus, brachioradialis muscle and tendon of biceps.

At the elbow, the radial nerve is blocked 2 cm lateral to the biceps tendon (medial to the brachioradialis muscle) on the intercondylar line, just superficial to the underlying bone.

○ **Which five nerve blocks are required for a complete ankle block?**

Tibial nerve, deep peroneal nerve, superficial peroneal nerve, sural nerve and saphenous nerve.

○ **A twenty-three year-old football player sustained fractures of the fourth and fifth metatarsal bones and presents for open reduction and fixation. An ankle block is performed. On incision over the fifth toe, the patient complains of pain. Which nerve is most likely to be inadequately blocked?**

The sural nerve (lateral dorsal cutaneous nerve) innervates the lateral edge of the foot to the fifth toe.

○ **What are the considerations in securing the airway in a patient with rheumatoid arthritis who is to undergo general anesthesia for total knee replacement?**

Ankylosis of the temporomandibular joint, if present, leads to limited mouth opening. Ankylosis and fixation of the cervical vertebrae will result in severely limited range of motion of the neck. Laxity or disruption of the cruciform ligament of the axis leads to mobility of the odontoid process within the spinal canal. Anterior atlantoaxial subluxation occurs in approximately 20% to 40% of patients. Posterior subluxation, occurring during neck flexion is far less common, and can result in severe neurologic injury, including quadriplegia. Arthritis of the cricoarytenoid joint is fairly common, which can present with a foreign body feeling and painful swallowing or speaking. It can progress to hoarseness and stridor, which may occur because of swelling and fixation of the vocal cords.

○   **During which orthopedic procedures is there a risk of venous air embolism?**

Venous air embolism may occur during any procedure where the operative field is above the level of the heart, especially if the distance is > 5 cm, (cervical spine surgery in the sitting position, shoulder surgery in the beach chair position, spine surgery in the prone position, and hip surgery in the lateral position), when sinuses are open (after bone cement removal during revision of total hip arthroplasty), with a large gravitational gradient and low central venous filling pressure and from the pressurization of the cement when it is placed at a site without protection of the circulation by pneumatic tourniquet (endoprosthesis insertions into the femur).

○   **What advantage may regional anesthesia provide over general anesthesia for total hip replacement?**

*   Lower total blood loss
*   Less risk of transfusion-related morbidity and cost
*   Lower incidence of deep venous thrombosis
*   Less acute postoperative confusion (not significant at 3 months postoperatively)
*   Hypotensive epidural anesthesia may improve the quality of the interface between methylmethacrylate and bone
*   May improve neutrophil activity

○   **How does hypotensive anesthesia affect the quality of cement bone fixation during total hip replacement?**

Hypotensive anesthesia has radiographically been demonstrated to improve the quality of cement bone fixation, as the quality of fixation at the cement-bone interface is improved if there is an absence of blood across the cancellous bone during application of the cement.

○   **How may profound hypotension and hypoxia result from the employment of polymethylmethacrylate cement and the insertion of a cemented femoral prosthesis during total hip replacement?**

Profound hypotension and circulatory collapse occurs in less than 5% of long stem and revision total hip arthroplasties. This occurrence may result from the solubilization of fat and embolization of fat, air or bone marrow following relocation of the hip joint and the unkinking of the femoral vein. Also possible but unproved is a direct action of the cement (monomer, and to a lesser extent the small-chain polymer), which may cause vasodilation and/or direct myocardial depression, degranulation of mast cells and the release of histamine.

○   **What are the systemic effects of tourniquet release during limb surgery under general anesthesia?**

Depending upon the duration of tourniquet inflation (especially longer than 30 minutes), and whether an upper or lower limb is isolated (the effect is significantly greater in the lower extremity), the following hemodynamic and metabolic effects may be noted:
-Transient drop in mean arterial pressure and CVP which may remain significantly depressed up to 15 minutes post release caused by: volume shift back to the limb on deflation of the tourniquet; post ischemic reactive vasodilatation with decrease in SVR; myocardial depression; bleeding from non-ligated vessels.
- Increase in heart rate 6-12 bpm
- Transient increase in cerebral blood flow and decrease in cerebral perfusion pressure
- Decrease in core body temperature of 0.7 °C within 90 seconds of deflation of lower limb tourniquet
- Release of vasoactive substances (lactate, prostaglandin and bradykinin)
- Reduction in pH and serum bicarbonate
- Elevation of potassium, lactic acid, lactic acid dehydrogenase and creatinine kinase
- Transient decrease in central venous oxygen tension, but systemic hypoxemia is unusual
- Acute rise in end-tidal CO_2, with peak levels observed within 1 minutes, persisting for 10 minutes
Changes in arterial pH, PaO_2, $PaCO_2$, lactate and potassium normalize within 30 minutes.

○   **Prior to tourniquet deflation in a trauma patient who may have associated blunt head injury, what considerations should be given to prevent secondary injury to the brain?**

Intravenous fluid administration with hyperventilation and vasopressor agents, as needed, for 10-15 minutes following tourniquet deflation may ameliorate the associated hypotension and hypercarbia which could produce an increase in cerebral blood flow and ICP, with a decrease in cerebral perfusion pressure that would worsen the cerebral injury.

○   **How does recovery of transient hypotension and hypercapnia after release of a pneumatic thigh tourniquet differ in general anesthesia with mechanically-controlled ventilation (CMV) when compared with regional anesthesia (epidural or spinal) with conscious spontaneous respiration?**

The recovery of hypotension is faster in general anesthesia with CMV than regional anesthesia with conscious spontaneous respiration. The reverse is true for recovery from hypercapnia.

○   **What is the explanation for a gradual increase in blood pressure during application of a pneumatic tourniquet for limb surgery?**

The mechanism is not completely understood. Tourniquet inflation mostly likely stimulates C fibers, which then activate N-methyl-D-aspartic acid (NMDA) receptors. The NMDA receptor activation increases blood pressure. Tourniquet-induced hypertension occurs in 11-66 percent of cases approximately 30-60 minutes after inflation of the cuff. It is more common with general anesthesia than with regional anesthesia.

○   **Describe tourniquet pain. What modalities of treatment have been proposed?**

Tourniquet pain is described as dull, burning, deep, poorly localized and aching pain that increases steadily until it becomes unbearable. It develops in up to 66% of patients during limb surgery under regional anesthesia, 30 to 60 minutes after cuff inflation. Suggested treatments include: sedation; IV opioids; double cuff with distal cuff over anesthetized area; intercostobrachial and subcutaneous blocks; sympathetic block; EMLA under the cuff; vibratory massager to inflate cuff; TENS; When tourniquet pain occurs most interventions are ineffective. *Supported prophylactic measures* include plain solutions of buivacaine for long duration spinals or epidurals and larger doses of LA for spinals. *Treatment* is symptomatic therapy, temporary use of a double tourniquet, general anesthesia; tourniquet release (relief of pain correlates with correction of metabolic abnormalities).

○   **What is the predominant cause of mortality following total joint replacement?**

Fatal pulmonary embolism; rates as high as 3% to 5% have been reported.

○   **An eight year-old male suffered a fractured right forearm and femur during a motor vehicle accident. His past medical history includes severe juvenile rheumatoid arthritis. What anesthetic considerations must be made for his medical condition?**

These pediatric patients are apt to develop fusion of the cervical spine and perichondrium of epiphyseal plates. Endotracheal intubation may therefore be complicated by a fixed neck and hypoplastic mandible. Axillary brachial plexus block may be difficult if this patient is unable to abduct his injured upper extremity. Conduction blockade may be technically difficult if he is frozen in a characteristic lumbar lordosis. Exaggerated neck flexion and inability of the patient to rotate his head may make placement of a central line via an internal jugular approach difficult to achieve.

○   **In general, what tourniquet pressures are required to prevent bleeding during orthopedic surgery?**

A cuff pressure 100 mm Hg above a patient's measured systolic pressure is adequate for the thigh, while 50 mm Hg above systolic pressure is adequate for the arm.

Arbitrary numbers like 250 mm Hg and 300 mm Hg are often selected. Should hypertensive episodes occur, cuff pressure should be increased accordingly. A general rule is to select a pressure between one and a half and two times the average anticipated systolic pressure. If the patient's systolic pressure exceeds the inflation pressure of the tourniquet, obstruction to venous outflow will occur (venous tourniquet). Inflation to very high pressures may create a bloodless field but cause disruption of the microvascular anatomy of the underlying muscle.

O   **What are contraindications of tourniquet use?**

Absolute contraindications
*   Sickle cell disease or other hemoglobinopathies that change configuration in response to acidosis or hypoxia
*   Severe peripheral vascular disease with arterial spasm or vasculitis
*   Ongoing ischemia in the operative limb

Relative contraindications
*   Existing peripheral neuropathy
*   Chronic vascular insufficiency of the limb
*   Synthetic or venous vascular graft for dialysis (thrombosis risk)
*   Existing venous insufficiency from either lymph node dissection (mastectomy) or vein harvest for revascularization or radiation therapy
*   Proven infection in the operative extremity, as both acute pulmonary edema and cardiac arrest have been reported after tourniquet
*   An extremity with a tumor where tumor cells may be introduced into the systemic circulation

O   **What is the safest maximum tourniquet time?**

The safest time is the shortest time. Current information suggests continuous application should not exceed 2 hours.

O   **How can postoperative ulnar neuropathy be avoided in a patient undergoing hand surgery?**

Padding and proper positioning of both the operative and non-operative upper extremity are important so that direct compression of the ulnar nerve immediately above the elbow and in the olecranon notch does not occur. Supination, as opposed to pronation of the forearm is desirable. Ongoing vigilance is mandatory, as movement caused by the surgery may alter correct positioning. However, all postoperative ulnar neuropathies are not preventable, and may occur without any evident cause.

O   **A seventy-eight-year-old female with severe, longstanding kyphoscoliosis is to undergo triple arthrodesis of the right foot under general anesthesia. What physiologic changes are suspected in this patient?**

Scoliosis impacts primarily the pulmonary and cardiovascular systems.

Pulmonary
*   Restrictive disease of the lungs with an associated reduction in lung volumes
*   Pulmonary hypertension (reactive and fixed)
*   Limited pulmonary reserve or respiratory failure; increase in normal postoperative pulmonary dysfunction which may require postoperative ventilatory support

Cardiovascular
*   Right ventricular dysfunction from chronic hypoxemia and pulmonary hypertension
*   Polycythemia (chronic hypoxemia)
*   Restrictive pericarditis and possible secondary pericardial effusion

○   **What is the concentration of epinephrine which corresponds to a 1:200,000 dilution?**

5 mcg/ml. 1 gm/ml = 1,000,000 mcg/ml = 1:1. Divide 1,000,000 mcg by dilution factor of 1:200,000 (1,000,000/200,000) = 5.

○   **A thirty-five year-old male is scheduled to undergo the removal of a protruding right fibular screw, originally placed 8 months prior, during an open reduction and internal fixation of the right ankle following a skiing accident. The area surrounding the protruding screw appears to be infected. Why is the injection of bupivacaine 0.25% around this area unlikely to produce an effective infiltrative nerve block?**

Local anesthetics are weak bases and cross nerve membranes to provide local anesthesia when in a lipid-soluble, nonionized form at physiologic pH. An injection into an acidic, infected area will provide poor quality anesthesia, as the predominant fraction of the anesthetic will exist in an ionized form which will not cross membranes.

○   **Why may significant hemodynamic changes result from an epidural blockade, but not from a subarachnoid block?**

Much larger doses of local anesthetic are utilized for epidural block. The proximity of the large venous plexus of Batson in the epidural space can provide transport of drug to the heart and the central nervous system.

○   **How is the function of the urinary bladder affected as a result of an epidural blockade?**

Temporary urinary bladder atony results from blockade of sacral segments S_2 to S_4. Catheterization of the bladder may become necessary until resolution of the block, especially if a continuous epidural technique is to be utilized intraoperatively and/or postoperatively. Overfilling may result in a neurogenic bladder. The incidence of urinary retention is related to the type of anesthesia (any central block), the surgical procedure (pelvic and major spine surgery will decrease the voiding reflex) and its duration.

○   **A seventy-eight year-old woman is undergoing left total knee arthroplasty. Twenty-five minutes following epidural blockade to the level of T_2 the patient becomes unconscious and apneic, requiring immediate intubation and mechanical ventilation. What is the most likely cause of this complication?**

High epidural blockade will result from the introduction of large volumes of local anesthetic solutions into the epidural space. Although rare, respiratory arrest most commonly results from extensive sympathetic blockade (which may develop over 25 to 30 minutes), reduced cardiac output, and reduced oxygen delivery to the brain.

Epidural blockade decreases pulmonary function proportionate to the level of motor block achieved (loss of abdominal muscles impairs active expiration; loss of intercostal muscles impairs inspiration and the ability to generate negative intrathoracic pressure; leaving the patient dependent on the diaphragm). In addition, high sensory blockade may blunt the respiratory response to hypercarbia. Contributory factors are more significant in patients with COPD.

○   **A sixty-two year old veteran male with long-standing insulin dependent diabetes and chronic obstructive pulmonary disease requires amputation of the right leg below the knee. If peripheral nerve blockade of the lower extremity is considered as the sole anesthetic, which nerves must be blocked to provide adequate regional anesthesia for this procedure?**

The femoral nerve and the sciatic nerve.

○   **Why does a motor block precede a sensory block when an axillary approach to a brachial plexus block is performed?**

The loss of motor function often preceding sensory block may be explained by the peripheral location of motor fibers along the peripheral nerves, despite the fact that motor fibers are larger in diameter than sensory fibers.

O   **Epidural anesthesia is chosen for a right above the knee amputation in a sixty-seven year-old male with peripheral vascular disease. Loss of resistance is obtained through a 17 gauge Tuohy needle with the patient in the lateral position. Immediately following the introduction of a 3cc test dose of local anesthetic solution containing epinephrine, clear fluid is noted to flow freely from the needle hub when the syringe is removed from the hub. How can you determine that the fluid is cerebrospinal fluid?**

If the immediate, free-flowing fluid is warm to the touch, it is likely to be CSF. A solution of local anesthetic just introduced into the epidural space is likely to still be near room temperature. If the returning fluid precipitates in a container of etidocaine solution, it is CSF. Local anesthetic solutions do not precipitate in etidocaine solution. CSF will also induce a positive color change on glucose test tape, while a solution containing local anesthetic will not.

O   **Why do elderly patients require less local anesthetic than young patients for the same spread of an epidural block?**

Narrowing of the intervertebral spaces in elderly patients. The decrease in dose requirement is magnified when larger volumes of anesthetic solution are used.

Extensive leakage of local anesthetic fluid has been demonstrated to occur through intervertebral foramina. While young patients have been shown to have largely patent intervertebral foramina, the intervertebral foramina of elderly patients have commonly been found to be blocked by areolar tissue.

O   **An active and otherwise healthy eighty-year-old female with osteoarthritis is to undergo general anesthesia with thiopental, rocuronium, isoflurane, N_2O, and O_2, for left hip replacement. Following induction and endotracheal intubation, the lungs are easily ventilated bilaterally. After she is placed in the right lateral decubitus position however, lung inflation requires high peak airway pressures. Upon auscultation, breath sounds are faint; wheezing is heard. What diagnoses do you entertain, and what immediate action(s) is (are) appropriate?**

Consider light anesthesia versus migration or mechanical obstruction of the endotracheal tube. The patient may also have underlying hyperactive airways disease.

Visually inspect whether the airway is patent as this is most likely from the description of little airway movement (breath sounds are faint). Listen to breath sounds bilaterally. If an obstruction/mainstem intubation is not immediately apparent, note the vital signs, and deepen the patient's anesthesia with the thought that bronchospasm is the result of light anesthesia. If that is insufficient, reposition the patient supine, reauscultate, and ensure patency and proper positioning of the endotracheal tube (fiberoptic inspection or extubate and reintubate).

O   **A fifteen-year old female with idiopathic thoracolumbar scoliosis is undergoing spinal instrumentation and fusion under general anesthesia with N_2O-O_2, narcotic, and muscle relaxant. What information is provided with the monitoring of somatosensory evoked potentials (SSEPs) intraoperatively?**

In this case SSEPs are elicited by stimulation of the common peroneal or posterior tibial nerve at the ankle. Characteristic electrical responses detected over the cortex indicate that the associated neural pathways along the spinal cord are intact. Baseline latency ("latency") of the response, and the magnitude of the response ("amplitude") are measured preoperatively. Values for latency and amplitude are then obtained nearly continuously intraoperatively, and compared with baseline values. The amplitude of the response is considered to be a more valid indication of the status of the nervous system than is the latency of the response.

O   **An eight-year old male with severe cerebral palsy presents for bilateral, femoral flexor tendon releases under general anesthesia. What are the pertinent anesthetic considerations?**

- Chronic malnutrition and dehydration
- Mild renal impairment
- Intravenous access may be difficult if contractures are severe, or if the patient is uncooperative
- An agitated or uncooperative patient may be dangerous to the health care team
- Positioning may be challenging
- Aspiration is a risk due to chronic gastroesophageal reflux, agitation and bulbar palsy with incompetent airway reflexes
- Chronic aspiration may lead to pulmonary dysfunction
- Succinylcholine in this case is not contraindicated
- Postoperative risk of respiratory depression from narcotics and residual anesthetic effects
- Nursing considerations related to limb spasticity

O   **An otherwise healthy sixteen-year old female with severe thoracolumbar scoliosis is to undergo spinal instrumentation under general anesthesia. Monitoring of SSEPs by stimulation of the posterior tibial nerve (PTN) at the ankle is planned. During the operation, what are likely causes for an increase in latency and decrease in amplitude of SSEPs with stimulation of the PTN?**

Provided that a preoperative, baseline response to PTN stimulation is normal, then pre-existing neuromuscular disease and other neurologic disorders, all of which can affect SSEPs, can effectively be ruled out. Surgical factors that will alter the latency and amplitude of SSEPs intraoperatively include direct trauma to the spinal cord, spinal cord ischemia, and the combination of externally applied pressure (such as that from instrumentation or bone fragments), and decreased spinal cord blood flow. Other factors important to the nurse anesthetist are hypoxia, hypercarbia, hypotension, hypothermia, and inhalation agents. Barbiturates, propofol, droperidol, diazepam, fentanyl, and morphine also have an effect on SSEPs. It is important for a steady state of anesthesia and physiologic variables to exist during critical monitoring phases to isolate the effect of surgery on the neural pathways.

O   **Of the approaches to blockade of the brachial plexus, which technique is most likely to result in inadvertent, intravenous injection of local anesthetic?**

The axillary approach to brachial plexus blockade is most likely to result in intravenous injection of local anesthetic because a major vein is underlying the nerves, and within the brachial plexus sheath at this level. The transarterial technique (high volume of local anesthetic injected posterior to the axillary artery) requires use of epinephrine for a vascular marker and injection in incremental doses, as the risk of intra-arterial injection is high.

O   **What is the mantle effect?**

When a peripheral nerve block is performed, a high concentration of local anesthetic surrounds the mantle of the nerve. Diffusion of local anesthetic into the bundle proceeds from the periphery, where the concentration is high, toward the "core", where the concentration will rise more slowly. Fibers located on the outside of the nerve bundle are anesthetized first, followed by fibers located at the "core" of the mantle. As peripherally located fibers innervate proximal structures in a limb, and centrally located fibers innervate more distal structures, anesthesia of the thigh for example, will precede anesthesia of the foot. This phenomenon has been termed the "mantle effect."

O   **Why should an interscalene approach to brachial plexus blockade not be considered the ideal choice in a sixty-two year old patient with moderate to severe COPD who is to undergo left shoulder replacement?**

An interscalene block is associated with unilateral phrenic nerve paralysis in virtually all cases causing an approximate 25% decrease in FEV_1 and FVC. Patients with pulmonary disease may not tolerate either the subjective dyspnea or the loss of functional residual capacity when respiratory function is driven by only one side of the diaphragm. Other complications include pneumothorax, high subarachnoid or epidural block, and an increased risk of dyspnea, hypoxia, and respiratory arrest.

❍   **A bed-ridden, eighty-three year old male with severe peripheral vascular disease, coronary artery disease, and history of congestive heart failure is to undergo a left above the knee amputation. What are the important anatomical landmarks for block of the obturator nerve as part of the peripheral nerve blocks adequate to provide regional anesthesia?**

Important landmarks for an obturator nerve block include the area two cm lateral and inferior to the pubic tubercle, and the horizontal ramus of the pubis. Alternatively, a 3-in-1 femoral block (inguinal ligament, femoral artery pulsation as landmarks) can also work.

❍   **What are complications reported with a supraclavicular approach to brachial plexus blockade?**

Pneumothorax is the most common complication, with an incidence of at least 1 percent if sought by x-ray (incidence is less if clinical signs are used for detection). Intravascular injection into the subclavian artery or vein is possible. Injury to the thoracic duct (left-sided block) and nerves of the brachial plexus are possible. Phrenic nerve paresis has been reported to occur in 28% to 80% of cases.

❍   **Which nerve block(s) is(are) frequently required for supplementation of an interscalene brachial plexus blockade for surgery of the proximal upper extremity?**

The intercostobrachial nerve and the median brachial cutaneous nerve. Thoracic innervation enters the arm, outside of the brachial plexus sheath, especially the skin surface innervated by C_2 to C_4, the medial thorax and the axilla.

❍   **Which peripheral nerves must be blocked to provide adequate regional anesthesia for arthroscopic knee surgery with the use of a tourniquet?**

The femoral, lateral femoral cutaneous, sciatic, and obturator nerves.

❍   **Which dermatomes correspond to the level of innervation by sympathetic cardiac accelerator fibers?**

Dermatomal levels T_1 through T_4.

❍   **Which dermatomes supply the inguinal region?**

Dermatomal levels T_{12} and L_1.

❍   **A four-year old boy with osteogenesis imperfecta and multiple long bone fractures is to undergo placement of bilateral femoral and tibial Sheffield expanding rods under general anesthesia. What are the considerations in securing this patient's airway?**

Head positioning for mask ventilation and intubation may be complicated by iatrogenic cervical fractures. Positioning of the head is furthermore made difficult by the likelihood that the patient may have an enlarged head and atlanto-axial instability. As these patients present with brittle teeth, placement of an oral airway, performance of laryngoscopy, and endotracheal intubation must be accomplished with great care, as teeth are easily broken.

❍   **How is a lateral femoral cutaneous nerve block performed?**

A needle is inserted 2.5 cm medial and 2.5 cm caudal to the anterior superior iliac spine, just below the inguinal ligament (fascia lata). Local anesthetic solution (10 to 15 cc) is then injected in a fan-wise direction.

❍   **What are contraindications to the use of an intravenous regional anesthetic?**

All contraindications and relative contraindications to the use of pneumatic tourniquets.

Intravenous regional anesthesia should be avoided in patients with severe peripheral vascular disease, and Raynaud's disease, where extended peripheral ischemia may occur. Sickle cell disease or trait is of concern, where sickling is promoted in acidic, hypoxemic, cold or ischemic environments. Patients with significant systolic hypertension, heart block, seizure disorder, hepatic disease, or cellulitis at the tourniquet site should also not be considered candidates for intravenous regional anesthesia.

LIVER SURGERY

Whoever Undertakes To Set Himself Up As Judge In The Field Of Truth And Knowledge Is Shipwrecked By The Laughter Of The Gods.
Albert Einstein

○ **What is the blood supply of the liver?**

The liver receives 25% of the cardiac output. Seventy five percent of the blood supply is derived from the portal vein and 25% from the hepatic artery. The hepatic oxygen supply, however, is derived approximately 50% from each.

○ **How does anesthesia affect liver blood flow?**

It depends on the type of anesthesia. Regional anesthesia has minimal effects on liver blood flow unless accompanied by hypotension. General anesthesia uniformly decreases liver blood flow by approximately 20-30%.

○ **What factors affect liver blood flow during anesthesia?**

Hypoxemia, hypocarbia, hypercarbia, hypovolemia and sympathetic stimulation. Surgical manipulation in the right upper quadrant can reduce hepatic blood flow up to 60% from sympathetic activation or direct compression of the vena cava and splanchnic vessels. Pneumoperitoneum significantly decreases hepatic blood flow during laparoscopic cholecystectomy compared with small incision gallbladder surgery.

○ **What are the effects of CO_2 on the liver blood flow?**

Hypocarbia decreases hepatic arterial blood flow. Hypercarbia reduces portal blood flow (sympathetic activation causing splanchnic vasoconstriction) and increases hepatic artery flow.

○ **What are the typical hemodynamic changes seen in cirrhosis?**

- Hyperdynamic circulation (high cardiac index and stroke volume, low systemic vascular resistance, low-to-normal mean arterial pressure, mild tachycardia)
- Central hypovolemia
- Hyporesponsiveness of the vasculature to pressor therapy
- Flow-dependent oxygen consumption
- Changes in the hepatic and splanchnic vasculature (portal hypertension, portal-systemic collateral circulation and decreased hepatic blood flow)

○ **What are the typical arterial blood gases seen in cirrhosis?**

Mild to moderate hypoxemia and respiratory alkalosis.

○ **What electrolyte changes are seen in patients with chronic liver disease?**

Typically, hyponatremia due to retention of water and impaired handling of sodium by the kidneys and hypokalemic metabolic alkalosis. Hypophosphatemia, hypocalcemia and hypomagnesemia are also seen.

○ **Why are patients with fulminant hepatic failure prone to hypoglycemia?**

Hypoglycemia is common due to failure of gluconeogenesis, insufficient insulin degradation and depletion of glycogen stores in the liver.

○   **Which are the vitamin K dependent coagulation factors?**

Factors II, VII, IX, X, and proteins C, S and Z.

○   **Is regional anesthesia contraindicated in patients with chronic liver disease?**

Coagulopathy and portal hypertension may contraindicate the use of regional anesthesia. Peripheral nerve blocks may pose less risk than a spinal or epidural technique if the nerve sheaths are located in a manually compressible space.

○   **Would you decrease the dose of local anesthetics in patients with liver disease?**

In theory, ester local anesthetics (procaine, chloroprocaine) can have a prolonged duration of action due to a decrease in plasma pseudocholinesterase levels. However, clinical duration of action is likely to be unaffected due to normal RBC esterase activity. Amide local anesthetic (lidocaine, bupivacaine, ropivacaine) doses need to be reduced due to decreased intrinsic clearance.

○   **A patient with massive ascites is scheduled for surgery requiring general anesthesia. How would you secure the airway?**

By rapid sequence induction (or awake intubation). Increase in intraabdominal pressure due to moderate or massive ascites and gastric and intestinal hypomotility increases the risk of aspiration.

○   **What is TIPS?**

Transjugular intrahepatic portosystemic shunt is an interventional radiologic procedure used in the management of variceal hemorrhage, which cannot be controlled with medical therapy or sclerotherapy. A communication is created between the hepatic and portal veins through the hepatic parenchyma by percutaneous placement of an expandable metallic stent via the internal jugular vein.

○   **A cirrhotic patient develops prolonged apnea after succinylcholine. What are the causes?**

Slightly prolonged duration of apnea is expected following succinylcholine in patients with liver disease due to a decrease in synthesis of pseudocholinesterase. A duration of longer than 10 minutes should alert one to the possibility of other causes.

○   **What drugs have a prolonged effect in pseudocholinesterase-deficient patients?**

Succinylcholine, mivacurium, ester local anesthetics (possibly) and trimethaphan.

○   **A cirrhotic patient undergoing portocaval shunt surgery has profuse surgical bleeding. Transfusion of red cells and fresh frozen plasma is in progress. The patient is hypotensive despite adequate replacement of intravascular volume. What is the most likely cause?**

Myocardial depression and peripheral vasodilation due to acute hypocalcemia from citrate toxicity, as citrate binds calcium. CPDA-1 (Citrate Phosphate Dextrose Adenine) is an anticoagulant preservative in blood. Citrate levels are high following rapid blood infusion (>1.5-2 ml/kg/min) and/or decreased metabolism due to hypothermia and/or states of absent or reduced liver blood flow. Ionized calcium levels < 0.56 mEq/L are likely to be associated with hypotension.

○   **How do you manage coagulopathy in patients scheduled for surgery?**

This includes administration of vitamin K (lack of response within 24 hours with PT ratio still >1.5 implies severe liver disease), FFP to correct PT within three seconds of normal, cryoprecipitate for fibrinogen levels below 100 mg/dl and transfusion of platelets to levels above 100,000 µL. Desmopressin may be efficacious. Prothrombin time is the best prognostic indicator for recovery of liver function and may be very resistant to attempted normalization with factor replacement therapy.

○   **A cirrhotic patient undergoing surgery for portocaval shunt is bleeding intraoperatively, in spite of administration of FFP, cryoprecipitate and platelets. What is your differential diagnosis?**

Suspect primary fibrinolysis and/or portal hypertension with excessive filling pressures. This may be demonstrated by thromboelastography or other laboratory tests and measurement of central filling pressures or stroke volume.

○   **What drugs are available to treat primary fibrinolysis in patients with liver disease?**

Epsilon aminocaproic acid, tranexamic acid or aprotinin.

○   **Is intraoperative administration of vitamin K indicated in a bleeding patient?**

Although peak effects may take as long as 24 hours, beneficial effects may be observed within hours after IM administration.

○   **Is DDAVP effective during intraoperative bleeding in cirrhotic patients?**

DDAVP may improve hemostasis by increasing factor VIII and von Willebrand factor. Desmopressin can cause hypotension, hyponatremia and increased platelet adhesiveness.

○   **Would you use halothane in a cirrhotic patient?**

Halothane is not contraindicated, but it should be avoided, as it is accompanied by the most prominent decrease in hepatic blood flow and oxygen supply and the greatest incidence of postoperative hepatic dysfunction of all available inhaled anesthetic agents. Anesthesia-induced hepatitis can occur on an immunologic basis with exposure to halothane, but this finding is rare and there is no evidence that cirrhosis is a predisposing factor.

○   **Is cisatracurium the drug of choice for neuromuscular blockade in patients with liver disease?**

Cisatracurium is ideal for muscle relaxation, being an intermediate-acting drug relatively independent of renal or hepatic function for elimination.

○   **Which muscle relaxants are largely eliminated by the liver?**

Vecuronium and rocuronium.

○   **What are the considerations if you choose to use pancuronium or vecuronium in patients with liver disease?**

The initial dose is increased due to increased volume of distribution. Repeat doses are dictated by elimination pathways: pancuronium has prolonged elimination; vecuronium < 0.15 mg/kg, the kinetics and duration of action are unaltered.

○   **What are the cardiovascular implications of alcoholic liver disease during anesthesia?**

Overt or subclinical cardiomyopathy and ventricular arrhythmias.

○   **What drugs are effective if spasm of the sphincter of Oddi is suspected?**

Atropine, glucagon, naloxone and nitroglycerin.

○   **What are the hemodynamic consequences of IVC cross-clamping?**

Clamping of the inferior vena cava decreases venous return, which results in a decrease in preload and cardiac output. This leads to hypotension, which causes a compensatory increase in SVR and heart rate.

○   **What is the half-life of albumin in plasma?**

The half-life of albumin is 20 days. Consequently, albumin levels will be normal in acute fulminant liver failure. Exogenous albumin lasts about 4 hours.

○   **Which plasma proteins are synthesized by the liver?**

All plasma proteins except factor VIII, von Willebrand factor and gamma globulins.

○   **How does severe parenchymal liver disease and biliary disease impair blood coagulation?**

The clotting factors V, VII, IX, X, prothrombin and fibrinogen are all dependent on the liver for synthesis. Parenchymal liver disease causes impaired formation of coagulation factors, fibrinolytic proteins and their inhibitors, as well as, defective hepatic clearance of activated fibrinolytic factors (tissue plasminogen activator). Thrombocytopenia and platelet dysfunction are also contributory. Biliary obstruction may decrease vitamin K absorption due to the absence of bile salts. In early stage cholestatic liver disease there may be TEG evidence of hypercoagulability due to increased levels of fibrinogen and preservation of platelet counts and function.

○   **What is the principal physiologic function of albumin?**

Albumin maintains normal plasma oncotic pressure and is the peripheral binding and transport protein for a large number of drugs. A serum albumin < 2.5 g/dL will clinically impact colloid oncotic pressure, placing the patient at risk for increased third space fluid shifts (edema and ascites) and significant alterations in protein-drug binding.

○   **List the major factors contributing to postoperative liver failure.**

Patients with pre-existing liver disease, massive blood transfusion, hepatic oxygen deprivation (hypoxemia, anemia, decreased arterial pressure or cardiac output and decreased hepatic blood flow), septicemia and drug toxicity.

○   **What is the most common cause of postoperative jaundice?**

If you ask a surgeon, halothane-induced hepatitis. If you ask an anesthetist, inadequate oxygenation of hepatocytes which is often due to multiple factors and difficult to diagnose.

○   **What factors are responsible for altered drug pharmacokinetics in patients with advanced liver disease?**

Impaired hepatocyte function (P450 cytochrome biotransformation, transport processes or biliary excretion), reduced hepatic blood flow, changes in free fraction of protein-bound drugs and altered volume of distribution.

○   **What are the best laboratory tests for evaluation of liver function?**

Parenchymal damage with failure of synthetic function:
• Prothrombin (PT)

- Albumin
- Aminotransferases: ALT (alanine) is the gold standard biomarker for hepatocellular injury
- AST (aspartate)

Cholestasis of obstructive liver disease:
- Bilirubin (total, conjugated and unconjugated)
- Alkaline phosphatase

Due to the liver's large functional reserve, routine laboratory values may be normal in the presence of significant underlying disease.

○ **Preoperative assessment of a patient scheduled for elective surgery is unremarkable except for an unexpected elevation in transaminase levels. What is the correct plan of action?**

Investigate prior to surgery and establish a diagnosis. For acute liver disease, surgery should be deferred until the condition improves. In patients with chronic liver disease either Child's class A or non-cirrhotic liver disease, proceed with surgery. In Child's class B and C cirrhosis, proceed with great caution or consider alternatives to surgery. Mortality rates are 30% and 75%, respectively.

○ **T/F: The perioperative mortality associated with acute hepatitis is the same in cases of acute viral hepatitis as those with acute alcoholic hepatitis.**

False. The surgical mortality rate in patients with alcoholic hepatitis is believed to be worse, in some series approaching 100%. The diagnosis is likely if the AST/ALT ratio exceeds 2:1.

○ **In acute viral hepatitis, what is the first sign of acute liver failure?**

Coagulopathy. INR > 1.75

○ **What are the risk factors associated with perioperative complications in cirrhotic patients?**

Male gender, high Child-Pugh score, ascites, cirrhosis other than primary biliary cirrhosis (especially cryptogenic cirrhosis), elevated serum creatinine, chronic obstructive pulmonary disease, preoperative infection, upper GI bleeding, ASA III or IV, high surgical severity score, surgery of the respiratory system and intraoperative hypotension.

○ **T/F: The odds ratio for perioperative mortality after cholecystectomy in patients with cirrhosis compared to patients without liver disease is 8.5.**

True. Liver disease markedly increases the risk of perioperative death. (odds ratio 8.47: 95% confidence interval, 6.34-11.33)

○ **Describe a patient with Child's C classification of liver disease.**

Bilirubin > 3 mg/dL (PBC and PSC patients > 10 mg/dL), albumin < 3 mg/dL, moderate ascites, advanced encephalopathy, poor nutrition, surgical risk mortality rate 50%. The Pugh Modification replaces nutrition with PT prolongation: C: PT > 6 sec over control or INR > 2.3.

○ **What is the Pringle maneuver?**

Interruption of hepatic vascular inflow by temporary occlusion of the portal triad (hepatic artery, portal vein and bile duct). The liver will tolerate 60 minutes of continuous vascular occlusion and 120 minutes of intermittent accumulated ischemia time.

○ **Which zone of hepatocytes surrounding a terminal afferent blood vessel is at risk for ischemia?**

Zone 3.

○ **What is a Phase I reaction?**

Functionalization reaction (90% oxidation) in the cytochrome P450 system or to a lesser extent mixed-function oxidases subject to enzyme induction, tolerance and competitive reactions. Susceptible to impairment due to disease; located in the ischemia-susceptible zone 3.

○ **What is the first pass effect?**

Clearance of drugs with a high ratio of hepatic extraction dependent on liver blood flow (lidocaine, morphine, verapamil, labetalol and propranolol).

○ **What is the best choice for general anesthesia in the cirrhotic patient?**

Sodium pentothal, succinylcholine, fentanyl, cisatracurium, oxygen and isoflurane – these drugs do not have altered pharmacodynamics in the cirrhotic, either due to termination of action via redistribution, or metabolism that is not liver-based. Avoid a reduction in hepatic blood flow due to hypotension, excessive sympathetic activation or high mean airway pressure. Maintain $PaCO_2$ 35-40 mmHg. Enlist a strategy for renal protection.

○ **Describe the proposed mechanisms of halothane-induced hepatoxicity.**

Hypoxia and hypoperfusion
Reductive metabolism
Altered calcium homeostasis
Immune-mediated (trifluoroacetylation of hepatocyte membranes leading to the production of IgG antibodies: anti-TFA antibody)

○ **What is the hepatitis risk from inhaled anesthetic agents?**

Halothane: 1:35,000; enflurane: 1:800,000; isoflurane: (six reported cases); desflurane: (one case); sevoflurane: (0 cases– no TFA proteins); nitrous oxide: (possibly one case).

○ **Following exposure to hepatitis C virus through a needle stick, what is the likelihood of becoming infected and what are the CDC guidelines for laboratory testing.**

The average incidence of anti-HCV seroconversion after unintentional needle stick from an HCV-positive source in 1.8%.

The only tests approved by the US FDA for diagnosis of HCV infection are those that measure anti-HCV (HCV EIA). Supplemental testing with a more specific assay (RIBA for anti-HCV, recombinant immunoblot assay) prevents reporting false-positive results. HCV RNA using gene amplification techniques (NAT, nucleic acid test for HCV RNA) can be detected in serum or plasma within 1-2 weeks after exposure to the virus and weeks before the onset of ALT elevations or anti-HCV appears. A negative test requires RIBA for anti-HCV prior to reporting results. The incubation period for HCV is 2 weeks to 6 months.

○ **What is the incidence of post-transfusion hepatitis from any cause?**

Negligible, and probably warrants a case report. Eighty-five percent of post-transfusion hepatitis from infective agents is caused by hepatitis C virus. Prior to 1990, there were no screening tests for HCV. The rate of post-transfusion HCV infection has since decreased from 8 to 10% to less than 1 chance per million units of blood or blood products transfused (CDC 2004).

○ **Define liver transplant terms: VVB, piggyback technique and reperfusion syndrome.**

VVB (venovenous bypass): an extracorporeal circulatory assistance device that improves venous return during the anhepatic stage. Non-heparinized blood flowing through cannulae inserted into the portal and/or femoral veins is returned to the right atrium via the axillary vein through a centripetal pump.

Piggyback technique: Hepatectomy in the recipient with preservation of the full length of the vena cava. The donor liver is then "piggy-backed" to the recipient IVC with the outflow venous anastomosis made end-to-side (donor IVC to recipient hepatic vein cuff) or side-to-side (donor IVC to recipient IVC).

Reperfusion syndrome: Hypotension (decrease in MAP > 30%) for at least one minute, within five minutes of reperfusion of the donor liver. Often accompanied by bradycardia, arrhythmias and, occasionally, cardiac arrest. Incidence: 30%. Etiology: unclear but likely systemic vasodilation and possibly myocardial depression from vasoactive substances, volume overload and transient hyperkalemia.

❍   **What are the consequences of hepatic enzyme induction?**

Exposure to many compounds stimulates microsomal zenobiotic-metabolizing activity in the liver through an increase in the cellular amount of RNA coding for the specific enzyme. Clinical effects are apparent when the rate-controlling step of drug detoxification or elimination is affected or with the formation of toxic intermediates.

TRANSPLANT SURGERY

Live As If You Were To Die Tomorrow. Learn As If You Were To Live Forever.
M.K. Gandhi

○ **Management of organ donors involves stabilization of a brain-dead patient. List common physiologic sequelae of brain death.**

Hypotension, arrhythmias, electrolyte abnormalities (hypernatremia, hypokalemia, hypomagnesemia and hypocalcemia), hypothermia, anemia, coagulopathies, hypoxemia and endocrine abnormalities (adrenal insufficiency, hypothyroidism, diabetes insipidus).

○ **What are the fluid management goals for the donor?**

Aggressive restoration and maintenance of the intravascular volume and the temporary use of vasoactive drugs, as needed. The specific organ(s) to be retrieved determines fluid management (colloid, crystalloid or blood products), ideal CVP and the choice of allowable maximum doses for pressor drug support (dopamine 1st, then phenylephrine, epinephrine or norepinephrine).

Targeted hemodynamic goals are described as the "rule of 100s". This includes maintaining a minimum systolic blood pressure of 90-100 mm Hg (mean arterial pressure of 65 mm Hg), CVP < 10 mm Hg, PCWP < 10 mm Hg, SVR < 1000 dynes/sec/cm^5 and heart rate < 100 beats/min with a urine output > 100 cc/hr.

○ **List the diagnostic criteria for brain death determination in the adult patient.**

- Coma or unresponsiveness
- No movement (spontaneous, elicited to pain, seizures or posturing)
- Absence of brain stem reflexes
- Apnea with an arterial PCO_2 of 60 mm Hg or greater.

"Brain death" is defined as irreversible cessation of all functions of the entire brain, including the brainstem. In patients with coma of undetermined origin, the patient must meet the clinical criteria, have an observation period > 24 hours, and have no cerebral blood flow or neuroimaging or CSF evidence of an acute CNS catastrophe that is compatible with brain death in the absence of confounding factors (hypothermia, sedation, shock, neuromuscular blocking agents, drug intoxication or poisoning and no severe electrolyte, acid-base or endocrine disorder).

○ **List the most common immunosuppressive protocol drugs.**

Cyclosporine , azathioprine, prednisone, OKT_3, mycophenolate mofetil, sirolimus and FK506.

○ **What is the current US Food and Drug Administration recommendation for prevention of transfusion-associated graft-versus-host disease in immunosuppressed patients.**

Gamma irradiation of whole blood and cellular blood components to 25 Gy (red cells and platelets) before transfusion.

○ **Describe a Child's C patient with cirrhosis according to the Child-Turcotte-Pugh (CPT) scoring system.**

Encephalopathy grade 3-4, ascites (at least moderate despite diuretic treatment), bilirubin > 3 mg/dl, albumin < 2.8 g/dL, prothrombin time > 6 seconds prolongation or INR > 2.3. For primary biliary cirrhosis, primary sclerosing cholangitis or other cholestatic liver disease, bilirubin > 10 mg/dl.

O   **What is the most accurate predictive scoring system for survival in adult patients undergoing a TIPS procedure (transjugular intrahepatic portosystemic shunt) or those listed and waiting for liver transplantation?**

MELD (model of end-stage liver disease)

O   **List the criteria used to calculate the MELD score in an adult patient.**

Creatinine, bilirubin and INR. (not etiology of liver disease or albumin; maximum score 40)

O   **Would you rather have a MELD score of 25 or 10?**

The predicted 6-month survival in a patient with a MELD score of 25 or greater is 25%, versus 100% survival in those with a MELD score of 10 or less.

O   **How does the pediatric model to predict survival in patients with end-stage liver disease differ from MELD?**

PELD (pediatric end-stage liver disease) score is calculated on the basis of age < one year, albumin, bilirubin, INR and growth failure < -2 standard deviations.

O   **Describe the causes of encephalopathy in liver transplant recipients.**

Portal-systemic encephalopathy (PSE) is the most common form and usually seen in patients with cirrhosis and portal hypertension. Arterial or CSF ammonia concentration or CSF glutamine levels correlate with the degree of CNS suppression. PSE is usually precipitated by ingestion of protein (meal or GI bleed), infection (spontaneous bacterial peritonitis) or dehydration due to overdiuresis.

Pseudo-PSE is difficult to distinguish clinically. It is caused by decreased clearance of sedatives, analgesics and tranquilizing drugs or metabolic abnormalities (alkalosis, acidosis or hypoglycemia).

O   **Describe the types of renal insufficiency seen in the liver transplant patient.**

- Pre-existing from the underlying process causing liver disease: hepatitis B, hepatitis C, analgesic overdose, amyloidosis, autoimmune disease.
- Pre-existing from other systemic illness: diabetes or hypertension
- Functional renal impairment from liver failure: mild sodium retention to hepatorenal syndrome.
- Management of encephalopathy and ascites: pre-renal secondary to hypovolemia from diuretic therapy.
- Immunosuppression-related complication: cyclosporine and FK506 nephrotoxicity.

O   **Why is adequate venous access so critical in liver transplantation anesthesia?**

Potential for major blood loss (liver surgery, clamping portal vein and vena cava, coagulopathy) and transfusion, maintain preload to the heart during caval clamping, allow veno-venous bypass during anhepatic period, route for administration of vasopressors/dilators and access for invasive monitoring and PA catheter insertion.

O   **Describe the hemodynamic changes associated with hepatic vascular occlusion.**

Hepatic vascular occlusion (HVE) combines portal triad clamping and occlusion of the inferior vena cava. The hemodynamic response to HVE is characterized by a 50% decrease in cardiac output, decrease in pulmonary artery pressure and increase in heart rate and systemic vascular resistance.

O   **What are the major problems associated with reperfusion of the new liver?**

1.   Post-reperfusion syndrome

2. Hyperkalemia (bradycardia, asystole, cardiac arrest, malignant ventricular arrhythmias)
3. Pulmonary embolism
4. Pulmonary hypertension (precipitating right ventricular failure)
5. Volume overload
6. Hypothermia
7. Hypotension (active bleeding, air or thrombus embolism, hyperkalemia, acidosis, hypocalcemia)
8. Hyperglycemia
9. Coagulopathy (especially primary fibrinolysis> donor heparin, low fibrinogen, factor deficiency, dilutional thrombocytopenia)
10. Primary nonfunction or delayed primary graft function

O Discuss intraoperative management of liver transplant patients with pulmonary hypertension.

Following insertion of a PA catheter and establishing an adequate level of anesthesia, if the mean pulmonary artery pressure exceeds 35 mm Hg, this is potentially a huge problem requiring management decisions (including canceling the case: normal MPAP < 25 mm Hg, normal PVR < 120 dynes.cm^{-5}). Evidence of response of PA pressures to therapy and preserved right ventricular function is essential. Pre-liver transplant combination of MPAP greater than 35 mm Hg and PVR greater than 250 dynes.cm^{-5} has been associated with a perioperative mortality rate of nearly 50%. Therapies for reduction of PA pressures include: nitric oxide 10-60 ppm (inhaled); IV: flolan (prostaglandin E_1 0.01-0.2 µg/kg/min), nitroglycerine (0.5-10 µg/kg/min). milrinone (0.375-0.75 µg/kg/min, bolus 50 µg/kg) and fenoldopam (0.03-0.6 µg/kg/min); PO: Viagra®.

O On induction of anesthesia for lung transplantation, patients with severe COPD are often hemodynamically unstable. Why?

This represents a transition from spontaneous breathing to controlled positive-pressure ventilation and loss of sympathetic tone.

Hemodynamic instability is due to a reduction in venous return and cardiac output from volume depletion, auto-peep secondary to air trapping, hyperinflation with "breath stacking", increase in intrathoracic pressure and possibly right ventricular dysfunction from increased pulmonary vascular resistance. These patients should be preloaded with a liter of crystalloid and ventilation adjusted to allow shallow tidal volumes and a long expiratory time (avoid high peak pressures, PEEP, auto-PEEP). In addition, chronotropic agents (to increase heart rate) and inotropic support (maintain systemic pressure for coronary perfusion) with pulmonary vasodilator drugs may be necessary.

O Explain why "permissive hypercapnia" is frequently unavoidable during lung transplant surgery?

Permissive hypercapnia is a technique of deliberate hypoventilation in which conventional positive-pressure ventilation is limited and the arterial PCO_2 is allowed to rise. Maintaining hemodynamic stability and normal ventilation are often mutually exclusive, as positive-pressure ventilation and air trapping may lead to pulmonary tamponade and circulatory arrest. Elevated $PaCO_2$s are accepted as long as the pH is maintained above 7.1. Intraoperative $PaCO_2$ values of 120 mm Hg may be tolerated with adequate oxygenation.

O What are the anesthetic considerations for induction of anesthesia in the cardiac transplant recipient?

1. Rapid-sequence induction due to aspiration risk (full stomach or gastroparesis due to gut hypoperfusion).
2. Low cardiac output state requires placement of invasive monitoring in the awake patient (availability of the TEE) and adjustment of drug dosages for a prolonged circulation time and reduced volume of distribution.
3. Unpredictable responses to sympathomimetic agents.
4. Vasoactive drugs are continued and adjusted accordingly to maintain adequate CO, coronary and cerebral perfusion pressures.
5. Avoid drugs and ventilatory maneuvers that will increase pulmonary vascular resistance.

❍   **What are the primary indications for heart-lung transplantation?**

Congenital heart disease and primary pulmonary hypertension.

❍   **Describe methods for minimizing increases in pulmonary vascular resistance (PVR) in the heart-lung transplant recipient during induction and the pre-bypass period.**

Pre-oxygenation is critical. Induction is generally accomplished with a high dose opiate and a small dose of a cardiostable induction agent such as etomidate or midazolam. Ketamine is relatively contraindicated because of its deleterious effects on PVR. Vasoactive drugs are frequently required. Useful combination therapies include prostaglandin E_1, milrinone, or nitroglycerine for PVR reduction combined with norepinephrine for increased systemic blood pressure and cardiac contractility. Nitric oxide may also be useful for selective pulmonary vasodilation. Avoid hypercarbia, hypoxemia and hypothermia.

❍   **What are the most important considerations in the preoperative assessment of the heart transplant patient scheduled for laparoscopic cholecystectomy?**

1. Functional evaluation of the graft
    •Early: detection of infection or rejection
    •Late: ischemia risk or the failing transplanted heart (diminished left ventricular ejection fraction or diastolic dysfunction)
2. Patient factors
    •Residual physiologic alterations
    •Coexisting systemic disease
    •Transplant surgery-related complications
    •Functional status
3. Immunosuppressive therapy
    •Pharmacology of cyclosporine, prednisone, mycophenolate mofetil, tacrolimus
    •Complications, toxicities and adverse effects

❍   **Describe the physiology of the transplanted heart.**

- •   Preload-dependent
- •   Afterload: a. cyclosporine-induced systemic hypertension
                                      b. delayed or blunted blood pressure response
- •   Sinus tachycardia: a. delayed and attenuated heart rate response
                                      b. beta-adrenergic and cholinergic supersensitivity
- •   dysrhythmias and SA node dysfunction
- •   normal cardiac output and contractility
- •   accelerated coronary artery disease, silent ischemia
- •   normal PAP and PCWP

❍   **Describe the physiologic consequences of acute denervation of the heart.**

Afferent denervation results in the lack of angina pectoris, alterations of peripheral autonomic responses (valsalva, carotid sinus massage, body position changes, heart rate variability and drug responses) and changes in sodium and water balance. Loss of efferent fibers results in an increase in the resting heart rate to 90 to 110 bpm (intrinsic rate of the heart) and a blunted chronotropic response to stresses such as exercise.

❍   **Describe the unique features of the SA node in a transplanted heart.**

The native SA node is isolated from the myocardium by the suture line, and does not influence the heart rate, although its P-wave may be visible on the EKG. The SA node from the donor heart controls the heart rate, with an intrinsic rate of 90 to 110 bpm due to denervation from sympathetic and parasympathetic modulation. Direct-acting chronotropic agents are preferred to increase heart rate. Heart rate responses are delayed and attenuated, with possible beta-adrenergic and cholinergic supersensitivity. There is evidence supporting autonomic reinnervation of the transplanted heart. Neostigmine may induce bradycardia or sinus arrest.

○ **In a patient undergoing renal transplantation, is succinylcholine contraindicated?**

No, if the baseline serum potassium is normal and the patient has no other condition that would suggest increased risk of an exaggerated hyperkalemic response with IV succinylcholine (any disorder in which there is proliferation of extrajunctional receptors ie: burns, muscular dystrophies, spinal cord injuries, upper and lower motor neuron disease). Case reports describe an exaggerated hyperkalemic response in patients with chronic renal insufficiency secondary to diabetes mellitus, with evidence of significant peripheral neuropathy and muscle wasting in the hands. Succinylcholine is a known trigger for malignant hyperthermia.

○ **In a patient undergoing renal transplantation are any of the nondepolarizing muscle relaxants absolutely contraindicated?**

No. Theoretically it would be best to avoid muscle relaxants with significant renal excretion (pancuronium, metocurine, doxacurium, tubocurarine).

○ **In a patient undergoing renal transplantation, in theory, which inhalational agent(s) should be avoided?**

Enflurane and sevoflurane. Methoxyflurane is no longer available.

Inorganic fluoride is a potentially nephrotoxic product of anesthetic metabolism. Fluoride-associated renal dysfunction may be a risk with methoxyflurane>>>enflurane and sevoflurane. Sevoflurane undergoes degradation producing compound A (pentafluoroisopropenyl fluoromethyl ether), which has been shown to cause nephrotoxicity in rats.

○ **What are some common systemic manifestations of end-stage renal disease that are important in the preoperative anesthetic assessment of the kidney transplant patient?**

Neurologic	Central: seizures, lethargy
	Peripheral: sensory and motor neuropathy, autonomic dysfunction
Respiratory	Hypocarbia
	Pleural effusion, edema, pneumonitis, infection
Cardiovascular	Indeterminate volume status, susceptible to fluid overload
	High cardiac output
	Hypertension, LVH
	Accelerated peripheral and coronary atherosclerosis
	Tachycardia, arrhythmias, and conduction disorders
	Attenuated reactivity of the sympathetic nervous system
	Reduced oxygen-carrying capacity, increased peripheral extraction of O_2
	Pericarditis, cardiac tamponade
Endocrine	Electrolyte disorders (hyperkalemia, hyponatremia, hypermagnesemia, hypocalcemia)
	Metabolic acidosis
	Secondary hyperparathyroidism
	Glucose intolerance
Gastrointestinal	Delayed gastric emptying and increased volume and acidity of gastric contents, aspiration risk
Musculoskeletal	Osteodystrophy, muscle wasting
Hematologic	Chronic anemia, right shift of hemoglobin dissociation curve
	Platelet dysfunction, coagulopathy
	Increased susceptibility to infection, carrier state for hepatitis B antigen and HIV

○ **Why is the hemoglobin level low in a renal transplant patient?**

Chronic anemia with hemoglobin levels of 5-7 gm/dl are a result of decreased production of erythropoietin and diminished red cell survival time. Iron absorption from the gastrointestinal tract may also be decreased in patients with ESRD leading to iron deficiency. Following kidney transplantation, immunosuppressive therapy (steroids, azathioprine and cyclosporine) may cause bone marrow depression resulting in various degrees of anemia, thrombocytopenia and lymphopenia. Hemoglobin levels may be normal in chronic renal failure patients treated with Procrit® (epoetin alfa).

O   **Is the renal transplant recipient at risk for pseudocholinesterase deficiency?**

Not due to chronic renal insufficiency. Plasma cholinesterase is produced in the liver.

O   **What are the most common causes of chronic renal failure?**

Diabetes mellitus > hypertension >> glomerulonephritis >>> cystic kidney (listed in order of incidence according to the US Renal Data System 2003).

O   **In a patient with end-stage renal disease is platelet function normal? Is there any treatment?**

The platelet count is often low and platelet function is abnormal (prolonged bleeding time, decreased platelet adhesiveness, and inhibition of secondary platelet aggregation from an increased plasma level of guanidino-succinic acid which causes a decline in platelet factor 3). Platelet function improves with dialysis and IV desmopressin 0.3 μg/kg.

O   **What are the causes of the bleeding diathesis seen in a patient with end-stage renal disease?**

Multifactorial. Platelet dysfunction, thrombocytopenia, decreased antithrombin III, excess heparin from dialysis and increased factor VIII and fibrinogen.

O   **What are some of the immediate postoperative complications following kidney transplantation?**

1. Residual neuromuscular blockade requiring continued mechanical ventilation.
2. Hypertension (myocardial ischemia, LV failure, pulmonary edema, hemorrhage at the vascular anastomosis or direct injury to the graft) and hypotension with fluid depletion.
3. Delayed primary function of the transplanted kidney (oliguria with adequate CVP), acute tubular necrosis or rejection.
4. Hyperglycemia and electrolyte disorders, persistent metabolic acidosis.
5. Complications of IV immunosuppressive therapy.
6. Pneumothorax from central line insertion.
7. Anemia requiring transfusion.
8. Surgical: arterial thrombosis, venous occlusion, graft hematoma or rupture, wound infection, urologic complications (urine leak or obstruction to flow) or loss of the graft.

O   **What are the hallmarks of clinical rejection in the transplanted kidney?**

Fever
Diminishing urine output
Fluid retention
Hypertension
Worsening renal function (increased BUN, creatinine, beta-2 microglobulins)
Enlargement and tenderness of the ectopic kidney

Diagnosis of rejection is difficult, requiring definitive renal biopsy. Causes of functional impairment of the transplanted kidney include: accelerated progression of an underlying disease process, cyclosporine nephrotoxicity, rejection (acute or chronic) and hypertension.

○ **What would be your choice for monitoring during renal transplantation, and why?**

Standard non-invasive monitors: EKG, non-invasive blood pressure, temperature, pulse oximetry and capnography. Urine output.

Invasive: intra-arterial blood pressure (anticipated hemodynamic instability ie: hypertension in retransplant or diabetic patient and sampling for arterial blood gases, hematocrit, glucose and electrolytes) and central venous pressure catheter to measure central filling pressure for volume loading and forced saline diuresis.

○ **What is the primary indication for isolated pancreas transplantation?**

Diabetes mellitus with severe neuropathy and labile diabetes (glycohemoglobin levels persistently > 10% despite insulin therapy or frequent hypoglycemia without attempts at strict control of glucose levels). Selected patients have been transplanted in an attempt to halt the progression of diabetic nephropathy.

○ **What are the intraoperative anesthetic considerations for pancreatic transplantation?**

1. Physiologic alterations and systemic manifestations of diabetes mellitus, most importantly assessment of cardiovascular and renal function, with predictable end-organ dysfunction.
2. Patients are at risk for aspiration requiring rapid sequence induction and intubation.
3. Maintain hemodynamic stability.
4. Strict perioperative control of glucose levels (70 to 100 mg/dl) with the administration of insulin. Hyperglycemia on reperfusion of the pancreatic graft should be anticipated.

○ **How does pancreatic islet transplantation differ from pancreas transplantation?**

Pancreatic islet transplantation is a form of selective transplantation since only the cells required by the recipient are transplanted. When only the islet cells are transplanted, complications related to the exocrine portion of the pancreas and immunologic reactivity are minimized.

OBSTETRICS

The Difference Between Genius And Stupidity, Is Genius Has Its Limits.
Albert Einstein

○ **What are the determinants of uterine blood flow (UBF) in pregnant women?**

Uterine blood flow is directly proportional to the change in blood pressure across the organ (mean arterial pressure minus central venous pressure) and inversely proportional to uterine vascular resistance. Flow = (UAP – UVP)/UVR. For example, during a contraction, uterine muscle tone increases, increasing uterine vascular resistance and decreasing flow.

Uterine arterial pressure (UAP), uterine venous pressure (UVP), uterine vascular resistance (UVR)

○ **Describe the autoregulatory curve for uterine blood flow.**

Uterine blood flow is not autoregulated but linearly proportional to mean arterial blood pressure.

○ **What are the effects of regional anesthesia on uterine blood flow (UBF) during labor?**

Regional anesthesia can increase UBF by reducing maternal pain and stress during labor, which decreases uterine tone and vascular resistance. In contrast, hypotension caused by regional anesthesia can decrease UBF. In the setting of severe preeclampsia, epidural anesthesia may increase intervillous blood flow.

○ **What is the effect of ketamine on uterine blood flow (UBF)?**

Ketamine, in intravenous doses up to 1mg/kg, is unlikely to alter UBF. Higher doses of ketamine (> 2 mg/kg) may decrease UBF due to increased uterine tone (UVR), however, in the setting of decreased intravascular volume, ketamine may help to maintain systemic blood pressure and thus maintain UBF.

○ **What effect do the following agents have on uterine tone?**

Volatile anesthetics	At 0.2 MAC minimal effect and beyond that dose-dependent reduction in uterine tone. Below 1 MAC uterine response to oxytocin is preserved.
Local anesthetics	Clinically insignificant effect at normal serum concentration
	Direct myometrial injection may cause uterine hyperstimulation
Ketamine	Dose dependent increase in uterine tone. Clinically insignificant effect with normal induction dose
Opioids	No effect
Nondepolarizing NMB's	No effect on smooth muscle
Succinylcholine	No effect on smooth muscle

○ **What are the determinants of placental transfer?**

- Maternal drug concentration
- Fetal drug concentration
- Placental factors (surface area, membrane thickness, and metabolism)
- Drug factors (lipid solubility, protein binding, molecular weight, and ionization)
- Placental blood flow

○ **Describe drug factors that favor drug transfer across the placenta.**

- Low molecular weight. A molecular weight of 1000 is a rough dividing line between those substances that cross the placenta by diffusion and those that are relatively impermeable by diffusion.
- Low protein binding
- High lipid solubility
- Low degree of ionization

○   **What is the relationship between the site of administration of local anesthetic drugs and maternal peak blood levels?**

For the various anesthetic techniques used in obstetrics, maternal peak blood levels from highest to lowest are as follows: Intravenous > intercostals > caudal > paracervical block > epidural > subarachnoid block.

○   **What is the P_{50} in the fetus and mother at term? (and what is a P_{50}??)**

P_{50} is the partial pressure of O_2 at which hemoglobin molecules are 50% saturated with oxygen. P_{50} values are 19 mm Hg and 30 mm Hg in the fetus and mother at term, respectively. P_{50} is 27 mm Hg in normal adults.

○   **Why is this difference in P_{50} important?**

The maternal-fetal P_{50} gap indicates that fetal hemoglobin has a greater affinity for oxygen than does maternal hemoglobin, encouraging maternal-fetal oxygen transfer.

○   **What is the normal Hct in the pregnant patient at term? Why?**

33-35%. Hct below 30% should be considered anemia. Hct above 35% may indicate hemoconcentration. During pregnancy, both RBC volume and plasma volume increase, but plasma volume increases more causing a dilutional effect.

○   **How does the requirement for local anesthetics used in regional anesthesia change during pregnancy?**

It decreases. Pregnant women need 25% - 30% less local anesthetic for regional anesthesia than do non-pregnant women. Distention of the epidural veins may decrease the epidural and intrathecal space and facilitate spread of epidural and spinal local anesthetics. Exaggerated lumbar lordosis may enhance cephalad spread of spinal local anesthetics. Increased progesterone during pregnancy may increase nerve sensitivity to local anesthetics or may enhance diffusion of the local anesthetics to the membrane receptor site.

○   **Why is inhalation induction of anesthesia faster in pregnant women than non-pregnant women?**

Decreased functional residual capacity (FRC) and increased minute ventilation result in a more rapid rise in alveolar concentration of anesthetic agent. Elevated cardiac output counteracts this effect somewhat, but the net effect remains that of increased rate of uptake in pregnancy.

○   **What effect does pregnancy have on the MAC of inhaled anesthetic agents?**

MAC is reduced by 30% during early pregnancy and returns to normal within the first three days following delivery.

○   **When does the cardiac output maximally increase in the parturient?**

In the immediate postpartum period, cardiac output can increase up to 75% above pre-labor values.

○   **What is "auto transfusion" during labor?**

Three to five hundred milliliters of blood will enter into the maternal circulation with each uterine contraction during labor. This "autotransfusion" can increase cardiac output and central blood volume by an additional 15% - 25%. When parturients receive effective analgesia, cardiac output and stroke volume are augmented to a lesser degree.

O   **Why is left uterine displacement (LUD) important in pregnant women in the supine position?**

In most term parturients, lying supine results in compression of the aorta and inferior vena cava (IVC) by the gravid uterus. This may result in elevated venous pressure in the lower extremities and decreased venous return to the heart, causing hypotension and reduced uteroplacental perfusion. When placed in the left lateral position, the weight of the uterus shifts off of the IVC and aorta.

O   **When does left uterine displacement become important?**

Supine aortocaval compression can be identified as early as the end of the first trimester, and is universally present by the 28th week.

O   **What is "supine hypotension syndrome"?**

Near term, approximately 8% of parturients experience hypotension when lying supine – the so-called "supine hypotension syndrome". Profound aortocaval compression causes a significant reduction in venous return to the heart resulting in hypotension which is not corrected by a compensatory increase in heart rate and SVR. If left untreated, bradycardia will develop and the patient will develop signs of shock - including hypotension, pallor, sweating, nausea, vomiting, and changes in mental status.

O   **What size of endotracheal tube should be used in obstetric patients?**

A 6.5 endotracheal tube is a good choice for most pregnant women. Small size cuffed endotracheal tubes (6.0 –7.0 mm ID) should be available. Nasotracheal intubation should be avoided and may lead to severe epistaxis.

O   **What physiologic factors predispose the parturient to hypoxemia during intubation?**

Decreased functional residual capacity (FRC) results in a diminished volume of alveolar oxygen available for absorption. Increased metabolic activity causes higher oxygen consumption and carbon dioxide production. Respiratory quotient remains unchanged. The net effect is a more rapid fall in PaO_2 during apnea.

O   **What are normal arterial blood gas values in the parturient at term?**

PH = 7.44, $PaCO_2$ = 30 mm Hg, PaO_2 = 103 mm Hg and bicarbonate = 20 mEq/ml; of course, the normal values are pH = 7.40, $PaCO_2$ = 40 mm Hg, PaO_2 = 100 mm Hg and bicarbonate = 24 mEq/ml. One can deduce that in the parturient there is a respiratory alkalosis with metabolic compensation.

O   **When should a parturient be considered to have a full stomach?**

Precautions against aspiration should be taken from as early as 12 weeks. After the first trimester, every parturient should be managed as a patient with a full stomach.

O   **How does plasma cholinesterase activity change during pregnancy?**

The plasma cholinesterase activity is reduced about 25%. After delivery there is a further reduction to less than 60% of the non-pregnant value. However, there is no clinically significant prolongation of action of succinylcholine or ester-type local anesthetics in the dosages generally given.

O   **When is the critical period of organogenesis?**

Between 15 and 60 days of gestation, however, the CNS does not fully develop until after birth.

○   **Is pain sensation different between the first stage and second stage of labor?**

Yes. During the first stage of labor, pain results from stretching of the uterus and cervix. Pain signals are transmitted through visceral afferents to $T_{10} - L_1$ nerve roots. This pain is often described as dull, aching, cramping and poorly localized. During the second stage of labor, pain results from stretching of the vagina and perineum as the fetal head descends. This pain is transmitted through somatosensory afferents to S_2-S_4 nerve roots and is described as sharp and well localized.

○   **What non-neuraxial techniques can be used to provide analgesia during the second stage of labor?**

Pudendal nerve block is an effective non-neuraxial technique for analgesia during the second stage. Pudendal nerve block is not effective, however, for mid-forceps deliveries, uterine manipulation, or repair of cervical lacerations. Paracervical and lumbar sympathetic blocks provide analgesia only for the first stage of labor.

○   **What are the concerns of performing regional analgesia/anesthesia for parturients?**

The main concern is maintaining uterine blood flow and fetal well being. Avoid maternal hypotension and treat it aggressively. Remember the absolute contraindications to regional analgesia: infection over the injection site, coagulopathy, marked hypovolemia, true allergy to local anesthetic drugs, and the patient's refusal of or inability to cooperate with regional anesthesia.

○   **Does epidural analgesia affect the course of labor?**

Studies have shown epidural analgesia does not slow the progress of labor in the first stage, however, the second stage of labor may be prolonged slightly (about 25 minutes). There is no evidence that this prolongation is harmful to the fetus.

○   **Why should an epidural be placed early in the morbidly obese pregnant patient?**

Lumbar epidural anesthesia is an excellent choice for labor and vaginal delivery. More than 50% of morbidly obese patients need cesarean section. Early epidural placement during labor decreases the likelihood of requiring general anesthesia for cesarean section. Epidural anesthesia reduces oxygen consumption and attenuates increases in cardiac output that occurs during labor and delivery.

○   **Is an epidural contraindicated for vaginal birth after cesarean section (VBAC)?**

No. The main concern is that the epidural may mask the pain of uterine rupture; however, pain from uterine rupture usually is sharp and unrelenting, not associated with contractions, in an unusual location for labor pains, and not relieved with additional epidural local anesthetic administration.

○   **Is major regional anesthesia for cesarean section contraindicated in patients with aortic stenosis?**

Spinal anesthesia is contraindicated. Epidural anesthesia can be used if administered slowly with appropriate hemodynamic monitoring to preserve preload, blood pressure, and SVR. It is best not to include epinephrine with test or therapeutic doses of local anesthetic.

○   **What is the major disadvantage of paracervical block?**

Fetal bradycardia (up to 33%). It may be related to decreased uterine blood flow secondary to uterine vasoconstriction from the local anesthetics applied closely to the uterine artery and direct cardiac toxicity due to high fetal blood levels of local anesthetic.

○   **Which local anesthetic may be a good choice for epidural anesthesia and fetal distress? Why?**

2-chloroprocaine. It is fast in onset and rapidly hydrolyzed by the fetus. Fetal acidosis does not promote fetal accumulation of the local anesthetic.

○ **What are the major disadvantages of using 2-chloroprocaine?**

The duration of drug action is approximately 45 minutes, so the epidural may need to be topped up with a longer-acting local anesthetic, depending on the length of the case. Chloroprocaine may also antagonize the activity of neuraxial morphine used for postoperative epidural analgesia.

○ **What is "ion trapping" of local anesthetics?**

Decreased fetal pH will increase the concentration of ionized local anesthetics (LA) in the fetal circulation. The ionization of the LA prevents diffusion across the placenta back to the maternal circulation. The unionized LA continues to move to the fetus down its concentration gradient. Thus local anesthetics can accumulate in fetal blood. This phenomenon is called "ion trapping" and explains the higher concentration of lidocaine in the fetus in the presence of fetal acidosis.

○ **What are the indications for insertion of a pulmonary artery catheter in severe preeclampsia?**

Hemodynamic monitoring and measurement of mixed venous oxygen saturation in the following clinical settings:
* Sepsis with refractory hypotension or oliguria
* Unexplained or refractory pulmonary edema, heart failure or oliguria
* Cardiovascular decompensation
* Massive blood and volume loss or replacement
* ARDS

○ **What techniques can be used to facilitate uterine relaxation following vaginal delivery?**

The obstetrician may request uterine relaxation for a patient with retained placenta or uterine inversion. Nitroglycerin can be administered either sublingually (400 mcg spray) or intravenously (100-200 mcg), while monitoring for accompanying hypotension. If relaxation is not sufficient, rapid sequence induction, endotracheal intubation and high concentrations of volatile anesthetic agents will provide profound uterine relaxation.

○ **What techniques are used in the treatment of uterine atony?**

The first line of treatment for uterine atony is drug therapy. Oxytocin is routinely administered intravenously following vaginal and cesarean deliveries. In non-preeclamptic patients, methylergonovine (Methergine®) is administered <u>intramuscularly</u> for continued atony. The third drug of choice is 15-methyl prostaglandin $F_{2\text{-alpha}}$. Obstetricians may administer prostaglandin E_2 rectal or vaginal suppositories as the last noninvasive measure. The second line of treatment involves invasive techniques such as uterine artery embolization or ligation, with hysterectomy as a possible last resort.

○ **What is the mechanism of action of oxytocin?**

Oxytocin is a polypeptide hormone produced in the posterior pituitary. Oxytocin acts directly on sodium channels in the uterine myofibrils, causing sodium influx, depolarization and smooth muscle contraction.

○ **What is the most important side effect of oxytocin?**

Systemic hypotension caused by peripheral vasodilatation.

○ **What is the mechanism of action of Methergine® (methylergonovine)?**

Uterine contraction mediated through activation of alpha-adrenergic receptors.

○   **What are the side effects of methylergonovine?**

Ergot alkaloids such as methylergonovine may cause nausea, vomiting, pulmonary hypertension, coronary artery vasoconstriction, and severe systemic hypertension (especially in patients with preeclampsia.)

○   **What is the mechanism of action of Hemabate®?**

Hemabate® (15-methyl prostaglandin $F_{2\text{-alpha}}$) increases uterine tone by increasing myometrial intracellular calcium concentration.

○   **What are the side effects of Hemabate®?**

Side effects of Hemabate® administration include bronchospasm, nausea, vomiting, and diarrhea. Increased pulmonary vascular resistance may lead to pulmonary hypertension, increased intrapulmonary shunting, and hypoxemia.

○   **Can methylergonovine be given intravenously for post partum hemorrhage?**

If hemorrhage is profound and maternal blood pressure is low, a small dose of 0.02 mg (dilution 10:1) can be given IV. Blood pressure should be rechecked before giving another dose 2-3 minutes later.   Routine methergine® dosing is recommended as 0.2 mg IM.

○   **How could general anesthesia for emergent cesarean section be administered without intravenous access?**

At least one case report has described using a sevoflurane inhalational induction by mask with cricoid pressure applied in a patient with no IV access and fetal distress. Placement of an intravenous catheter, either peripheral or central is essential.

○   **Why should excessive mechanical hyperventilation ($P_{ET}CO_2 < 24$ mm Hg) be avoided?**

Hypocapnia may reduce maternal cardiac output and uterine blood flow, resulting in fetal hypoxemia and acidosis.

○   **How quickly should the baby be delivered under general anesthesia?**

Prolonged skin incision-to-delivery (> 8 minutes) and uterine incision-to-delivery times (> 180 seconds) have been associated with fetal hypoxia and acidosis, regardless of the type of anesthesia.

○   **Does the parturient's height determine the requirement of local anesthetic for spinal anesthesia for cesarean section?**

No. The spread of hyperbaric spinal bupivicaine administered for cesarean section is unaffected by the parturient's age, height, weight or body mass index (weight/height in m^2). For most patients (except the very short (<5-ft/150-cm) or very tall (>6-ft/180-cm)), 12 mg of bupivacaine will achieve a T_4-T_6 level, which is necessary to ensure adequate anesthesia for cesarean section.

○   **What is the average anticipated blood loss for vaginal delivery and cesarean section?**

500-600 ml for vaginal delivery and 1000 ml for cesarean section. A more recent report observed 320-400 ml for vaginal delivery and 500 ml for cesarean section.

○   **Explain the causes of fetal deceleration patterns.**

Early –benign: due to fetal head compression during uterine contractions
Late – indicates uteroplacental insufficiency
Variable—usually benign: caused by cord compression

O   **What are normal values for fetal blood gases?**

Umbilical artery at birth: pH > 7.2, PaO_2 > 50 mm Hg, $PaCO_2$ < 48 mm Hg

The pH of the scalp sample lies between the pH of arterial and venous blood. Fetal scalp pH values of 7.25 or more are classified as normal and indicate that a patient may continue with labor. If the pH is < 7.20 delivery should be expedited. A pH between 7.20 and 7.25 warrants a second scalp pH determination.

O   **Briefly describe the Apgar Score.**

The Apgar scoring system for newborns is comprised of five parameters evaluated at 1 and 5 minutes following birth. Each is assigned a score from 0-2, for a possible total score ranging from 0 (the worst) to 10. Think about the ABCs. Respiratory rate, color (oxygenation), heart rate, and then muscle tone and reflex irritability. Parameters given 1 point are the hardest to remember: slow irregular respirations, HR <100 beats per minute, pink trunk with blue extremities, arms with some flexion, and face grimaced.   An all pink, actively moving, and vigorously crying infant should get a perfect 10!

O   **What are the indications for positive pressure ventilation in a neonate?**

Apnea, gasping respirations, persistent central cyanosis on 100% oxygen, HR < 100 beats per min.

O   **Which drugs are effective when administered via the endotracheal tube during neonatal resuscitation?**

Lidocaine, epinephrine, atropine, and naloxone (L-E-A-N). Recommended intratracheal doses are approximately two times higher than intravenous doses to ensure adequate absorption. Dilution with normal saline to a volume of 1-2 ml is recommended. Surfactant may be given through the ET tube to premature neonates with respiratory distress syndrome.

O   **What are the differences in cardiopulmonary resuscitation (CPR) between pregnant and non-pregnant patients?**

Avoid aortocaval compression by maintaining left lateral uterine displacement during CPR. If CPR is ineffective to resuscitate the mother it may be necessary to deliver the baby by emergent cesarean section. Maternal and fetal outcomes are best when cesarean section is performed within 5 minutes of maternal arrest. If cardiac arrest occurs before 24 weeks gestation (onset of fetal viability) the only concern should be saving the mother. Beyond 24 weeks, maintain LUD while placing the patient on a hard surface.

O   **Why is rapid cesarean delivery an important part of maternal resuscitation?**

Delivery of the fetus relieves aortocaval compression. With uterine contraction after delivery, auto transfusion may help increase venous return. Cardiac output produced by chest compression may be more effective without the fetus.

O   **How does management of the difficult airway differ for the pregnant patient?**

Two main concerns in establishing a difficult airway in obstetric patients are: (1) fetal considerations: with failed intubation and fetal distress, if we can ventilate, maintain cricoid pressure and deliver the fetus; if no fetal distress, waken the patient and (2) full stomach precautions must be observed with all parturients regardless of NPO status.

O   **What are the side effects of magnesium sulfate?**

Therapeutic serum levels are considered 6-8 mg/dL. Side effects of magnesium administration may include chest pain and tightness, palpitations, nausea, transient hypotension, blurred vision, sedation, pulmonary edema, respiratory depression, cardiac conduction defects (widened QRS, increased P-R interval) and cardiac arrest. Neonatal side effects include hypotonia, drowsiness, decreased gastric motility and hypocalcemia.

○   **How does cocaine use during pregnancy affect the fetus?**

Cocaine use during pregnancy can cause 1) uterine contractions resulting in preterm labor, 2) placental abruption, 3) intrauterine growth retardation and 4) fetal death. Cocaine can directly affect the fetus by 1) cerebral vasoconstriction, 2) teratogenic and developmental disturbances, 3) neurobehavioral abnormalities and 4) subarachnoid and intraventricular hemorrhage.

○   **When is the best time to perform elective surgery during pregnancy?**

All elective surgeries should be postponed until after delivery. Urgent surgeries are best deferred until the second or third trimester unless maternal health is in danger.

○   **At what gestational age is continuous fetal heart rate (FHR) monitoring feasible during surgery in the pregnant patient?**

18 weeks gestational age. Technical problems may limit the use of continuous FHR monitoring early on and accurate interpretation of the tracing is essential.

○   **What are the indications for fetal heart rate (FHR) monitoring in pregnant women undergoing non-obstetric surgery?**

FHR monitoring should be carried out during surgery whenever possible. The greatest value of intraoperative FHR monitoring is that it identifies a need to improve fetal oxygenation if the fetus shows signs of compromise. A change in FHR mandates evaluation of maternal position, blood pressure, oxygenation, acid-base status, and inspection of the surgical field.

○   **What strategies may prevent fetal compromise during non-obstetric surgery?**

Maintain uteroplacental perfusion and fetal oxygenation by: 1) left uterine displacement, 2) administration of a higher inspired concentration of oxygen, 3) maintain normal PaO_2 and $PaCO_2$, 4) augmentation of maternal circulating blood volume, and 5) pharmacological treatment of hypotension.

○   **For non-obstetric surgery during pregnancy, what is the best anesthetic technique?**

No study has documented that any anesthetic agent or technique is associated with a higher or lower incidence of preterm labor or improved fetal outcome. The anesthetic management of the parturient during surgery should focus on avoidance of hypoxemia, hypotension, acidosis, and hyperventilation.
The type and location of the operation are the only factors that correlate with preterm labor.

○   **Can laparoscopic procedures be done during pregnancy?**

Yes. The Society of American Gastrointestinal Endoscopic Surgeons has issued "Guidelines for Laparoscopic Surgery during Pregnancy," which recommends the following: 1) deferring surgery until the second trimester, 2) using intermittent pneumatic compression devices to prevent thrombosis resulting from lower extremity venous stasis, 3) monitoring fetal and uterine status and maternal end-tidal CO_2 and arterial blood gas measurements, 4) using an open technique to enter the abdomen, 5) avoiding aortocaval compression, 6) maintaining low pneumoperitoneum pressures (not to exceed 15 mm Hg), and 7) obtaining preoperative obstetric consultation.

○   **What are the adverse effects of CO_2 pneumoperitoneum on a pregnant patient?**

1) Uterine or fetal trauma, 2) fetal acidosis from systemic absorption of carbon dioxide, and 3) decreased maternal cardiac output and uteroplacental perfusion.

❍ **What is the normal PaCO$_2$ in pregnancy?**

About 32 mm Hg. Chronic mild hyperventilation is presumably a result of a progesterone-effect increasing respiratory rate, tidal volume and minute ventilation.

❍ **What is the predominant change in the lung volumes in pregnancy?**

Decrease in functional residual capacity, by as much as 15-25%.

❍ **T/F: The elevated diaphragm reduces tidal volume.**

False. Tidal volume actually increases and accounts for much of the increased minute ventilation and mild respiratory alkalosis.

❍ **What effect does preeclampsia have on the intravascular volume status?**

Although parturients with preeclampsia are edematous and have elevated total body water, the intravascular volume is often normal or diminished. Pulmonary capillary wedge pressure (PCWP) in preeclampsia is often in the range of 1-5 mmHg, compared to 6-12 mmHg in normal parturients.

❍ **How should oliguria be treated in the parturient with preeclampsia?**

Oliguria in most patients with preeclampsia is caused by low intravascular volume and can be treated with cautious administration of intravenous crystalloid or colloid. In patients with severe preeclampsia, before administering large volumes of fluid, monitoring of central venous pressure may be necessary.

❍ **What is the most common presenting sign of uterine rupture?**

Fetal distress is the most reliable sign of uterine rupture. In fact, abdominal pain has been shown to occur in only 10% of patients with uterine dehiscence or true uterine rupture. Other signs include vaginal bleeding, maternal hypotension, and cessation of labor.

❍ **What are risk factors for uterine rupture?**

Risk factors include multiparty, fetal malpresentation, and use of oxytocin to augment labor. Uterine rupture is rare in the absence of previous uterine surgery, and hemorrhage from rupture of a classical scar is more severe than that of a low transverse scar.

❍ **Why is the incidence of thromboembolic events increased in pregnancy?**

The risk is 5-6 times greater than that for non-pregnant patients. The mechanism is venous stasis from uterine pressure on the inferior vena cava, vascular injury during delivery, and an increase in clotting factors. There is elevated platelet activation, clotting, and fibrinolysis, representing a state of accelerated but compensated intravascular coagulation.

❍ **What are some additional risk factors for thromboembolism in pregnancy?**

Previous embolus in pregnancy, underlying genetic hypercoagulable states, cesarean section, multiparity, bed rest, obesity, increased maternal age and surgical procedures.

❍ **How does amniotic fluid enter the maternal circulation?**

Through uterine tears or injury and endocervical veins.

○   **What are the major consequences of amniotic fluid embolism?**

Hypotension, cardiac arrest, pulmonary edema, ARDS, and disseminated intravascular coagulation are all common sequelae.

○   **What are the potential mechanisms of cardiorespiratory collapse following embolism?**

The early phase consists of transient (but intense) pulmonary vasospasm. This may account for the right heart dysfuntion that is often fatal. Low cardiac output leads to increased V/Q mismatch, hypoxemia, and hypotension. A second phase of left ventricular failure and pulmonary edema occurs in those women who survive the initial insult.

○   **How can amniotic fluid embolism be diagnosed?**

By demonstrating fetal squamous cells in the maternal pulmonary circulation or lanugo and mucin in pulmonary arterial blood. These tests lack specificity and a search for more sensitive markers is ongoing.

○   **What is the treatment of amniotic fluid embolism?**

Supportive care. The differential diagnosis includes: venous air embolism, thromboembolism, concealed placental abruption, local anesthetic toxicity, septic shock, and complications of severe preeclampsia.

○   **What is the mortality rate in amniotic fluid embolism?**

First-hour maternal mortality may be as high as 65%, and overall maternal mortality rate is 60-80%.

○   **What is the classic presentation of venous air embolism?**

Chest pain or dyspnea and sudden onset of hypotension with a mill wheel murmur audible over the precordium. Other features include: cyanosis, low SpO_2, low end-tidal CO_2 and cardiac dysrhythmias.

○   **What is the incidence of venous air embolism during cesarean section?**

Venous air embolism (VAE) can be detected in up to 67% of cesarean sections performed under neuraxial anesthesia using precordial Doppler monitoring. These are hemodynamically significant in only 0.7- 2 % of cesarean sections. Clinical suspicion of VAE should be high in the case of cardiopulmonary collapse during or immediately following cesarean section.

○   **What factors increase the risk of venous air embolism during cesarean section?**

Steep Trendelenburg (head-down) position which places the operative site above the heart and low central venous pressure.

○   **What are the factors in pregnancy increasing the risk of aspiration of stomach contents?**

Increased intragastric pressure from the gravid uterus, progesterone-induced relaxation of the lower esophageal sphincter, delayed gastric emptying in labor, and depressed mental status from analgesia. The placenta secretes gastrin which promotes hypersecretion of gastric acid.

○   **What is the general outcome of asthma in pregnancy?**

The course of asthma in pregnancy may be the same, worse, or better.

O   **T/F: An arterial PCO$_2$ of 36 mm Hg does not represent severe asthma in the pregnant woman.**

False. When interpreting arterial blood gases, remember that a normal PaCO$_2$ during pregnancy ranges from 32 to 34 mm Hg. This benign looking PCO$_2$ may actually indicate that the patient is getting tired.

O   **What is the major pulmonary complication of tocolytic therapy?**

Tocolytic-induced pulmonary edema.

O   **Which agents are associated with this syndrome?**

Terbutaline, ritodrine and magnesium sulfate.

O   **What are the proposed mechanisms for tocolytic-induced pulmonary edema?**

Fluid overload, myocardial toxicity, cardiac failure secondary to tachycardia and down regulation of cardiac β-receptor due to chronic β agonist exposure.

O   **What is the therapy for terbutaline-induced pulmonary edema?**

Stop the tocolytic, supportive care, restrict fluids, administer oxygen, diuresis and intubate, as needed.

O   **What factors should be taken into consideration during intubation of a pregnant patient?**

Anatomic and physiologic changes of pregnancy increase the risk of failed intubation. Always observe full stomach precautions.

O   **Which anticoagulant is safe for use in pregnancy.**

Heparin. Risks of heparin administration include: maternal thrombocytopenia, osteoporosis, hemorrhage, abruptio placentae, and spontaneous abortion. A plan for discontinuation is essential when epidural anesthesia is planned. Warfarin is usually avoided, especially during the first trimester. Low molecular weight heparin (LMWH) has been used safely, as it does not cross the placenta. Careful coordination of epidural placement/removal and anticoagulant dosing is necessary to minimize the risk of epidural hematoma.

O   **How can the anesthetist help facilitate breech vaginal delivery complicated by fetal head entrapment?**

The goals are (1) relaxation of cervical smooth and skeletal muscle and (2) analgesia for forceps delivery with external suprapubic pressure. Cervical smooth muscle relaxation is achieved with sublingual or intravenous nitroglycerin. Cervical and perineal skeletal muscle relaxation and analgesia are achieved with epidural local anesthetic.

O   **What is the treatment for acute fatty liver of pregnancy?**

Treatment consists of stabilization of electrolyte and coagulation abnormalities, followed by delivery of the fetus. Maternal condition improves within 24 hours of delivery, and there are no long-term hepatic sequelae. The most common anesthetic concern is management of significant peripartum hemorrhage that frequently occurs as a result of coagulopathy.

O   **Which nerves are most frequently injured as a result of obstetric rather than anesthetic complications during vaginal delivery?**

Obstetric injuries usually involve compression injuries to the obturator, femoral and lateral femoral cutaneous nerves. These injuries are typically unilateral, have a dermatomal distribution corresponding to a peripheral nerve and may involve sensory and motor deficits (i.e. foot drop)

NEONATAL ANESTHESIA

I Am Not Young Enough To Know Everything.
Oscar Wilde

○ **Until what age is an infant considered a neonate?**

1 month.

○ **Until what age is a child considered an infant?**

1 year.

○ **What are normal vital signs for a full-term neonate?**

Blood pressure 65 mm Hg systolic, heart rate 130-160 beats-per-minute, respiratory rate 45-60 breaths-per-minute.

○ **What are normal arterial blood gas values for a healthy full-term newborn?**

The pH will be about 7.21, p_aO_2 about 50 mm Hg, and the p_aCO_2 about 40-50 mm Hg.

○ **How does the blood gas of a healthy term infant change in the first hour of life?**

The pH increases from 7.21 to 7.33 in the first hour, the p_aCO_2 decreases to 30-40 mm Hg in the first hour, and the p_aO_2 increases from 50 mm Hg at birth to 65 mm Hg at one hour and usually stabilizes at about 75 mm Hg by 24 hours.

○ **How does the fetal circulation differ from the extrauterine circulation?**

The fetal circulation basically excludes the lungs, whereas in the extrauterine circulation, the pulmonary and systemic circulations occur in parallel. In the fetus, pulmonary vascular resistance is relatively high because of the low PO_2 and small lung volumes. The placental circulation forms the low-resistance circuit in the fetus but in extrauterine life, the pulmonary circuit has the lower resistance. Consequently, since blood follows the path of least resistance, in fetal life it preferentially flows from the pulmonary artery to the systemic arteries (aorta) via the ductus arteriosus. Because of the relatively high pulmonary vascular resistance in fetal life, right ventricular pressures tend to be elevated as well. Consequently, blood flows from the right to the left atrium via the foramen ovale, which closes in extrauterine life as the right ventricular and atrial pressures fall.

○ **What features characterize persistent pulmonary hypertension of the newborn (PPHN).**

In many ways, PPHN mimics the fetal circulation. There is increased pulmonary vascular resistance, increased pulmonary artery pressure, decreased pulmonary blood flow and right to left shunting across foramen ovale and ductus arteriosus.

○ **What causes persistent pulmonary hypertension of the newborn?**

PPHN is caused by any condition that prevents the normal transition from fetal to neonatal circulation. Most commonly this is caused by conditions that increase pulmonary vascular resistance, most notably acidosis and hypoxemia.

○   **What are the common neonatal abdominal emergencies?**

Omphalocele, gastroschisis, intestinal atresias, imperforate anus, malrotation and volvulus. Others include congenital diaphragmatic hernia, biliary atresia, incarcerated inguinal hernia and exstrophy of the bladder.

○   **What are the common non-abdominal neonatal emergencies?**

Myelomeningocele, tracheoesophageal fistula and bilateral choanal atresia.

○   **What are the differences between gastroschisis and omphalocele?**

Omphalocele involves herniation of abdominal contents into an abdominal wall defect at the umbilicus. Umbilical hernia is a very mild form of omphalocele. The herniated abdominal contents (which may include abdominal organs other than bowel) are contained within a sac consisting of peritoneum that protects the organs from irritation by amniotic fluid. The peritoneal covering can rupture at birth, exposing abdominal contents to the environment. Omphalocele is often associated with other congenital anomalies.

In gastroschisis there is an abdominal wall defect to the right of the normal umbilicus through which abdominal contents herniate. Since they are not contained within a peritoneal sac, the herniated abdominal contents are exposed directly to amniotic fluid in utero. Gastroschisis outcomes are somewhat worse than those seen with omphalocele because of the amount of time the abdominal contents spend being bathed in irritating amniotic fluid. Recovery of bowel function is slower in gastroschisis, and the bowel tends to be inflamed and edematous, often making primary closure more difficult. Gastroschisis is usually found in isolation and occurs more commonly in premature infants.

○   **When should primary closure of gastroschisis or omphalocele be attempted?**

Primary closure of omphalocele or gastroschisis may cause circulatory, ventilatory and/or renal dysfunction, as well as bowel necrosis if the abdominal pressure is too high upon closure. Primary closure should only be attempted when the intragastric pressure is < 20 cm H_2O, the central venous pressure does not increase by 4 mm Hg or more, and adequate ventilation can be maintained as the abdominal viscera are replaced into the abdominal cavity.

○   **If primary closure is not attempted in gastroschisis or omphalocele patients, how is the abdominal wall closed?**

A silastic sheet can be fashioned into a chimney or silo to contain the bowel. The silo volume is decreased over the course of a few days. Once the height of the silo is level with the rest of the abdominal wall, the infant can return to the operating room for surgical abdominal wall closure.

○   **List three major goals in the perioperative management of gastroschisis/omphalocele?**

1. Management of fluid and heat losses from exposed abdominal contents
2. Protection of herniated organs
3. Antibiotics to minimize the risk of sepsis

○   **Describe the developmental history of congenital diaphragmatic hernia.**

Typically the abdominal viscera herniate through a defect in the left hemidiaphragm into the left hemi- thorax. The presence of abdominal contents in the thoracic cavity prevents adequate growth and development of both lungs, but the ipsilateral lung in particular is affected with resultant pulmonary hypoplasia. Right-sided diaphragmatic hernias occur but are less common (10-15%).

○   **What findings are present on physical examination of neonates with congenital diaphragmatic hernia?**

Scaphoid abdomen, bowel sounds in the chest, displaced heart sounds, and poor air entry. At birth, these infants often exhibit the classic triad of respiratory distress, cyanosis and apparent dextrocardia.

❍   **What is the underlying cause of the respiratory failure associated with left-sided congenital diaphragmatic hernia?**

Left lung hypoplasia and pulmonary hypertension.

❍   **What is the mortality associated with congenital diaphragmatic hernia?**

40-50%.

❍   **What are the major goals in the perioperative management of neonates with congenital diaphragmatic hernia?**

To prevent the occurrence of hypoxemia and acidosis (which can contribute to a return to a fetal circulation pattern) by optimizing ventilation, maximizing oxygenation and minimizing metabolic perturbations. Low pressure, high frequency ventilation is preferred to minimize barotrauma (and resulting pneumothorax), especially to the more compliant contralateral lung.

❍   **Describe the clinical course of neonates with congenital diaphragmatic hernia if hypoxemia and acidosis persist despite therapy.**

Hypoxemia and acidosis induce pulmonary vasoconstriction, leading to increased pulmonary vascular resistance. Increased pulmonary vascular resistance produces an elevation in pulmonary artery, right atrial and right ventricular pressures. Elevated right-sided pressures and resistances, in turn, induce a return to the fetal circulatory state, with reopening of the foramen ovale and the ductus arteriosus with right to left shunting and subsequent cyanosis. This persistent fetal circulation, usually directly due to persistent pulmonary hypertension, induces further hypoxemia and acidosis, eventually resulting in multiple organ dysfunction and death.

❍   **If a fetal circulatory pattern persists in a neonate with congenital diaphragmatic hernia despite optimized ventilatory and pharmacologic support, what alternative therapy is available?**

Extracorporeal Membrane Oxygenation (ECMO)

❍   **Which bowel segments are typically involved in intestinal atresias?**

Duodenum, jejunum, terminal ileum and anus.

❍   **Which bowel segment obstruction presents earliest?**

Duodenal atresia usually presents within the first 12 hours of life. Other intestinal obstructions may not present until 2-7 days after birth, but usually occur within the first two weeks of life.

❍   **What chromosomal anomaly is associated with duodenal atresia?**

Trisomy 21 (Down Syndrome).

❍   **What is meconium ileus?**

Meconium ileus is small bowel obstruction caused by inspissated meconium that was never passed. This form of bowel obstruction is pathognomonic for cystic fibrosis (although only 20% of cystic fibrosis patients have a history of meconium ileus).

❍   **At what age is pyloric stenosis most commonly seen?**

The average age of onset is 3-4 weeks, with a range of 1-12 weeks.

○   **What physical findings are characteristic of pyloric stenosis?**

The "olive." This is a firm mass usually palpable just to the right of the midline in the epigastric area.

○   **What non-invasive diagnostic test can reliably confirm the diagnosis of pyloric stenosis?**

Ultrasound.

○   **What are the metabolic disturbances typically seen in infants with pyloric stenosis?**

Dehydration, hyponatremia, hypokalemia, and a hypochloremic metabolic alkalosis.

○   **T/F: Pyloric stenosis is a surgical emergency.**

FALSE. Rehydration and correction of electrolyte and acid-base abnormalities should be completed first.

○   **What anesthesia-related precaution is particularly important to observe in the infant undergoing pyloromyotomy?**

These patients should always be treated as if they have a full stomach. Intravenous access should be established and the stomach should be emptied with a large-bore sump tube before induction of anesthesia. Some anesthetists prefer to intubate the infant awake but there is evidence that an IV induction (rapid sequence) may be better. The trachea should not be extubated at the end of the procedure until the infant's airway reflexes are intact.

○   **What is the most common form of congenital tracheoesophageal fistula?**

Proximal esophageal atresia - distal fistula. This form occurs in more than 90% of cases.

○   **Tracheoesophageal fistula is a feature of which syndrome?**

VATER syndrome. This consists of _v_ertebral anomalies; _a_nal anomalies, such as atresia; _t_racheoesophageal fistula or _e_sophageal atresia; and _r_adial or _r_enal anomalies. Roughly 20-25% of these children also have congenital heart disease (most commonly ventricular septal defect or tetralogy of Fallot) and the term VACTER is then used. Another 10% have midline facial clefts as well, such as cleft lip and palate.

○   **T/F: Tracheoesophageal fistula a surgical emergency.**

True. The stomach must be decompressed and the fistula closed in order to prevent pulmonary aspiration of stomach contents.

○   **Describe a technique for inducing anesthesia for a right thoracotomy to repair a tracheoesophageal fistula?**

[1] The proximal esophageal pouch should be emptied with a sump tube. [2] With the infant in a semi-upright position, a gas induction with sevoflurane (or halothane) and oxygen should be performed with the patient breathing spontaneously. [3] After airway reflexes are sufficiently obtunded, the trachea should be intubated. [4] The endotracheal tube should be advanced carefully into a mainstem bronchus, confirmed by loss of breath sounds over one hemithorax. [5] The endotracheal tube should then be pulled back slowly until breath sounds can just be heard bilaterally. [6] The endotracheal tube should be rotated so that the Murphy eye and the bevel are not facing posteriorly toward the fistula. [7] Spontaneous ventilation or gentle assist should be maintained until the chest is opened, at which time ventilation must be controlled. Until the fistula is isolated, it is best to minimize the ventilatory pressure. If the patient undergoes a decompressive gastrostomy prior to

thoracotomy, the gastrostomy tube will act as a low resistance vent that can decrease ventilation to the lungs. If this occurs, the gastrostomy tube can be partially or fully clamped. Note: the most likely location of the fistula is 2 cm above the carina on the posterior trachea.

○ **What problems do children with a history of tracheoesophageal fistula repair encounter as they grow?**

Obstructive and restrictive lung disease later in life and frequent respiratory infections. Other problems include tracheomalacia, weak tracheal wall at the fistula site, esophageal stricture and esophageal dysmotility.

○ **What is the most significant difficulty in inducing anesthesia in an infant with myelomeningocele?**

Care must be taken to avoid direct pressure or trauma to the defect. Intubation can be accomplished in a lateral position. Alternatively, if placed supine for induction, padding should be placed around the outside of the meningocele sac to protect it. Elevation of the occiput and shoulders should then be used to position the patient for laryngoscopy and intubation.

○ **A neonate presents with respiratory distress, cyanosis and apnea that improves if the baby cries. What is the likely diagnosis?**

Bilateral choanal atresia, resulting in nasal obstruction. This occurs because infants are obligate nasal breathers.

○ **Until what age are infants obligate nose breathers?**

3 to 5 months.

○ **Explain why infants desaturate more quickly than adults when apneic under anesthesia.**

In infants, the cartilaginous ribcage and immature thoracic musculature result in a highly compliant chest and relatively poor outward recoil of the chest wall. The inward recoil of the lung, on the other hand, is only slightly less than in adults. As a result, the inward forces outweigh the outward forces and a reduction in functional residual capacity occurs with apnea. In addition, oxygen consumption is higher in infants than in adults. Both these phenomenon contribute to a more rapid desaturation when apneic under anesthesia.

○ **What is retinopathy of prematurity?**

This is a vascular disorder of the developing retinal circulation that can result in complete retinal detachment and blindness in extreme cases. The principle etiologic factor is thought to be increased pO_2 in the developing retinal artery. Infants are thought to be at risk of retinopathy of prematurity until 44 weeks post-conceptual age when the retinal vessels are fully mature. Until that time, the minimum oxygen tension required to maintain adequate organ perfusion should be the goal. An arterial pO_2 of 60-80 mm Hg should be adequate in most cases. Elective surgery should be delayed until the infant is no longer at risk.

○ **What is the most common cause of bradycardia in the neonate?**

Hypoxia. Therefore, when an infant becomes bradycardic, the *first* thing to do is to ensure adequacy of ventilation and oxygenation.

○ **T/F: In the neonate, cardiac output depends mostly on stroke volume.**

False. The neonatal heart is less distensible than the adult heart and is therefore less able to increase stroke volume. Consequently, heart rate is the most important factor in the determination of cardiac output in neonates. CO = SV X HR

○   **Which neonates are at risk for hypoglycemia?**

Premature infants, small for gestational age infants and infants of diabetic mothers.

○   **What is the definition of hypoglycemia in neonates?**

Blood glucose ≤ 25 mg/dL in preterm infants on the first day of life; ≤ 35 mg/dL in term infants; and ≤ 45mg/dL thereafter.

○   **T/F: Neonates experience a slower induction with *inhaled* anesthetic agents compared to older children?**

False.   The ratio of minute ventilation to functional residual capacity is higher in neonates compared to older children.   Therefore, the gas in the alveolar space equilibrates more quickly and induction occurs more rapidly.

○   **Does fetal hemoglobin (Hb F) have a higher or a lower P_{50} than adult hemoglobin (Hb A)?**

The P_{50} of fetal hemoglobin (19 mm Hg) is lower than the P_{50} of Hb A (26 mm Hg).   This represents an adaptation to intrauterine life since Hb F more readily binds molecular oxygen than Hb A, at the low oxygen tensions in utero.

○   **What is *physiologic anemia*?**

Over the first few months of life, the high level of fetal hemoglobin seen at birth decreases, reaching its lowest level at 2-3 months of age.   A normal hematocrit at this age is 33%.   The P_{50} increases rapidly during the neonatal period so that tissue oxygen delivery is still adequate despite less hemoglobin.   As adult hemoglobin replaces fetal hemoglobin, this anemia resolves.

○   **A full term newborn is flaccid, blue, with no respiratory effort, and has a heart rate of 90 bpm after the first minute of life.   What is the Apgar score?**

The Apgar score is 1.

○   **What is the FIRST thing you do for this infant?**

Airway! Ventilate with 100% oxygen either by bag and mask or via endotracheal intubation.

○   **At what rate should ventilation be performed during neonatal resuscitation?**

40-60 breaths per minute.

○   **What is the initial lung inflation pressure required for positive pressure ventilation in the newborn infant?**

30-40 cm H_2O.   Some may require 50 cm H_2O.   A lower pressure (20 cm H_2O) is usually sufficient for subsequent breaths.

○   **Which clinical signs are indicative of an improvement in the neonate's status during resuscitation?**

Increasing heart rate, spontaneous respiration and improvement in color.

○   **When should chest compressions be initiated during resuscitation of a neonate?**

When the heart rate is below 60 beats/minute or is 60-80 beats/ minute and is not increasing after 15-30 seconds of positive pressure ventilation with 100% oxygen.

○   **If this infant does not clinically improve (Apgar score of > 2 after two minutes of life) what is the next step?**

Obtain vascular access (umbilical or venous) and treat with epinephrine and volume expanders. Consider congenital heart disease, narcotic-induced depression, and hypoglycemia.

○   **T/F: Neonates are more sensitive to non-depolarizing neuromuscular blockers than are adults and older children.**

True. However, since infants generally have a higher volume of distribution for these drugs, clinical doses are similar to adults on a mg/kg basis.

○   **T/F: Infants require less neostigmine than adults for reversal of neuromuscular blockade?**

True. The standard dose of neostigmine in infants is 0.05 mg/kg.

○   **At what vertebral level does the spinal cord terminate in neonates?**

The spinal cord terminates at L_3 in neonates. It recedes to the adult level (L_1) by one year of age.

○   **T/F: Fluid loading prior to spinal anesthesia in infants is essential in preventing hypotension?**

False. Hypotension is rarely seen in infants undergoing spinal anesthesia. Many practitioners will even place the intravenous catheter in the foot after the block has been placed.

○   **T/F: The duration of spinal anesthesia is shorter in infants compared with adults?**

True. Relatively higher cardiac output and regional blood flow result in greater uptake of drug and a shorter duration of block.

○   **What factors contribute to an infant's difficulty in maintaining body temperature when exposed to a cold environment?**

Infants have a high surface area to volume ratio, increased thermal conductance, and immature central thermoregulatory mechanisms.

○   **What unique method do neonates utilize to maintain body temperature?**

Nonshivering thermogenesis occurs primarily through the metabolism of brown fat. It makes up about 5% of an infants body weight. Brown fat differentiates around 26-30 weeks gestation and so may not be available to some premature infants.

○   **Water accounts for what percentage of body weight in premature neonates?**

80%.

○   **Water accounts for what percentage of body weight in full-term neonates?**

70%.

○   **What is the estimated blood volume of a premature neonate?**

90-100 ml/kg.

O   **What is the estimated blood volume of a full-term neonate?**

80-90 ml/kg.

O   **What is the maximum concentration of urine possible in a neonate?**

600-700 mOsm/L. The kidneys are not capable of concentrating to the adult maximum of 1400 mOsm/L until the end of the first year of life.

O   **How does the immaturity of the neonatal kidney contribute to problems with the regulation of intravascular volume?**

The inability of the neonatal kidney to fully concentrate urine makes the neonate less able to protect intravascular volume in the face of hypovolemia.

O   **What size and at what depth should an oral endotracheal tube be taped in a full term neonate?**

A 3.0 tube secured at 9 cm at the lips is a good guideline. Bilateral breath sounds should always be confirmed. A depth of three times the internal diameter is a useful guideline for infants.

O   **How does the position of the larynx differ between neonates and adults?**

In premature infants, the larynx lies at the third cervical vertebra (C_3). In term neonates, the larynx is usually at C_{3-4}. In adults, the larynx has descended to C_{4-5}.

O   **How does the shape of the epiglottis differ between neonates than in adults?**

In neonates, the epiglottis is relatively long, omega-shaped and stiff. In adults, it is often flat and short and less obstructive on laryngoscopic view.

O   **If thick meconium is noted at delivery, what steps should be taken with the neonate?**

The neonate should be intubated and suctioned using a special adapter (a meconium aspirator). Mechanical suction should be set no higher than –100 mm Hg.

O   **During anesthesia, a neonate's heart rate is 200 bpm. Does this indicate a problem?**

Although tachycardia may represent a response to surgical stimulation, high heart rates in neonates are often indicative of intravascular volume depletion. A fluid challenge of 10 ml/kg of crystalloid or colloid solution will often slow the heart rate.

O   **Until what age are premature infants at increased risk for post-operative apnea?**

The answer to this question is somewhat controversial. The available literature suggests that post-operative apnea may be a risk in infants 44 to 55 weeks post-conceptual age or younger. The implication of this risk is that elective procedures requiring general anesthesia should be delayed, if possible, until these age criteria are met. If surgery is necessary before then, the infants should be admitted and monitored overnight.

O   **What will the cardiovascular evaluation of a newborn with a patent ductus arteriosus reveal?**

A machine-like continuous murmur at the left upper sternal border, bounding pulses and a widened pulse pressure.

O   **Does the ductus venosus carry oxygenated or deosygenated blood in fetal life?**

Oxygenated blood from the placenta.

○ **What is the main ionizing group on local anesthetics and narcotics?**

Local anesthetics and narcotics are weak bases with an amine group as the main ionizing group.

○ **What is fetal ion trapping of local anesthetics and narcotics?**

This describes the situation where local anesthetics and narcotics become more ionized in the fetal circulation (lower pH) and then can't diffuse back across the placenta into the maternal circulation in this charged form. They are then "trapped" in the fetal circulation.

○ **Why is thiopental not subject to fetal ion trapping?**

Thiopental's main ionizing group is the carboxyl group, which becomes neutral at lower pH.

○ **When does fetal ion trapping become clinically significant?**

In the case of an asphyxiated infant who is acidotic. In this case local anesthetic toxicity and opioid toxicity can become evident due to fetal ion trapping.

○ **Which carries blood highest in oxygen tension and lowest in carbon dioxide tension, the umbilical vein or the umbilical artery?**

The umbilical vein.

PEDIATRIC ANESTHESIA

Great Spirits Have Always Found Violent Opposition From Mediocre Minds.
Albert Einstein

○ **What is the most common cause of death due to trauma in children?**

Serious head injury.

○ **What is the most commonly injured intra-abdominal organ in childhood trauma?**

Spleen.

○ **T/F: A splenectomy is usually necessary after splenic trauma?**

False. Ninety-seven percent of injured spleens can be treated conservatively if no other abdominal organ damage is suspected.

○ **Acute renal failure, Coomb's negative hemolytic anemia and thrombocytopenia comprise the triad for which syndrome?**

Hemolytic-Uremic Syndrome (HUS).

○ **What is the most common cause of Superior Vena Cava Syndrome in children?**

Mediastinal malignancies, most commonly lymphomas.

○ **Aplastic crisis in sickle cell disease is associated with what infectious agent?**

Parvovirus (the causative agent in fifth disease). The primary erythropoietic failure during aplastic crisis can result in a life-threatening anemia in these patients with a significantly decreased RBC life span.

○ **What are the features required to make the diagnosis of Guillain-Barré' Syndrome?**

Progressive motor weakness and areflexia.

○ **What are the main precipitating factors of status epilepticus in children?**

Intercurrent infection, sleep deprivation, toxic or metabolic disorders or anticonvulsant drug withdrawal.

○ **The most feared complication associated with Extra Corporeal Membrane Oxygenation (ECMO) is?**

Intracranial hemorrhage (ICH).

ICH occurs in 13% of neonates, 5% of children, and 4% of cardiac patients who require ECMO and is the most frequent cause of death in newborns managed with this technique. Although the cause of the hemorrhage is multifactorial, the necessary use of systemic heparinization during ECMO contributes to the often-unusual extent and location of hemorrhage.

○ **What are the hemodynamic findings of decompensated shock?**

Hypotension and low cardiac output. Tachycardia is often present. Bradycardia, if present, is an ominous sign and suggests impending cardiac arrest.

O   **The lower limit of systolic blood pressure for a child older than one year of age can be estimated by using which formula?**

70 mm Hg + (2 x age in years).

O   **In a child younger than ten years what is the narrowest point of the airway?**

The cricoid cartilage.

O   **What is the most common cause of shock in children?**

Hypovolemic shock. It is usually associated with dehydration or hemorrhage but can also occur due to massive extravascular fluid shifts such as those seen in sepsis or extensive burns.

O   **When should atropine be used for the treatment of bradycardia?**

Only after adequate ventilation and oxygenation have been established, since hypoxemia is a common cause of bradycardia.

O   **T/F: Cervical spine injury is less common in pediatric than in adult trauma?**

True. The child's spine is more elastic and mobile than that of the adult and the softer pediatric vertebrae are less likely to fracture. Fewer than 10% of spinal cord injuries occur in children.

O   **Which drugs are contraindicated for infusion through an intraosseous route?**

None. The intraosseous route can safely administer any intravenous drug or fluid required during the resuscitation of children.

O   **List the major complications associated with intraosseous cannulation and infusion?**

Tibia fracture, compartment syndrome, skin necrosis and osteomyelitis. This has been reported in less than 1 % of patients.

O   **A child presents with sepsis and rash (maculopapular and petechial) involving the palms and soles. What are the possible etiologies?**

Meningococcemia and Rocky Mountain spotted fever.

O   **What is the cause of the majority of intracerebral hemorrhages seen in children?**

Congenital abnormalities of the cerebral blood vessels. The most common of these are arteriovenous malformations.

O   **Acute myocardial infarction in children is associated with which pediatric diseases?**

Kawasaki disease and anomalous origin of the left coronary artery. It can also occur as a consequence of perinatal stress, blunt chest wall trauma, cardiac transplantation and arterial switch procedures.

O   **Ingestion of gasoline is associated with what major complication?**

Pulmonary aspiration. Dyspnea, cyanosis and respiratory failure usually occur within the first 24 hours.

○ **Describe the blood gas analysis characteristic of a patient triggering with malignant hyperthermia?**

Metabolic and respiratory acidosis.

○ **What is the treatment protocol for malignant hyperthermia?**

Discontinuation of triggering agent(s), hyperventilation with 100% oxygen, dantrolene 2.5 mg/kg and repeated doses as needed, active cooling, and symptomatic treatment of electrolyte abnormalities and blood gas derangements.

○ **A two-year-old sickle cell patient presents with pallor, weakness, tachycardia and abdominal fullness. What diagnosis should you suspect?**

Acute splenic sequestration. This disorder is caused by acute and massive splenic enlargement due to sequestration of a large portion of the sickle cell patient's blood volume. This is an emergency since acute hypovolemia can result from so much blood being trapped within the spleen.

○ **What should the treatment plan for this patient include?**

Colloid and whole blood transfusions to correct hypovolemia and anemia

○ **What is the most common age range for esophageal foreign bodies?**

1 to 6 years of age.

○ **What are the most common esophageal foreign bodies?**

Coins.

○ **During airway foreign body extraction, at what point is complete immobility of the patient crucial? Why?**

As the endoscopist is delivering the foreign body across the glottis. If the patient coughs or moves during this phase of the procedure, the foreign body can be dislodged and fall into the airway.

○ **T/F: Most airway foreign bodies are radiopaque.**

False. Airway foreign bodies are usually radiolucent (most commonly food).

○ **What is the preferred maintenance fluid for infants?**

5% dextrose in 0.2% saline. The immature kidney is less able to handle a solute load.

○ **What is the preferred crystalloid for replacement of extracellular fluid or "third space" losses?**

Lactated Ringer's, normal saline, or other similar fluid.

○ **What complications can occur when hypotonic maintenance fluids are used for volume resuscitation?**

Hyponatremia and hyperglycemia.

○ **What is malignant hyperthermia?**

The hallmark of malignant hyperthermia is hypermetabolism induced by exposure to halogenated anesthetic agents and/or succinylcholine. Malignant hyperthermia produces a true hypermetabolic crisis characterized by hypercapnia, tachycardia, acidosis and usually (but not always) rapidly rising body temperature. Treatment includes dantrolene and supportive therapy.

○ **T/F: Masseter spasm after IV succinylcholine heralds malignant hyperthermia.**

False, but the answer to this question is somewhat controversial. Currently, there is no clear evidence to suggest that all patients who experience masseter spasm in response to IV succinylcholine will develop a full blown malignant hyperthermia crisis. In fact, most patients who receive succinylcholine experience muscle contracture to some degree before relaxation occurs. Masseter spasm after succinylcholine may represent an exaggerated contracture response brought on by high circulating catecholamine levels. Therefore, patients who experience masseter spasm after succinylcholine should not be labeled as malignant hyperthermia susceptible until further evaluation is undertaken, particularly in the absence of a family history of malignant hyperthermia susceptibility or previous anesthesia-related problems suggestive of malignant hyperthermia. Despite this, without further work-up, an episode of masseter spasm suggests use of a non-triggering anesthetic technique for subsequent operations.

○ **A child with a platelet count of 30,000/mm³ from idiopathic thrombocytopenic purpura is scheduled for splenectomy. Should this child receive a preoperative platelet transfusion?**

No. Transfused platelets are fairly rapidly consumed in this disorder and generally should not be given prophylactically. Platelet transfusions should be reserved for acute therapy to treat serious, life-threatening bleeding. Administration is usually delayed until after the splenic pedicle has been clamped. Patients that have been treated with gamma-globulin infusions (IVIG), should have 1g/kg per day administered IV once daily on the two days before surgery. The increase in platelet count evoked by IVIG may be maintained for 2 to 3 weeks.

○ **The end-tidal CO_2 in a T-piece breathing circuit depends upon what factors?**

The fresh gas flow and the minute ventilation.

○ **What are the disadvantages of a T-piece breathing system?**

They require high fresh gas flows (to prevent rebreathing) and use large volumes of volatile anesthetics.

○ **Are T-piece breathing systems classified as semi-open or semi-closed?**

Semi-open, because rebreathing of alveolar gas occurs . In a semi-closed system, rebreathing of alveolar gas does not occur due to the presence of a CO_2 absorber and valves separating the inspiratory from the expiratory limbs.

○ **A 4 year old child presents with sudden onset of stridor, fever and mild respiratory distress. The child appears anxious, sitting up, drooling and holding on to its mother. What is the most likely diagnosis?**

This is a classic presentation of epiglottitis.

In general, epiglottitis involves the acute onset (6-24 hours) of a bacterial inflammation of the epiglottis that can rapidly lead to airway obstruction. Although a lateral x-ray of the neck may confirm epiglottic enlargement, if the diagnosis is suspected, immediate intubation for airway control is the first priority. Routine pediatric vaccination for *Haemophilus influenzae*, type B has dramatically decreased the incidence of acute epiglottis.

○   **How can croup and epiglottitis be clinically differentiated?**

Croup is more common in infants, whereas epiglottis tends to occur in 2-6 year old children. Epiglottitis is associated with a high fever, toxic appearance, and abrupt onset of respiratory distress and stridor. Croup, however, is usually more subacute in onset with lower fevers and is characterized by a barking cough.

○   **What is the treatment for epiglottitis?**

Tracheal intubation under general anesthesia in the operating room after direct laryngoscopy, followed by intravenous antibiotic treatment. The patient is usually ready for extubation within 36-72 hours of starting antibiotic therapy.

○   **What is the narrowest point in the airway of a child less than 10 years of age?**

The cricoid cartilage.

○   **What is resistance to airflow in the airway inversely proportional to?**

The fourth power of the radius of the airway (when laminar air flow is present during quiet breathing). A smaller radius means higher resistance. This is Poiseuille's Law.

○   **What is the formula to estimate endotracheal tube size?**

Endotracheal tube size = (age in years / 4) + 4.

○   **At what age are infants no longer obligate nose breathers?**

3-5months

○   **Describe the unique characteristics of the infant airway.**

Neonates have soft, easily collapsible tissue in the airway. The larynx is located more anterior and cephalad (C_{3-4}). The epiglottis is large.

○   **What symptoms are commonly found in a patient with an airway foreign body?**

Lower airway: localized wheezing, dyspnea, fever, and cough. Upper airway: dyspnea, stridor, cough, and cyanosis.

○   **What are the most common objects aspirated by children?**

Food items such as peanuts, popcorn, and carrots. Less common are plastic and metal parts of toys.

○   **What types of airway foreign bodies typically produce the greatest inflammatory response?**

Food items, peanuts in particular.

○   **Why do peanuts pose a special risk when aspirated?**

During bronchoscopy and extraction, the peanut may break apart spreading particles into distal lung segments. Spread may also occur to both lungs rather than being confined to one. The oil in peanuts can also cause a local tissue reaction.

○   **Why does a patient often not improve immediately after removal of an airway foreign body?**

Depending on the type of foreign body and the duration of impaction, the airway mounts an inflammatory response that may persist well beyond the point of removal. Local swelling may decrease the cross-sectional area of the airway lumen and continue to limit airflow. Systemic inflammatory mediators may increase airway smooth muscle reactivity causing generalized bronchospasm.

O   **A child with hemoglobin SS disease (sickle cell anemia) is scheduled for cholecystectomy. His hematocrit is 20%. Is transfusion necessary?**

These children are at increased risk for perioperative sickling and stroke in the presence of hypoxemia, hypothermia, hypovolemia and acidosis. Steps should be taken both to minimize these triggers and to reduce the concentration of Hemoglobin S (HbS) through either exchange transfusion or by simple transfusion of packed red blood cells. A target goal for HbS concentration is less than 30-50%, with the hematocrit approximately 30%. Hemoglobin electropheresis measuring HbS should be performed to follow response to therapy.

O   **Children, particularly infants, have larger volumes of distribution for many drugs compared to adults. Why?**

Infants, especially neonates, have lower protein binding to act as a drug reservoir. Also, total body water, extracellular fluid volume, and blood volume are relatively higher in children than in adults.

O   **How does a larger volume of distribution affect the pharmacokinetics of a drug?**

More drug may be required (on a mg/kg of weight basis) to achieve the desired clinical effect.

O   **T/F: Children with cerebral palsy are at increased risk for hyperkalemia after succinylcholine.**

False.

O   **What is the most common congenital heart defect associated with Trisomy 21 (Down syndrome)?**

Endocardial cushion defect (A-V Canal).

O   **What are the four classic cardiac features of tetralogy of Fallot?**

Right ventricular hypertrophy, ventriculoseptal defect (VSD), infundibular pulmonary stenosis, and an overriding aorta.

O   **What is a "TET" spell?**

In a patient with tetralogy of Fallot, a hypercyanotic or "TET" spell results from spasm of the subpulmonary infundibulum causing increased resistance to blood flow in the right ventricular outflow tract. This results in decreased pulmonary blood flow and an increased right-to-left shunt across the VSD with subsequent cyanosis.

O   **During general anesthesia, how do you treat a hypercyanotic spell in a patient with tetralogy of Fallot?**

Management is aimed at reducing right-to-left shunting by increasing SVR and decreasing resistance in the pulmonary outflow tract. Methods of treatment include: administration of intravenous volume (boluses of 10 ml/kg), ventilation with 100% oxygen, and boluses (1-10 μg/kg) or an infusion (0.05-0.2 μg/kg/min) of phenylephrine to increase systemic vascular resistance.

The primary reason for hypoxemic spells under general anesthesia is hypovolemia. Fasting should be minimized and IV fluids should be administered preoperatively whenever possible.

○ **Why is succinylcholine contraindicated in children with muscular dystrophy?**

It can cause an exaggerated hyperkalemic response and cardiac arrest.

○ **How do platelet transfusions affect the platelet count in children?**

1 unit/5 kg of body weight should increase the platelet count by $20,000 - 70,000/mm^3$.

○ **Which children are at risk for infective endocarditis and require antibiotic prophylaxis prior to surgery?**

Children with any kind of congenital heart disease (repaired or unrepaired) except repaired secundum atrial septal defect or repaired patent ductus arteriosus more than 6 months post-op. Also included are children with a history of rheumatic heart disease, infective endocarditis, or known valvular dysfunction.

○ **A 5-year-old presents for tonsillectomy. He has a runny nose and a cough, but no fever. Is a general anesthetic safe for this patient?**

There is no true consensus regarding the safety of anesthetizing children who have an upper respiratory infection (URI). Most of the literature does suggest an increased risk of perioperative pulmonary complications in the setting of a URI. However, most of these complications are mild and do not usually result in significant morbidity. Importantly, children with reactive airways disease have a much greater risk than otherwise healthy children. The type of procedure, necessity of intubation and general health of the child should all be considered in deciding whether to delay elective surgery.

○ **What pediatric surgical procedures have a high incidence of post-operative nausea and vomiting?**

Strabismus repair, adenotonsillectomy, middle ear surgery and genital procedures. Use of narcotics and a history of motion sickness are also associated with this complication.

○ **T/F: Intraoperative use of nitrous oxide is associated with post-operative nausea and vomiting.**

True. Eliminating nitrous oxide has been associated with less post-operative nausea and vomiting. This issue is still debated.

○ **Why are T-piece breathing systems considered useful in pediatric anesthesia?**

They have minimal dead space and no valves which reduces the resistance to breathing.

○ **T/F: Infants and children have a longer induction time with inhaled anesthetic agents compared to adults?**

False. Although tidal volume per unit of body weight is constant (6 cc/kg) throughout life, infants and children have relatively higher alveolar ventilation compared to adults and a lower relative functional residual capacity (FRC). This increased ratio of minute ventilation to FRC results in a more rapid uptake of inhaled anesthetics. The effect is less pronounced for less blood soluble agents.

○ **T/F: Infants and children with cyanotic congenital heart disease (right-to-left shunt) have a longer induction time with *inhaled* anesthetic agents compared to children with normal hearts?**

True. With right-to-left shunt, a portion of the blood returning to the heart bypasses the lung and therefore is not exposed to anesthetic, slowing the induction of anesthesia. A large shunt will slow induction more than a smaller shunt. This effect is more pronounced with less soluble agents.

❍   **T/F: Infants and children with cyanotic congenital heart disease (right-to-left shunt) have a longer induction time with *intravenous* drugs compared to children with normal hearts?**

False. Intravenous induction actually occurs slightly more quickly in children with cyanotic congenital heart disease since venous blood containing drug returns to the right atrium and a portion is shunted directly to the left heart and carried to the brain, bypassing the pulmonary circulation. With fast-acting induction agents, the clinical relevance of this effect is questionable though.

❍   **T/F: Infants and children with left-to-right shunt have a slower induction with *inhalation* anesthetics?**

Unless the shunt is very large (>80%), left-to-right shunt produces negligible change in the induction time with inhaled anesthetics.

❍   **What is the first sign of hypovolemia in children under general anesthesia?**

Tachycardia. Hypotension usually does not occur in children until there is a 20-25% loss of circulating blood volume.

❍   **List the possible complications of caudal anesthesia in children.**

Intravascular injection, dural puncture, intraosseous injection of anesthetic agents, muscle weakness, and urinary retention.

❍   **What is laryngospasm?**

Laryngospasm represents the involuntary closure of the glottis by intrinsic laryngeal muscles that bring the vocal cords to the midline. It is a normal, protective reflex to prevent pulmonary aspiration.

❍   **How is laryngospasm managed in pediatric patients?**

Initial therapy includes initiation of positive pressure to the airway by mask with 100% oxygen. The spasm often ceases with this maneuver after 30-45 seconds.   If spasm continues and oxygen saturation falls, muscle relaxant can be administered. Succinylcholine is classically used although non-depolarizing agents such as rocuronium can be considered. A full intubating dose is not normally required to break laryngospasm. Since bradycardia often accompanies hypoxemia in children, atropine use should be strongly considered when the laryngospasm does not resolve quickly.

❍   **What conditions are associated with postoperative apnea in infants?**

Premature infants (defined as born at less than 37 weeks) are most prone to apnea, especially those who receive general anesthesia (or any sedatives), have ongoing apnea, or are anemic.

❍   **What is the preferred method of anesthesia for premature infants?**

There is no consensus that one anesthetic technique is better than another. Although regional anesthesia has been recommended in the past, there is no conclusive evidence that it is "safer." Even those infants who have regional anesthesia should be monitored in the hospital postoperatively.

❍   **What drug may be effective in the prevention of postoperative apnea in premature infants?**

Intravenous caffeine (10mg/kg) may have beneficial effects that can last several days.

❍   **Describe the anesthetic implications of Pierre-Robin syndrome.**

Children with Pierre-Robin syndrome can be difficult to intubate due to facial anomalies. These include mandibular hypoplasia and cleft palate.

○ **What signs would you expect to find on examination of a child with a patent ductus arteriosus (PDA)?**

Tachycardia, systolic murmur, bounding peripheral pulses and radiographic evidence of increased pulmonary blood flow.

○ **Do most infants with patent ductus arteriosus require surgery?**

No. Ductal closure is usually accomplished with medical therapy using indomethacin. Surgery occurs if this fails and the patient remains symptomatic.

○ **T/F: Cyanosis is a common feature of patent ductus arteriosus?**

False. The pulmonary vasculature usually has a lower resistance than the systemic circulation, so flow across the ductus arteriosus is usually left-to-right.

○ **How does minimum alveolar concentration (MAC) change with age?**

MAC is highest in infants at term to 6 months of age and decreases with both increasing age and prematurity.

○ **Why is sevoflurane favored for use in pediatric anesthesia?**

Sevoflurane has a low blood solubility (blood:gas partition coefficient 0.47, at 37 °C)which provides for a rapid inhalational induction and awakening. It is non-pungent and less irritating, so better tolerated by children. Also, it has excellent cardiovascular stability by primarily decreasing SVR while tending to support cardiac output.

○ **Compare and contrast the cardiovascular effects of sevoflurane and halothane.**

Sevoflurane tends to maintain blood pressure with an increase in heart rate, whereas halothane maintains or lowers heart rate with a fall in systolic blood pressure.

○ **What is the most common cardiovascular side effect of succinylcholine in children?**

Bradycardia, especially with a second dose. Atropine administration (20 mcg/kg) may help to minimize this side effect.

○ **For healthy children undergoing elective procedures, what are appropriate fasting guidelines?**

According to the American Society of Anesthesiologists, regardless of age, the appropriate minimum fasting times are 2 hours for clear liquids, 4 hours for breast milk, and six hours for a light meal, formula or non-human milk.

○ **Calculate maintenance fluids in a 35 kg child.**

Maintenance is 75 cc/hr. Calculation: 4 cc/kg for the first 10 kg, 2 cc/kg for the next 10 and 1 cc/kg thereafter.

○ **During surgery, a 12 kg child becomes acidotic with a pH of 7.0, serum bicarbonate 15 mEq/L and a base deficit minus 10 (-10). How much bicarbonate would you need to give to correct this deficit?**

Bicarbonate deficit is calculated by the formula: Wt (kg) x 0.3 x base deficit. You should give half the calculated amount and recheck the arterial blood gas pH in 20-30 minutes.

○   **What are the possible side effects of bicarbonate administration?**

Bicarbonate can cause paradoxical acidosis when it is converted to carbon dioxide. It can also cause hypernatremia, hyperosmolality (which may contribute to intraventricular hemorrhage in premature infants), and a left shift of the oxygen hemoglobin dissociation curve secondary to alkalosis.

○   **What is the most common initial sign of respiratory distress in an infant?**

Tachypnea. Neonates (both full-term and premature) respond to hypoxemia with an initial increase in respiratory rate followed by sustained respiratory depression. By three weeks of age, full-term infants respond to hypoxemia with sustained hyperventilation (as do older children and adults). Newborn infants respond to hypercapnea with increased ventilation as well, although this effect is less pronounced compared to older children and adults.

○   **Describe the differences between pediatric and adult lung function.**

The pediatric lung is less compliant. Chest wall compliance on the other hand, is greater in children due to the cartilaginous structure of the ribcage. Airway resistance is also greater in children since this resistance is a function of the forth power of the radius of the airway lumen (Poiseuille's law). Functional residual capacity is smaller and alveolar ventilation is higher in infants and small children compared to adults. Resting tidal volume is the same on a per kilogram basis for both adults and children.

○   **T/F: Body surface area to mass ratio is greater in children compared to adults.**

True.

○   **Why is an infant at risk for hypothermia?**

Their losses are greater because infants have poor central thermoregulation, higher minute ventilation, thin insulating fat and increased body surface area to mass ratio. Shivering is an ineffective mechanism for heat production because of limited muscle mass and nonshivering thermogenesis significantly increases oxygen consumption. A cold-stressed infant is at risk for developing cardiovascular depression and lactic acidosis.

○   **What are the effects of hypothermia in neonates and infants?**

- Apnea and bradycardia
- Respiratory depression
- Coagulopathy
- Vasoconstriction
- Altered drug clearance

GERIATRIC PATIENTS

"I intend to live forever, or die trying"
Groucho Marx

○   **The response of an elderly patient to premedication is unpredictable. Why?**

Doses of narcotics and benzodiazepines should be reduced 20-40% in elderly patients. Contributing factors include; an increase in CNS sensitivity, decrease in volume of distribution, and decrease in liver blood flow producing high initial plasma levels and prolonged drug effects. Narcotic administration may produce apnea and episodic respiration, predisposing to airway obstruction.

○   **What is the elimination half-life of diazepam in the elderly population?**

The elimination half-life of diazepam in hours approximates the patient's age in years. It could be as long as 80-90 hours.

○   **In spite of the age-related decline in renal function, the serum creatinine of the elderly remains within normal limits. Why?**

A decrease in skeletal muscle mass leads to decreased production of creatinine which parallels the decline in creatinine clearance.

○   **What is the cause of mild elevations in the serum potassium levels in the elderly?**

Renovascular changes that occur in the juxtaglomerular apparatus cause decline in the production of renin and aldosterone. Functional hypoaldosteronism leads to decreased renal excretion of potassium. This is offset by a loss of lean body mass and reduction in exchangeable potassium.

○   **How is cerebral autoregulation of blood flow affected in a healthy elderly patient?**

It is unaffected in the healthy elderly patient.

○   **Even though anesthetic agents such as propofol, methohexital, ketamine and etomidate are eliminated by hepatic metabolism, the clinical effects of these drugs are not significantly prolonged in the elderly. Why?**

For induction doses, the termination of the clinical effects of these drugs occurs when they are redistributed from the vessel rich organs to vessel poor groups. Once redistribution sites are saturated with larger doses or prolonged infusions, metabolism does affect clinical length of action.

○   **What is the cause of a slow heart rate response to hypotension in the elderly?**

This reflects the slower autonomic reflex responses.

○   **What is the most important physiologic effect of aging on the heart of a healthy patient?**

Aging makes patients volume-dependent yet volume-intolerant due to an increase in cardiac chamber stiffness (decrease in ventricular compliance) such that hemodynamic function is optimal only within a narrow range of end-diastolic pressure and volume.

Additional functional changes include decreased arterial compliance, reduction of maximal cardiac output due to reduction of maximal heart rate and prolongation of time required for both myocardial contraction and relaxation.

○   What EKG findings should lead to further investigation in an elderly patient prior to elective surgery?

Left anterior bundle branch block, atrioventricular conduction delays and atrial flutter or fibrillation suggests underlying cardiac disease and requires further investigation. Disturbances in cardiac rhythm associated with aging and not necessarily indicative of pathology include: sick sinus syndrome, right bundle-branch blocks and premature ventricular and supraventricular beats.

○   What are two significant predictors for the presence of coronary artery disease in the elderly?

Peripheral vascular disease and cerebrovascular disease.

○   What is the effect of age on ventilatory response to imposed hypoxia and hypercarbia?

The ventilatory response is smaller in magnitude and delayed in onset. Moment-to-moment regulation of ventilation is unimpaired.

○   How are the pharmacokinetics of spinal anesthesia affected by age?

Anticipate a higher level of spinal anesthesia, with faster onset of action and prolonged duration due to; decreased blood flow to the subarachnoid space resulting in slower absorption of anesthetic solutions, increased cephalad spread due to a smaller volume and higher specific gravity of the cerebrospinal fluid and exaggerated lumbar lordosis or thoracic kyphosis. The incidence of postdural puncture headache is lower.

○   Are geriatric patients prone to develop exaggerated reductions in blood pressure with spinal anesthesia compared to younger patients?

Yes. This is due to lower residual inherent vascular tone and lack of adequate compensatory reflexes with reduced β-adrenergic responsiveness. Age also influences the level of spinal anesthesia, with greater cephalad spread per injected dose, especially when larger volumes of anesthetic solution are used.

○   Is spinal anesthesia better for the elderly patient's postoperative mental function?

No! The incidence of cognitive dysfunction is equivalent between general and regional anesthesia. There may be a benefit if the patient does not receive any sedation.

○   T/F: The American Society of Anesthesiologists (ASA) physical status classification takes into consideration the age of the patient.

False. The ASA classification is a preoperative physical status classification of patients taking into consideration severity of systemic disease, functional limitations and the need to proceed as elective or emergency surgery.

○   A 74-year-old patient with a history of non-insulin dependent diabetes mellitus is scheduled for peripheral vascular surgery. He has a normal resting EKG. Does he need further cardiac evaluation?

Yes. Myocardial ischemia is often silent in diabetic patients. Patients with two or more intermediate predictors of clinical risk as defined by the American Heart Association would benefit from further noninvasive cardiac testing. This includes presence of prior MI by history or EKG, angina pectoris, compensated or prior CHF, and/or diabetes mellitus. Consideration of functional capacity and level of surgery-specific risk are also determinants.

○ **How does aging affect heart rate and blood pressure?**

Maximal heart rate and beta-adrenergic responsiveness is decreased. Systolic blood pressure is increased and diastolic blood pressure is unchanged or reduced producing a widening of the arterial pulse pressure.

○ **Are systemic and pulmonary vascular resistance affected by advancing age?**

SVR and PVR are elevated due to decreased elasticity and arterial compliance.

○ **How would you calculate the expected PaO_2 for a given age?**

PaO_2 (mm Hg) = 102 – age/3.

○ **What is the effect of aging on vital capacity (VC) and total lung capacity (TLC)?**

VC is progressively reduced as residual volume increases, with TLC remaining relatively unchanged (10% reduction by age 80) unless physical stature is reduced.

○ **What are the possible detrimental effects of hypothermia in the elderly?**

Delayed emergence; prolongation of neuromuscular blockade (reduced metabolism) and the effects of inhaled anesthetic agents (decreased MAC); postoperative shivering and tachycardia (increased oxygen consumption, increased myocardial oxygen demand, ischemia, myocardial depression or ventricular arrhythmia); cold diuresis (hypovolemia); hypoxemia (V/Q mismatch) and impaired coagulation (platelet dysfunction or reduced clotting factor activity). Elderly patients are at risk for hypothermia due to impaired autonomic vascular control.

○ **Are elderly patients at greater risk for aspiration? Why?**

Yes, due to reduced responsiveness of protective airway reflexes, delayed gastric emptying, increased incidence of hiatal hernia, greater residual anesthetic effects, sensitivity to narcotics and sedatives and postoperative delirium.

○ **How are cerebral autoregulation and the cerebrovascular response to hyperventilation altered in the elderly?**

Both autoregulation of cerebrovascular resistance in response to changes in arterial blood pressure and cerebral vasoconstrictor response to hyperventilation remains intact in elderly patients free of cerebrovascular disease.

○ **T/F: The induction dose of barbiturates should be reduced in elderly patients because their CNS is more sensitive to the hypnotic action of these drugs.**

False. The induction dose of barbiturates should be reduced, but for pharmacokinetic and not pharmacodynamic reasons. A smaller initial volume of distribution and altered distribution of cardiac output result in a slower intercompartmental transfer and redistribution of the drug from the central compartment. This results in apparent drug sensitivity due to a transiently higher initial plasma concentration of the injected drug.

○ **What happens to the elimination half-life (t 1/2) of benzodiazepines in the elderly?**

The t 1/2 of midazolam is almost doubled when compared to younger adults. The t 1/2 of diazepam increases with age. A rule of thumb is that the t 1/2 of diazepam in hours equals the patient's age in years.

○   **T/F: Propofol causes less hypotension in the elderly when compared to younger adults.**

False. Hypotension is more marked in the elderly. Termination of clinical drug effect depends on the rate constant for intercompartmental drug transfer, similar to thiopental. The induction dose should be reduced by 20 to 40 percent in elderly patients, and administered slowly. Remember: "Start low and go slow".

○   **Is the presence of peripheral vascular disease a predictor of coronary artery disease in the elderly?**

Yes. The incidence of cardiovascular disease is 50 to 65% in the elderly, and may be found in patients that are completely symptom-free.

○   **What percentage of myocardial infarctions in the elderly are "silent"?**

Almost 50%. Elderly patients with EKG findings that support the diagnosis of ischemic heart disease and those with decreased exercise tolerance for unclear reasons or with unreliable histories should be referred for further cardiac evaluation

○   **How do elderly patients increase their cardiac output in response to exercise?**

By increasing stroke volume (Frank-Starling mechanism) rather than increasing heart rate or stimulation of β-adrenergic agonists.

○   **T/F: The dose of succinylcholine should be reduced in the elderly.**

Some elderly men demonstrate an increased sensitivity to succinylcholine due to reduced plasma cholinesterase enzyme activity and therefore require a dose reduction. In most elderly patients the impact is clinically insignificant.

○   **What changes occur in the kidneys with aging?**

The kidneys become smaller with age. Glomerulosclerosis results in a progressive reduction of renal mass, with as much as 30% lost by the age of 70 years. Consequently there is a reduction in both renal blood flow (RBF) and glomerular filtration rate (GFR). RBF decreases 10 percent per decade in the adult years with relative sparing of the renal medulla. GFR decreases at the rate of approximately 1 mL/min/1.73 m^2/year or 1-1.5% per year. Creatinine clearance decreases by 1% per year after age 40 and can be estimated using the equation: creatinine clearance = (140-age) X wt (kg)/ 72 X serum creatinine. Serum creatinine levels remain within normal limits despite the reduction in GFR because of reduced muscle mass and less creatinine production.

Elderly patients have a reduced ability to concentrate the urine (less responsive to ADH) and to excrete acid load, with impaired ability to conserve sodium.

○   **How is the myocardium affected by aging?**

Reduced elasticity in the peripheral vasculature causes increased afterload and leads to left ventricular hypertrophy, dilation of the aorta and elevated systolic blood pressure. This thickening and stiffening of the heart results in loss of contractility and adversely affects diastolic relaxation. The role of atrial contraction in ventricular filling becomes increasingly important, with the onset of atrial fibrillation adversely affecting cardiac output.

Disturbances in cardiac rhythm are associated with fibrosis of the sinoatrial node, atrophy of conduction pathways and loss of normal pacemaker cells. Common findings include: sick sinus syndrome, left anterior hemiblock, bundle-branch blocks, supraventricuar and ventricular ectopic beats.

Changes in autonomic function leave the elderly in a state of *physiologic beta blockade*. Patients have reduced chronotropic and inotropic response to beta-adrenergic agonists, lower maximal heart rates in response to stress and diminished heart rate response to hypotension.

○ **How is cardiac output affected by aging?**

Elderly patients who exercise regularly and maintain their skeletal muscle mass show little or no change in cardiac output at rest and during moderate exercise. Maximal cardiac output does decrease 1% per year after age 30 years due to a progressive decrease in maximum heart rate.

Aging produces ventricular hypertrophy and diastolic dysfunction; therefore, cardiac output is more dependent on the atrial contribution to ventricular filling. The elderly increase cardiac output by increasing stroke volume (Frank-Starling mechanism) rather than increasing heart rate or by stimulation of β-adrenergic agonists.

○ **A 69-year-old, otherwise healthy patient with no significant past medical history is scheduled for repair of an inguinal hernia. He has good exercise tolerance, but a routine 12-lead EKG shows a RBBB (right bundle branch block). What further cardiac evaluation is indicated?**

None. An isolated right bundle branch block in an elderly patient, who is otherwise asymptomatic, does not appear to be associated with an increased incidence of cardiac disease. Further evaluation would be justified if there were; Q waves or evidence of prior myocardial infarction, left anterior hemiblock, atrioventricular conduction delays and atrial flutter or fibrillation.

○ **What are the predominant changes in the respiratory system in the elderly patient?**

Decreased lung volumes and reduced gas exchange, with a decrease in resting PaO_2.

The PaO_2 is decreased and the alveolar-arterial oxygen gradient is increased primarily due to mismatching of ventilation and perfusion and reduced alveolar surface area. FRC and CC both increase with age, but CC increases to a greater extent until they overlap at 44 years of age (supine), and 66 years of age (standing). When CC>FRC, airway closure occurs during normal tidal breathing leading to air trapping and uneven inhaled gas distribution. Changes in PFTs include: decreased TLC, VC and FEV_1; increased residual volume, FRC, CC and dead space. In the elderly the ventilatory responses to hypoxia and hypercapnia are markedly reduced in the awake state. These patients are at increased risk for apnea, episodic respiration and airway obstruction in the recovery room. In addition, there is a general loss of muscle mass in the airways resulting in a reduced responsiveness of protective airway reflexes with increased risk of aspiration.

Chest wall mechanics is altered due to fibrosis and calcification of the rib cage and declining respiratory muscle strength. Diminished elastin and an increase in connective tissue reduces elastic recoil of the lungs. There is an increase in lung compliance, however, total pulmonary compliance changes are minimal.

○ **T/F: Advancing age has a clinically significant adverse effect on liver metabolism?**

False. The liver becomes smaller with age, but has a wide margin of functional reserve. Enzymatic function is preserved, so drug metabolism will be minimally affected given the loss of liver mass and parallel decrease in liver blood flow. There is a slight decrease in the clearance of drugs extensively dependent on first-pass drug extraction.

○ **How does body composition change with aging?**

Body mass index and the proportion of body fat is increased, skeletal muscle mass is decreased approximately 10% and there is a reduction in intracellular water, with maintenance of intravascular volume in healthy individuals.

○ **How is energy production changed by the structural changes described above?**

Energy expenditure gradually decreases 1 to 2% from the ages of 20 to 80 years. Increased levels of norepinephrine reflect increased basal sympathetic activity in the aged, however, sympathetically mediated metabolic responses are blunted. This is seen with the decreased responsiveness of maximal heart rate and β-adrenergic activity. It has been postulated that the elderly's blunted thermogenic response may be a manifestation of this phenomenon and result in increased fat stores. Loss of skeletal muscle results in a decrease in maximal and resting oxygen consumption and diminished production of body heat. Combined with less insulating subcutaneous tissue and diminished reflex cutaneous vasoconstriction to prevent heat loss, body temperature may be difficult to control in older patients.

○   Summarize the affect of aging on baroreceptor function?

Advancing age is associated with impairment of baroreflex responsiveness and increased risk of orthostatic hypotension. Baroreceptors are stretch receptors located in the aortic arch and carotid sinus. The decrease in arterial compliance associated with aging can reduce the ability to transduce changes in pressure at the baroreceptors, diminishing the magnitude of the reflex.

○   Compare and contrast the cardiovascular effects of thiopental and propofol in the elderly.

Thiopental IV produces peripheral vasodilation with a moderate reduction in blood pressure. In the elderly patient with a diminished baroreceptor reflex and increased vascular wall stiffness, thiopental can cause a significant hypotension. As a result of an increased volume of distribution at steady state the elimination half-life of thiopental is twice as long in the elderly (13-25 hours) as compared to the young patient In addition the thiopental dosage requirement decreases 25-75 % in the geriatric patient and it may take longer to induce unconsciousness. In the elderly patient the induction dose of propofol is half that of the younger patient. Propofol clearance is reduced in the elderly patient, resulting in reduced dose requirements for maintenance. The cardiovascular depression seen with propofol is greater than that seen with thiopental. These effects can be minimized if propofol is injected slowly.

○   Do anesthetic requirements increase or decrease with aging?

The minimum alveolar concentration (MAC: minimum alveolar concentration of an inhaled anesthetic) decreases 4-5% each decade after the age of 40 years. ED_{50} (median effective dose of an intravenous drug) is also reduced. The physiologic basis for these changes is unclear.

○   Is cerebral autoregulation and the cerebrovascular response to hyperventilation altered in the elderly?

Both autoregulation of cerebrovascular resistance in response to changes in arterial blood pressure and cerebral vasoconstrictor response to hyperventilation remain largely intact in elderly patients that are free of cerebrovascular disease.

Cerebrovascular autoregulation may however be somewhat impaired especially in the elderly patient with systolic hypertension. Impaired autoregulation and baroreceptor dysfunction may lead to episodic cerebral hypoperfusion during sleep and in the postprandial period. There may be an association between episodic hypotension, impaired autoregulation and silent strokes in the elderly.

○   Does an elderly patient need a larger or smaller volume of local anesthetic solution injected into the epidural space to achieve the same level of block compared with younger patients? Why?

Smaller local anesthetic dose.

Segmental dose requirements for epidural anesthetics are reduced with the injection of large volumes resulting in a markedly exaggerated cephalad spread of the solution. Injection of small volumes of local anesthetic solutions produces no significant change. Reduced overall compliance of the epidural space, and a decrease in the size of the intervertebral foramina limiting lateral drug loss may explain these phenomena.

○   **How are the pharmacokinetic profiles of nondepolarizing muscle relaxants altered in the elderly?**

Decreased volume of distribution (reduced skeletal muscle mass) and reduced clearance.

Nondepolarizing muscle relaxants are required in about the same quantity in elderly and younger patients to provide the same degree of paralysis, but their duration of action is prolonged if they require hepatic or renal elimination and/or biotransformation. Antagonism of neuromuscular blockade with neostigmine is not altered, but the incidence of arrhythmias is higher in the elderly with cardiovascular disease.

○   **Is beta-adrenergic receptor sensitivity increased or decreased in the elderly?**

β-adrenergic responsiveness is reduced to both agonists and antagonists, the so-called endogenous "β-blockade of aging". The receptor density is unchanged.

○   **Are elderly patients more sensitive to the effects of opioids?**

Yes. Pharmacodynamic changes are primarily responsible for the increased potency of opioids in the elderly. In addition, reduced central volume of distribution and clearance produce a high peak plasma concentration after a bolus dose and prolonged drug effect. Dose requirements should be reduced 30 to 50%.

○   **How is the speed of anesthetic induction affected by aging?**

Intravenous induction is prolonged in the presence of reduced cardiac output which increases arm-brain circulation time. In contrast, inhalational induction may be faster than in young adults, because a decrease in cardiac output results in decreased anesthetic uptake and faster increase in alveolar anesthetic partial pressures and a greater percentage of cardiac output going to the brain.

OUTPATIENT SURGERY

We Are Made Wise Not By The Recollection Of Our Past, But By The Responsibility For Our Future.
George Bernard Shaw

○   **Most shoulder surgeries are performed on an outpatient basis. Discuss postoperative pain management.**

Regional anesthesia as a sole anesthetic or used in combination with general anesthesia is ideal. Blocks may be performed preoperatively or postoperatively using either a single shot, continuous infusion, or patient-controlled pain pumps. The addition of clonidine or the mixed agonist-antagonist opioid compounds to local anesthetic has been shown to prolong analgesia for brachial plexus blocks. Adjuvant therapy includes: oral, IV, IM and IV PCA opioids, NSAIDs, acetaminophen, agonist-antagonist analgesics and ice to minimize pain and swelling.

○   **What is the benzodiazepine-specific antagonist?**

Flumazenil 0.2 mg (Romazicon) IV repeated every 60 seconds to 1 mg reverses all CNS effects including sedation-hypnosis, amnesia, muscle relaxation and EEG changes but has a relatively short half-life of 0.7 to 1.8 hours. Therefore re-sedation is possible.

○   **Is midazolam acceptable for outpatient anesthesia?**

Yes. A 5 mg dose produces amnesia in 1 to 2 minutes, which lasts for at least 30 minutes. Recovery may be as long as 2 to 4 hours before discharge, requiring that postoperative instructions be given in writing.

○   **What are some important ways in which diazepam differs from midazolam?**

Diazepam	*Midazolam*
Water-insoluble	Water soluble
Long-acting ($T\beta_{1/2}$ = age in years)	Short-acting: ($T\beta_{1/2}$ = 1 to 4 hours)
Less potent	2 to 4 times more potent
Pain on injection and venous thrombosis (propylene glycol and sodium benzoate)	No local irritation
Liver metabolized to active metabolites (prolonged by H_2-blockers)	Liver metabolized to active metabolites (not altered by H_2-blockers)
Protein-binding ++	Protein-binding ++

○   **Does midazolam cause anterograde or retrograde amnesia?**

Anterograde.

○   **What role might oral clonidine play in the preoperative period?**

As an alpha 2-adrenergic agonist, oral clonidine ($3\mu g/kg$) can reduce anesthetic requirements by virtue of its analgesic effects, and has been used to provide sedation and anxiolysis while reducing the lability of intraoperative blood pressure.

○   **What is the standard endocarditis prophylactic regimen for dental, oral, or upper airway procedures in adult patients at risk?**

Amoxicillin, 3.0 g orally, 1 hour before the procedure; and 1.5 g 6 hours after initial dose.

○   **If the patient is amoxicillin/penicillin-allergic, what would be an alternate choice for SBE prophylaxis?**

Erythromycin ethyl succinate 800mg, or erythromycin stearate 1.0g orally 2 hours before the procedure then half the dose 6 hours after the initial dose. Or clindamycin 300mg orally 1 hour before procedure then 150mg 6 hours after the initial dose.

○   **What are the relative contraindications to using a laryngeal mask airway (LMA)?**

1) When pulmonary aspiration of gastric contents is probable, and 2) where controlled ventilation is likely to require a high inflation pressure (> 20 cm H_2O).

○   **What electrolyte abnormality is a risk factor for precipitating digitalis toxicity?**

Hypokalemia (K^+ < 4 mEq/L). Other factors that predispose to digitalis toxicity include: hypercalcemia, hypoxia, drugs (propranolol, amiodarone, verapamil, quinidine), hypothyroidism, advanced age and renal insufficiency. Since magnesium is a cofactor of the Na^+/K^+-ATPase pump, alterations of its concentration will affect the pump's actions. (not really increased toxicity).

○   **List three types of medications that generally should be discontinued or withheld before general anesthesia?**

Oral hypoglycemic agents (1 day) all anticoagulants (Coumadin 3-5 days, heparin 4 hours, Lovenox – low molecular weight heparin 24 hours) and anti-platelet drugs like Plavix (clopidogrel bisulfate) 5-7 days. MAO inhibitors (some still say hold for two weeks), amiodarone, ACEI (angiotensin-converting enzyme inhibitors eg: enalapril), and ARA (angiotensin II receptor antagonists eg: irbesartan) are still controversial issues.

After warfarin therapy is stopped, it takes about four days for the international normalized ratio (INR) to reach 1.5 in almost all patients. If a patient's INR is between 2.0 and 3.0, four scheduled doses of warfarin should be withheld to allow the INR to fall spontaneously to 1.5 or less before surgery. Warfarin should be withheld for a longer period if the INR is normally maintained above 3.0 or if it is necessary to keep it at a lower level (i.e., <1.3). The INR should be measured a day before surgery to ensure adequate progress in the reversal of anticoagulation..

○   **What are the recommended indications for preoperative hemoglobin testing?**

Any procedure commonly associated with major blood loss, pregnancy, any suspicion of anemia, renal disease, malignancy, patients older than 75 years, neonates, smoking history of greater than 20 pack/yr, and patients with cardiovascular disease.

○   **What are the recommended indications for preoperative liver function testing?**

Patients with liver disease, a remote history of hepatitis or exposure to hepatitis, and known metastatic malignancy.

○   **In the review of systems of a 70 year old male with multiple cardiac risk factors, what piece of information is particularly important in deciding whether the patient requires further cardiac evaluation or to proceed with surgery?**

The patient's functional capacity. The patient's suitability for surgery is determined by exercise tolerance (climbing a flight of stairs), clinical predictors of increased perioperative cardiac risk and the surgery-specific risk.

○   **What advantage does exercise thallium imaging offer over exercise electrocardiography?**

Exercise thallium imaging is another noninvasive test that can be used in patients who have abnormal electrocardiograms suggestive of ischemic heart disease. It increases the sensitivity and specificity of the exercise ECG. Thallium is taken up by the coronary circulation and distributed to the myocardium. Fixed perfusion defects indicate infarcted myocardium and poorly perfused areas that later refill indicate areas at risk for ischemia.

○ **Why is history alone a poor method of assessing coronary artery disease in diabetic patients?**

There is a high incidence of silent (painless) myocardial ischemia and infarction in diabetic patients with hypertension and diabetic autonomic neuropathy (early satiety, lack of sweating, reduced sinus arrhythmia and beat-to-beat variability of the heart rate, orthostatic hypotension, impotence, resting tachycardia, nocturnal diarrhea, peripheral neuropathy). The type II diabetic patient has the same risk of fatal or non-fatal MI and death from cardiovascular causes as a non-diabetic with prior MI.

○ **How does the decision to intubate influence the perioperative risk of respiratory problems in a infant with a mild upper respiratory infection?**

Infants with upper respiratory infections who undergo *intubation* are at significant risk of developing major adverse respiratory events (i.e. postoperative croup) versus older children. The reason is that edema secondary to intubation results in a greater reduction in cross sectional area of the trachea.

○ **How does age affect postoperative apnea in the premature infant?**

As the post-conceptional age of the premature infant increases, postoperative apnea decreases proportionately.

○ **What is at the top of your differential diagnosis if 8 hours after general endotracheal anesthesia, the mother of a 4 year old with Down syndrome reports the child can not ambulate?**

Cervical spinal cord injury secondary to ligamentous laxity and subluxation at the atlantoaxial joint (C_1-C_2) (seen with laryngoscopy or positioning of the head for central line placement). The incidence atlantoaxial dislocation is 20% in Down patients and most are asymptomatic which accounts for the recommendation of routine screening at age 5 years or before participation in the Special Olympics.

○ **What is the course of preoperative evaluation if you highly suspect atlantoaxial subluxation?**

The "Down series" consists of flexion, extension and neutral lateral radiographs of the cervical spine. If atlantoaxial instability exists (5 mm or greater distance between the posterior and inferior aspects of the anterior area of the atlas and adjacent surface of the odontoid process), further evaluation with CT and myelography is indicated. Through-the-mouth odontoid views may also be helpful.

○ **What are the high risk perioperative periods for inducing atlantoaxial subluxation in children with Down syndrome?**

The high risk perioperative periods for flexion-extension as well as rotation include laryngoscopy and tracheal intubation, mask ventilation, positioning (central line placement), transport, tracheal suctioning, and radiograph plate placements.

○ **How does infant formula and breast milk affect gastric emptying?**

Both have a high fat content and will result in delayed emptying. Hence the recommendation of no breast milk within 4 hours of surgery.

○ **T/F: Breast milk is not considered a solid food.**

False. Breast milk should be regarded as similar to a solid.

The 1999 ASA practice guidelines recommend a minimum fasting period for non-human milk and infant formula of 6 hours and for breast milk 4 hours.

O   **What are two adverse medical consequences of prolonged fasting in children?**

Hypoglycemia and/or hypovolemia.

O   **Children may have unlimited clear liquids up to how many hours prior to scheduled anesthetic induction?**

2 hours.

O   **What is the role of preoperative metoclopramide?**

Metoclopramide is a gastrointestinal stimulant (decreasing aspiration risk possibly) and antiemetic agent. It has been shown to decrease the gastric residual volume and increase lower esophageal sphincter tone. It is not the most efficacious agent as a prophylactic antiemetic.

O   **What is the disadvantage of giving a non-particulate antacid to buffer gastric acidity?**

It can potentially increase gastric residual volume.

O   **What are some adverse effects of extended fasting times prior to elective surgery?**

Long fasting prior to an elective operation is not only uncomfortable for the patient but has detrimental effects. It causes thirst, hunger, irritability, noncompliance, and resentment in adult patients. Prolonged fasting is especially deleterious in children since it may also produce dehydration, hypovolemia, and hypoglycemia.

O   **Are patients who take clear liquids closer to their surgery at greater risk of aspiration syndrome?**

No, it appears that patients who have been drinking are at no greater risk of aspiration syndrome should regurgitation occur.

O   **Between ondansetron, droperidol , and metoclopramide, which is the best antiemetic prophylaxis for a 22 year old healthy female scheduled for a therapeutic abortion?**

Eight milligrams of intravenous ondansetron appears to be superior to 10 mg of metoclopramide or 1.25 mg of droperidol in preventing postoperative vomiting after general anesthesia for minor gynecologic surgery. 1.25 mg of droperidol is as efficacious as 4 mg of ondansetron with a similar incidence of side effects.

O   **What is the presumed mechanism of action of the perioperative antiemetic effect of ephedrine?**

Ephedrine increases sympathetic tone, and therefore is thought to minimize postoperative nausea and vomiting that is secondary to a high degree of vagal tone. Intestinal motility may decrease as an adrenergic side effect. Ephedrine corrects hypotension-induced nausea and vomiting seen with spinal anesthesia.

O   **What type of patients would you not give ephedrine to as an antiemetic?**

Any patient that would be adversely effected by the hypertension and tachycardia associated with the use of ephedrine. Patients on MAO inhibitors.

O   **How are extrapyramidal reactions to droperidol classified?**

Extrapyramidal reactions to droperidol are mediated via central dopaminergic receptor blockade involved in motor function. Three major categories include: 1) *Acute dystonic reactions* that involves spasm of muscles of the tongue, face, neck, and back (this can also include oculogyric crisis and episodes including sweating, tachypnea, and vasodilation); 2) *Parkinsonian signs* and symptoms, which include bradykinesia, rigidity, masklike facies, drooling, cogwheel rigidity and tremor; and 3) *akathisia*, which are feelings of motor restlessness.

○ **What advantages might there be to maintaining anesthesia with propofol instead of volatile agents in pediatric ambulatory patients?**

Propofol induction and maintenance of anesthesia in pediatric outpatients has been shown to be associated with less postoperative emesis. Not only is this drug safe in children, but it appears to be associated with a decreased incidence of airway obstruction. Thus, propofol is a useful alternative to volatile agent anesthetics in pediatric anesthesia.

○ **What is a reliable alternative induction technique in a 5 year old struggling child who refuses the mask and cannot be managed by an IV induction because of lack of accessible veins?**

Ketamine 4-8 mg/kg IM has been shown to be a useful drug for induction of the uncooperative child (2-4 mg/kg IM is the sedation and analgesia dose). The onset time is short, and the recovery time is not prolonged unless larger doses of ketamine (>5 mg/kg) are combined with a volatile anesthetic. Recurrent illusions, vivid dreams and flashbacks have been reported several weeks after ketamine administration in children. However, dysphoric symptoms are less common in pediatric compared to adult patients. (Pediatric IV induction dose of ketamine: 1-2 mg/kg).

○ **After a dose of oral midazolam (0.5mg/kg) for premedication, when is it appropriate to separate children from their parents?**

Within 10 to 20 minutes.

○ **What type of patients may be best suited for oral ketamine?**

The oral administration of ketamine (or IM) either for analgesia or to induce anesthesia is a recognized technique in situations that may be hazardous for staff to approach a patient or when the patient is distressed (i.e. severely mentally handicapped individuals who are frightened, unruly and uncooperative). The use of small volumes of attractive fluid to camouflage ketamine (10mg/kg) may help to overcome the problem, especially thirsty patients who have been fasting.

○ **What could be the result of an intraarterial injection of thiopental?**

Intraarterial injection causes red cell hemolysis, platelet aggregation, blockage of small arterioles by acid crystals and local norepinephrine release causing vasospasm, resulting in thrombosis and severe ischemia of the extremity.

○ **What is the therapy for intraarterial injection of thiopental?**

Therapy involves intravascular dilution, perivascular infiltration with local anesthetic, sympathetic blockade of the extremity to reduce vasoconstrictor tone and limit the area of ischemic injury, and anticoagulation with heparin. Supportive care includes narcotics for analgesia, elevation of the arm and antibiotics for gangrene.

○ **When flumazenil (Romazicon) is administered in the postoperative period, what effect does it have on intraoperative amnesia?**

None.

○ **What are three reasons for such widespread popularity of propofol in ambulatory anesthesia?**

1) Shortest time to recovery of all IV induction agents. 2) It has a lower incidence of postoperative nausea and vomiting. 3) It has a high degree of patient satisfaction, due to the rapid return to a clear-headed state, minimal side effects, and elation produced by the drug.

○ **What are the cardiovascular effects of propofol?**

Hypotension (decrease in blood pressure 15 to 20%). Propofol causes cardiovascular depression by a combination of direct myocardial effects and vasodilatation. These effects are more pronounced in elderly patients.

○ **What pharmacokinetic property of nitrous oxide makes both induction and emergence with this agent rapid?**

Low blood gas solubility (blood/gas partition coefficient 0.47).

○ **Describe the second gas effect of nitrous oxide?**

The ability of nitrous oxide to increase the uptake of other concurrently administered volatile anesthetics.

○ **List at least 3 advantages of nitrous oxide?**

Low solubility, nonflammable, easy to administer, inexpensive.

○ **List some disadvantages of nitrous oxide?**

It can diffuse readily into air-containing spaces in the body expanding them, potentially could contribute to postoperative nausea and vomiting, and it has a low potency when used alone (MAC 105). Prolonged exposure may result in bone marrow depression (megaloblastic anemia) and neurologic deficiencies (peripheral neuropathies and pernicious anemia). Teratogenic effects have been reported. May exacerbate pulmonary hypertension. Diffusion hypoxia.

○ **What is the onset of action of fentanyl after an intravenous injection?**

One arm-brain circulation (45 seconds to1 minute), after IV administration.

○ **What is the duration of analgesia of fentanyl?**

Approximately 45 minutes. Despite its short duration of action, recovery and discharge times have been reported to be no different using fentanyl or morphine for postoperative analgesia after ambulatory surgical procedures.

○ **Bradycardia can be seen with all opioids except which one?**

Meperidine. Tachycardia is due to atropine-like structure and reflex response to hypotension.

○ **How do the pharmacokinetics of remifentanil compare to other opioids commonly used in the OR?**

Remifentanil is an ultrashort-acting opioid analgesic, with a terminal half-life of 8 to 10 minutes and a context-sensitive half-life of 4 minutes regardless of the duration of infusion. Alfentanil has a context-sensitive half-life of 58 minutes and depends on its small volume of distribution for short elimination half-life. Remifentanil's analgesic potency is similar to that of fentanyl.

○   **How is remifentanil metabolized?**

Nonspecific esterases.

○   **Among the currently available potent inhaled agents, which ones have a pleasant odor and are not irritating to the airway?**

Halothane and sevoflurane.

○   **How may the use of halothane lead to the occurrence of arrhythmias?**

All volatile agents sensitize the myocardium to epinephrine. Isoflurane, sevoflurane and desflurane all require 3-6 fold greater doses of epinephrine to cause dysrrythmia when compared with halothane. Epinephrine 1μg/kg during halothane anesthesia is unlikely to produce PVCs. The ED_{50} for subcutaneous epinephrine causing PVCs is 2.1 μg/kg for halothane, 3.7 μg/kg when lidocaine is added to halothane anesthesia, 6.7 μg/kg with enflurane and 10.9 μg/kg with isoflurane. Children appear to tolerate epinephrine better than do adults. Unlike isoflurane, enflurane and desflurane which increase heart rate, halothane may cause no change or decrease heart rate.

○   **Which potent inhaled agent is associated with seizure activity at higher concentrations?**

Enflurane. Seizures can be produced at 1.5 to 2 MAC of enflurane, especially when combined with hypocarbia.

○   **How do the pharmacokinetics of desflurane differ from isoflurane?**

Desflurane has significantly lower blood-gas (0.42 versus isoflurane 1.4) making induction and emergence very rapid and lower blood-tissue coefficients, which means less drug is deposited in peripheral tissues and less hangover after prolonged cases.

○   **What effect does desflurane have on the sympathetic nervous system?**

Rapid changes in inspired desflurane, whether at induction or during the anesthetic, result in sympathetic nervous system discharge producing tachycardia (more pronounced at deeper levels of anesthesia) and hypertension. Desflurane is a potent vasodilator, with a reduction in systemic vascular resistance causing hypotension.

○   **Is the blood-gas partition coefficient of sevoflurane high or low?**

Sevoflurane has a low blood-gas partition coefficient (0.69).

○   **What receptor does succinylcholine target?**

The postjunctional nicotinic cholinergic receptor.

○   **What patient population might have a decreased amount of pseudocholinesterase enzyme prolonging the effects of succinylcholine?**

This may be seen in ambulatory patients taking anticholinesterase medications for glaucoma or myasthenia gravis, or patients taking chemotherapeutic drugs, as well as in patients with a genetically atypical enzyme.

○   **Name at least 5 adverse side effects of succinylcholine.**

Cardiac arrhythmias, hyperkalemia, postoperative myalgia, myoglobinuria, increased pressures (intraocular, intragastric, intracranial), trismus, allergic reactions, phase II blockade, rhabdomyolysis, prolonged apnea, and trigger for malignant hyperthermia.

❍   **How is atracurium metabolized?**

It undergoes spontaneous degradation (Hofmann elimination) at body pH and temperature, in addition to undergoing ester hydrolysis.

❍   **Which neuromuscular blocking agent might be best in an ambulatory patient with significant renal or liver disease?**

Cis-atracurium, because it undergoes spontaneous degradation.

❍   **What is the shortest acting available nondepolarizing neuromuscular blocking agent of the benzylisoquinoline group?**

Mivacurium

❍   **How is mivacurium metabolized?**

Mivacurium is hydrolyzed by plasma cholinesterase, at a rate approximately 70% to 88% that of succinylcholine. Prolonged recovery has been reported in patients homozygous for atypical pseudocholinesterase enzyme.

❍   **Which nondepolarizing neuromuscular blocking agent might be best in an ambulatory patient who might be particularly sensitive to blood pressure changes?**

Vecuronium and cis-atracurium are the only neuromuscular blocking agents essentially devoid of cardiovascular side effects.

❍   **List at least 5 factors that predispose to postoperative nausea and vomiting (PONV)?**

There are patient, surgery and anesthetic technique factors. Female gender, infants and small children, history of motion sickness, history of PONV, obesity, and surgery during menstruation and ovulation are patient factors. Surgical factors include certain operations - strabismus/laparoscopy/middle ear/T&A/abortion/female reproductive organ surgery. Anesthetic technique factors include, inexperienced operator of mask and bag ventilation, nitrous oxide (possibly), high total narcotic dose, general anesthesia versus other techniques, early oral intake in the PACU, postoperative hypotension and early ambulation.

❍   **What are the benefits of intraoperative analgesics?**

The intraoperative use of analgesic drugs improves hemodynamic stability, decreases the anesthetic requirement, and provides for a more rapid emergence from anesthesia and decreases postoperative pain and discomfort. Adequate pain control achieved prior to entry to PACU decreases discharge times.

❍   **How do nonsteroidal anti-inflammatory drugs work?**

Nonsteroidal anti-inflammatory drugs act primarily through peripheral inhibition of prostaglandin synthesis. The cyclo-oxygenase enzyme is inhibited, reducing the conversion of arachidonic acid to cyclic endoperoxide, a prostaglandin and thromboxane precursor. Decreased production of arachidonic metabolites limits inflammation and perceived pain while avoiding opioid chemoreceptor stimulation and attendant side effects.

❍   **What are the advantages of using propofol instead of thiopental for induction and/or maintenance in pediatric patients undergoing ambulatory surgery?**

It has been shown that the continuous infusion of propofol is a well-tolerated anesthetic technique in children. The speed and quality of recovery after propofol is superior to that observed after thiopental and/or halothane administration, and is associated with an extremely low incidence of vomiting.

○   **What type of economic benefits are there for using a MAC (propofol sedation with an ilioinguinal-hypogastric nerve block) technique versus general (LMA, propofol, sevoflurane, nitrous oxide/oxygen) or spinal (bupivacaine-fentanyl) anesthesia in ambulatory patients having unilateral inguinal herniorrhaphy?**

The use of peripheral nerve block with propofol sedation results in shorter time-to-home readiness, lower pain scores at discharge, greater patient satisfaction and lower associated, anesthetic-related institutional costs compared general and spinal anesthesia.

○   **Why is it that despite the low blood:gas solubility of sevoflurane, that the washout compared to other volatile inhaled anesthetics is essentially the same?**

Although the blood:gas partition coefficient is considerably lower for sevoflurane compared with halothane, the solubility in other tissues, e.g., muscle, is very similar. Thus, when the inspired concentration of the inhaled drug is abruptly reduced to zero at the conclusion of an anesthetic, muscle will continue to release the drug back to the blood (for delivery to the lungs for exhalation) at an essentially similar rate for both drugs and therefore prolongs the washout of sevoflurane in spite of its low blood:gas solubility.

○   **Are there advantages in administering morphine instead of fentanyl for postoperative pain in ambulatory patients?**

Morphine has been shown to produce a better quality of analgesia (lower pain scores and less oral analgesic use) than fentanyl in ambulatory surgical patients, with no difference in recovery times or discharge times. Morphine is associated with increased nausea and vomiting, especially after discharge.

○   **What are the consequences of administering remifentanil to patients with pseudocholinesterase deficiency?**

The circulating esterases responsible for remifentanil metabolism are distinct from those enzymes which metabolize succinylcholine or acetylcholine, and the short duration of remifentanil may even be preserved in patients with deficiency of pseudocholinesterase activity or in patients taking medications which inhibit plasma pseudocholinesterases (e.g., echothiophate). In fact, the pharmacokinetics of remifentanil in patients with impaired hepatic or renal function appear to be unchanged.

○   **What muscle relaxant is a good alternative to succinylcholine if rapid onset is desired?**

Rocuronium.

Intubating conditions are satisfactory and similar to that observed after succinylcholine, 60 to 90 seconds after rocuronium 0.6 mg/kg IV (0.6 mg is 2 x ED 95)   It also depends on what other drugs were administered with rocuronium. In the vast majority of patients receiving alfentanil 15ug/kg, followed by propofol, 2.0 mg/kg, and rocuronium 0.45 mg/kg, good to excellent conditions for intubation will be present 75 to 90 seconds after the completion of drug administration. The intermediate duration of action associated with an intubating dose of rocuronium provides adequate surgical relaxation for most outpatient cases.

○   **What are some anesthetic considerations for pediatric cases in remote locations of the hospital?**

1) The anesthetic technique must provide predictable, brief anesthesia of adequate depth and an immobile patient; 2) the anesthetics must be able to be safely given repeatedly with portable equipment; 3) a rapid awakening with short recovery time is desirable; 4) maintenance of a patent airway in a variety of body positions and during transport is mandatory; 5) provisions for standard monitoring are required for general anesthesia remote from the patient; and 6) minimizing psychological and physical trauma during the repeated procedures is desirable.

O   **How can you decrease the incidence of toxic symptoms and increase the percentage of successful blocks while performing intravenous regional anesthesia?**

A successful block can be achieved by elevating the arm and exsanguinating with an elastic Esmarch bandage applied from distal to proximal, inflating the upper arm tourniquet to a pressure of a least 300 mmHg, and then injecting a low concentration and high volume of local anesthetic (e.g. 0.5% lidocaine at 3 mg/kg) over at least 90 seconds, into a vein on the distal dorsum of the hand.

Patient safety depends on the integrity of the pneumatic tourniquet, which must be inflated and maintained for a safe interval (> 30 minutes), regardless of the duration of the surgery (usually one hour or less). Use of a double tourniquet is ideal. Care must be taken in deflating the tourniquet to minimize the CNS toxicity from a bolus release of local anesthetic into the venous system. For short surgeries, the tourniquet should be deflated for one to two seconds and then re-inflated, checking for CNS signs between each deflation-inflation sequence, only if done less than 30-40 minutes due to lack of time for diffusion to occur out of vasculature. Drug choice is usually 0.5 % lidocaine, avoiding the more cardiotoxic agents ie: bupivacaine. Lidocaine 0.5% should be prepared from a 1% solution by dilution with normal saline, avoiding dextrose-containing solutions which increase the incidence of thrombophlebitis. Midazolam IV should be used as a sedative given its anxiolytic and anticonvulsant properties that raise the seizure threshold.

O   **What is the best tourniquet deflation technique after intravenous regional anesthesia to minimize the peak blood level of local anesthetics?**

Cyclic deflation-reinflation techniques have been shown to be superior to single deflation in minimizing local anesthetic toxicity. Although cyclic techniques do not reduce the peak plasma concentration of local anesthetics, they significantly prolong the time to reach peak concentration. If cuff is released after 10 min, about 30% of the dose is released immediately in the first flush. After 45 min, drug release is much slower; 30% of the total dose release takes almost 4 min. Drugs released must first pass through lungs, protecting the CNS and heart (extravascular pH of lung < plasma causing ion trapping)

O   **What is the purpose of preoperative screening in the ambulatory pediatric patient?**

To ensure that the child has no active respiratory tract infection or other preexisting condition that requires additional investigation or treatment.

O   **T/F: Every child with a runny nose should be canceled for surgery.**

False. The child who has a fever, rhonchi that do not clear with coughing, wheeze, abnormal chest x-ray, elevated white count, purulent productive cough and/or nasal secretions, decreased level of activity or "off their feeds" should be rescheduled. Most nurse anesthetists would proceed with surgery with a child if the upper respiratory tract infection is uncomplicated and resolving, unless the child has a history of asthma or other significant pulmonary disease. Chronic nasal discharge is usually noninfectious in origin and caused by allergy or vasomotor rhinitis.

O   **What are the effects of viral URI's on lung function?**

The risk of pulmonary complications is 9 to 11 times greater up to 2 weeks after an upper respiratory tract infection, especially if the patient is intubated. Studies in adults evaluating PFTs before and following a RTI have shown changes in small airway hyper-reactivity that persists up to 7 weeks and general respiratory muscle weakness up to 12 days. Similar PFT changes have been demonstrated in children ages 6 and older with a URI. Underlying abnormalities include: increased airway reactivity with wheeze (decreased PEFR and MMEF), decreased diffusion capacity for oxygen, decreased compliance and resistance, decreased closing volumes (decreased FEV_1 and FVC), increased shunting and increased incidence of hypoxemia.

O   **What are some systemic symptoms that are considered contraindications to elective surgery by most anesthesia providers?**

Fever, purulent rhinorrhea, wheeze, and productive cough.

○   **Define prematurity.**

Gestational age less than 37 weeks or weight less than 2,500 g at birth.

○   **Define gestational age.**

Number of weeks from conception to the time of birth.

○   **Define postnatal age.**

The age from birth to the present.

○   **Define postconceptual age.**

The sum of gestational age and postnatal age (weeks).

○   **In general, what type of problems are common in premature babies?**

Neurological: intraventricular hemorrhage, hydrocephalus, retinopathy of prematurity, seizures, delayed development, impaired temperature regulation.
Respiratory: apnea and bradycardia, bronchopulmonary dysplasia, respiratory distress syndrome, bullae, pneumonia, reactive pulmonary vasculature, subglottic stenosis, tracheomalacia.
Cardiac: patent ductus arteriosus, cardiomyopathy.
Endocrine: hypoglycemia, metabolic acidosis, and malnutrition.
Gastrointestinal: necrotizing enterocolitis, GE reflux, and poor gag reflex.
Genitourinary: chronic renal failure, renal tubular acidosis.

○   **Until what age should infants be admitted and monitored for postoperative apnea?**

Former premature infants should be admitted for observation unless they are over approximately 54 weeks postconceptual age without anemia, ongoing apnea, or other significant medical problems; the anesthetic and recovery room period need to have proceeded uneventfully to allow consideration of discharge.

○   **What lab test in a patient with congenital heart disease is indicative of chronic hypoxemia?**

Hemoglobin or hematocrit level.

○   **What are four questions that must be answered in a patient with congenital heart disease before proceeding with surgery?**

Functional status, anatomy of lesion including whether there right or left ventricular outflow obstruction, direction of blood flow (left-to-right with pulmonary hypertension or right-to-left shunt with cyanosis, and associated anomalies.

○   **What are some advantages of regional anesthesia?**

Outcome differences relate primarily to the epidural technique most studied - decreased graft thrombosis in peripheral revascularization, decreased bleeding and DVTs in hip surgery, better post-operative pain control if the technique is continued into the postoperative period following major abdominal/thoracic/orthopedic surgery, possible reduction in phantom limb pain if used prior to amputations, improved pulmonary function following thoracic surgery with thoracic epidural pain relief. It bypasses many of the potential sources of minor or major morbidity associated with general anesthesia. For example, trauma to the lips, teeth, pharynx, vocal cords; bronchospasm; aspiration; prolonged somnolence; prolonged paralysis; and potential allergy and adverse responses to other anesthetic agents. Also protracted nausea and vomiting are less common.

O   **What are the advantages of using intravenous regional anesthesia (Bier's block)?**

Advantages include that it is easily performed, reliable, safe, high degree of patient satisfaction and it rapidly resolves with tourniquet release.

O   **What peripheral nerve of the brachial plexus can be potentially spared after performing an interscalene block?**

Ulnar.

C_8 to T_2 roots are often missed: ulnar, medial brachial and antebrachial cutaneous nerves, certain radial and thoracodorsal nerves and the medial aspect of the upper and lower arm, hand and fingers.

O   **What peripheral nerve of the brachial plexus is most commonly spared after performing an axillary block?**

Musculocutaneous.

O   **What is the origin of the brachial plexus?**

It arises from the anterior primary divisions of the fifth cervical through first thoracic nerves.

O   **The interscalene block is performed at what level of the brachial plexus?**

Roots.

O   **After performing an axillary block why might the medial aspect of the upper arm occasionally be spared?**

The medial aspect of the upper arm may not be anesthetized by a brachial plexus block as it is innervated by the intercostobrachial and medial brachial cutaneous nerves ($T_{1,2}$) which are not part of the brachial plexus. This requires injection a subcutaneous ring of local anesthetic solution in the upper arm along the axillary fold.

O   **How do you test motor block of the median nerve?**

Opposition of the thumb (opponens pollicis).

O   **How would you test motor block of the musculocutaneous nerve?**

Flexion of the elbow (biceps, brachialis and coracobrachialis) and supination of the forearm.

O   **The sciatic nerve divides distally at the popliteal fossa, into what two nerves?**

Tibial and common peroneal (common fibular) nerves.

O   **The common peroneal nerve encircles the head of the fibula laterally and divides into what two nerves?**

Deep and superficial peroneal nerves.

O   **The sural nerve arise from branches of what two nerves?**

Tibial (medial sural cutaneous nerve) and common peroneal (communicating branch of the common peroneal nerve) nerves.

○   **List at least 3 advantages of spinal anesthesia over lumbar epidural anesthesia in the outpatient setting.**

It is technically easier and more rapidly performed, faster onset time, has a higher success rate, is less likely to be associated with intravascular injection and toxicity, and it is more reliable in achieving complete sensory block, especially sacral segments.

○   **The spinal cord typically ends at what level?**

At the level of the L_1 or L_2 vertebra in 90% of people.

○   **What are the landmarks to performing a midline lumbar spinal block?**

The iliac crest, L_4 and L_5 spinal processes (and/or L_3 spinous process).

○   **What would be the indication of a subarachnoid or subdural injection while test dosing an epidural with local anesthetic?**

The rapid onset of significant sensory block within 2 minutes of subarachnoid injection.

○   **List at least 4 complications associated with spinal anesthesia.**

Hypotension, bradycardia, unexpected cardiac arrest, postdural puncture headache, high spinal (hypotension and hypoventilation), nausea and vomiting, urinary retention, backache (incidence 25%), and neurologic sequelae.

○   **At what level does the subarachnoid space terminate in children?**

The dural and arachnoid sacs usually terminate at the level of the 2nd sacral vertebrae in adults, but may extend to the 3rd or 4th sacral levels in infants.

○   **The retrobulbar block ablates sensation of the eye by blocking what nerve?**

The nasociliary nerve (via the short ciliary nerves), a branch of the ophthalmic nerve.

○   **The retrobulbar block prevents movement of the globe by blocking what nerves?**

Cranial nerves II, III and VI (cranial nerve IV lies outside the muscle cone).

○   **What is the purpose of blocking the facial nerve in conjunction with a retrobulbar block?**

To prevent movement of the orbicularis oculi muscle.

○   **What are the potential clinical manifestations of retrobulbar hemorrhage?**

Retrobulbar hemorrhage usually manifests as motor block of the globe with proptosis, closing of the upper lid and increased intraocular pressure. Subconjunctival hemorrhage and eyelid ecchymosis develop as the hemorrhage extends anteriorly.

○   **What are some advantages of continuous spinal over single-dose spinal and continuous epidural anesthesia?**

Advantages include the following: 1) facilitation of the surgical schedule if the catheter is placed in the preinduction area, 2) the potential for positional hypotension is minimized since the patient may be fully anesthetized after being positioned, 3) the possibility of systemic toxic reactions are virtually eliminated due to the ability to titrate small amounts of local anesthetics, 4) titratability increases the likelihood of obtaining exactly the right level of anesthesia and decreases the likelihood of cardiovascular instability during induction, 5) employing a short-acting local anesthetic shortens the recovery period, 6) the duration of anesthesia can be prolonged indefinitely, 7) A definite end point (aspiration of CSF) assures the catheter is in the correct place therefore enhances the likelihood of successful anesthesia, 8) subarachnoid narcotics may be administered during a surgical procedure or continued into the recovery period to provide long-lasting postoperative analgesia.

O   **What are some disadvantages of continuous spinal anesthesia?**

Cauda equina syndrome associated with small-bore continuous spinal anesthesia and the use of hyperbaric lidocaine, especially 5%.

Other disadvantages include: 1) additional time required for placement of the catheter, 2) postdural puncture headache, 3) possible catheter breakage, and 4) a potential for infection, neurologic changes, and hemorrhage.

O   **What are the goals of regional anesthesia for cataract extraction with intraocular lens implantation?**

Goals include: globe and conjunctival analgesia; globe, lid and periorbital muscle akinesia; and orbit and globe hypotension.

O   **What is context-sensitive half time?**

The time for the plasma concentration to decrease by 50% from an infusion that maintains a constant concentration, with the context being the duration of the infusion.

O   **What happens to the dose requirement of propofol when an opioid is used in conjunction with it?**

The concomitant use of an opioid reduces propofol requirements significantly.

O   **Which radiological procedure has more scatter radiation, fluoroscopy or CT?**

Fluoroscopy.

O   **What safety precautions can nurse anesthetists take to prevent excessive radiation exposure?**

Lead aprons, thyroid collars, and lead glass screens or treated glasses and goggles.

O   **What distance away from a radiation source is a bystander considered safe?**

6 feet of distance, equivalent to 2.5 mm of lead.

O   **What signs and symptoms might you see after contrast media administration?**

These hyperosmolar solutions may cause flushing, tachycardia, and nausea by releasing vasoactive substances.

During cerebral angiography---Neurotoxic reactions: dizziness, convulsions, coma, hemiplegia, blindness and aphasia. Allergic reactions: pruritus, burning on injection, mild skin rashes, wheezing, dyspnea, syncope and cardiovascular collapse.

During coronary angiography---myocardial depression, coronary vasodilation, decrease in blood pH, increase serum osmolarity and allergic reactions (limit to 5 mL/kg).

Contrast agents may also cause osmotic diuresis, volume contraction, high urine osmolality, and nephropathy.

○ **How safe are patients with spinal fusion rods and limb prostheses in the MRI scanner?**

The concern would be attraction of ferromagnetic objects to the magnet.

Generally these types of implants are not a problem, although temperature increases may be noted around metallic implants. Detailed lists of each manufacturer's implantable devices and their ferromagnetic properties have been published and should be consulted.

○ **What effect do magnetic fields have on pacemakers?**

The effects are variable. Potential problems include possible reed switch closure or damage, pacemaker inhibition or reversion to an asynchronous mode. Programming changes, torque on the pacemaker itself or development of voltage across the pacemaker inhibiting its discharge may also occur. MRI may deactivate implanted automatic cardiac defibrillators.

○ **Where should the pulse oximetry probe be placed in a patient having an MRI scan?**

The extremity as far as possible from the scanner (usually the foot) with the cable in a straight line and wrapped with aluminum to minimize RF artifact in the MRI image. Metal parts of the sensor have been known to cause patient burns, especially if the cable is wrapped around an extremity, increasing the strength of the magnetic field. All leads must be properly insulated, not permitted to loop within the magnetic core and separated from the patient's skin by thermal insulating padding. Pulse oximetry manufacturers have incorporated RF filters, ECG-locking facilities and fiberoptic signal linking between the sensor and monitor.

○ **What are some advantages to the use of total intravenous anesthesia in remote locations?**

The difficulty of transporting an anesthesia machine to multiple locations is eliminated since there is no need to scavenge anesthetic gases, and a rapid emergence for prompt recovery and discharge can be anticipated.

○ **What are major anesthetic challenges for ultrasound-assisted lipoplasty?**

Estimating blood loss, fluid and electrolyte imbalances, pulmonary edema, pulmonary embolism and determining the appropriate time for discharge home or to a 23-hour observation unit. With tumescent and super-wet techniques 30 to 35 mg/kg of tissue can be safely removed.

○ **How might spinal or epidural anesthesia be a disadvantage in patients having liposuction (ultrasound-assisted lipoplasty)?**

When the anticipated volume of aspirate exceeds 1 liter, an estimation of the patient's volume status is essential and inadequate volume status may be complicated by the sympathetic blockade. However, with adequate fluid loading, epidural anesthesia may be the anesthesia of choice for patients undergoing UAL as the incidence of nausea and vomiting is reduced and discharge is facilitated by a return of motor and sensory functions within 30 to 45 minutes of completion of the surgery if 1.5% lidocaine and 3% chloroprocaine are the local anesthetics used.

○ **What are the requirements in order to have an airway fire?**

Ignition source, oxidizing agents, and combustible material.

○ **What can be done to minimize the risk of pharyngeal fires?**

The goal is to limit laser beam contact with flammable materials and high concentrations of gases that support combustion.

Strategies include: (1) Reduce the flammability of the airway by decreasing the oxygen concentration (oxygen-helium mixture) and covering tissues with moist occlusive pharyngeal packs and (2) remove flammable materials from the airway by using metallic Venturi jet ventilation cannulas or by ventilating with intermittent extubation. Others advocate using a PVC endotracheal tube wrapped with metallic tape.

❍   **What risk do lasers pose to patients and healthcare providers?**

Damage to eyes and skin from reflection of laser light by surgical instruments, electrical shock, fire and explosion, and contamination of the atmosphere (smoke and diseased particulate matter).

❍   **What effect can CO_2 laser have on the eyes?**

The nature of the ocular damage depends on the wavelength of the laser light. Exposure to a 10,600 nm wavelength produced by the CO_2 laser can cause corneal opacification because energy is largely absorbed on the surface of the eye. Nd:YAG lasers cause damage to the retina.

❍   **Give several examples of stimuli capable of provoking laryngospasm.**

Presence of bloody secretions or vomitus in the airway: visceral pain; chemical irritation of laryngeal or pharyngeal mucosa; and tracheal intubation or extubation during inappropriate depth of anesthesia.

❍   **What drug might you give prior to the extubation to decrease the chance of laryngospasm?**

Lidocaine IV or injected down the endotracheal tube.

❍   **What is the initial treatment of laryngospasm?**

Remove the stimulus if possible, provide jaw-thrust and positive pressure by mask with 100% oxygen.

❍   **What is the mechanism of postobstructive pulmonary edema or negative pressure pulmonary edema?**

Extremely negative pulmonary interstitial fluid pressure pulmonary edema is multifactorial.

Probably, forced inspiration against a closed glottis causes large negative intrapleural and transpulmonary pressure gradients promoting transudation of edema fluid from the pulmonary capillaries into the interstitium.

Causes include vigorous spontaneous ventilation against an obstructed airway (upper airway mass; laryngospasm; infection, inflammation, edema, vocal cord paralysis, strangulation), rapid re-expansion of lung or vigorous pleural suctioning (thoracentesis, chest tube).

❍   **If proper treatment is instituted what is the usual course of postobstructive pulmonary edema?**

The pulmonary edema typically resolves within 24 hours, if not sooner.

❍   **Clinically how would vocal cord edema present differently than croup?**

Vocal cord edema is characterized by inspiratory stridor, whereas croup is characterized by expiratory or biphasic stridor.

❍   **What are some factors implicated in producing post extubation croup?**

Tight-fitting endotracheal tube, traumatic or repeated intubations, coughing while intubated, passive head repositioning, a previous history of post extubation croup, prolonged intubation and high pressure-low volume cuffs, patient age 1-4, non-humidified gases.

○   **What is the treatment for edema induced by partial glottic or subglottic airway obstruction?**

Therapy consists of humidified oxygen, adequate hydration, and if necessary corticosteroids alone or in combination with nebulized racemic epinephrine.

○   **What is usually the etiology for serious reactions to local anesthetics?**

Inadvertent intravascular injections of large volumes causing CNS and rarely cardiac toxicity.

○   **What topical anesthetics have been known to induce methemoglobinemia?**

Prilocaine (500 to 600 mg), benzocaine, lidocaine and procaine.

○   **At what methemoglobin levels are patients usually symptomatic?**

Although cyanosis may appear with methemoglobin levels as low as 15%, acquired methemoglobinemia is only rarely symptomatic when levels are below 20%.

○   **What is the treatment for methemoglobinemia?**

Treatment consists of administration of IV methylene blue, 2 mg/kg (1 to 5 mg/kg) over 5 minutes, or less successfully with ascorbic acid, 2 mg/kg.

○   **What maximal doses of cocaine is recommended for nasal procedures?**

Cocaine's maximum dose is 3 mg/kg.

○   **In what patients and with what medications should the use of cocaine for topicalization be avoided?**

In hypertensives and patients taking adrenergic modifying drugs such as guanethidine, reserpine, tricyclic antidepressants, and monoamine oxidase inhibitors. A combination of these drugs may produce a hypersympathetic response. Ketamine, because of its sympathomimetic effects may also exaggerate hypertension.

○   **Which inhalational agent is the worst offender in terms of sensitizing the myocardium to catecholamines?**

Halothane.

○   **Why should cocaine-induced cardiovascular instability be treated with labetalol and not propranolol.**

Labetalol offers the distinct advantage of both an alpha and beta-adrenergic receptor blockade, whereas a lethal hypertensive exacerbation has been attributed to the unopposed alpha stimulation following propranolol.

○   **List common problems associated with middle ear surgery.**

Nitrous oxide-induced changes in middle ear pressure, bleeding, facial nerve injury, cervical spine injury secondary to improper head positioning, nausea, vomiting, and vertigo.

❍   **What type of sedation should children with sleep apnea be given preoperatively?**

None. No sedative premedication should be given to children with a history of sleep apnea, intermittent airway obstruction, or those with extremely hypertrophied tonsils.

❍   **What are some signs of ongoing bleeding after T&A in the PACU?**

Frequent swallowing, tachycardia and hypotension (or occasionally hypertension). Aspiration of large amounts of blood can produce intrapulmonary shunting and hypoxemia. The child may be hypovolemic, anemic, agitated and or in shock.

❍   **If hemorrhage is going to occur after tonsillectomy, when is it most common?**

Most post-tonsillectomy bleeding occurs within the first 6 hours after surgery.

❍   **Name the 4 types of lasers available for clinical use.**

Carbon dioxide, argon, krypton, Nd:YAG, and Nd:YAG-KTP (neodymium:yttrium-aluminum-garnet: potassium-titanyl-phosphate).

❍   **What is the disadvantage of using PVC, red rubber, or silicone endotracheal tubes during laser surgery?**

Each of these tubes can be ignited by the carbon dioxide laser in an environment of 100% oxygen. PVC tubes are the least flammable.

❍   **What is the appropriate management of an airway fire?**

Immediately stop ventilation, disconnect the oxygen source, remove the endotracheal tube, flood the surgical field with saline, ventilate the patient by mask with 100% oxygen, reintubate, examine the extent of damage and remove debris by laryngoscopy /bronchoscopy, ventilate with humidified oxygen and continue monitoring in critical care setting for 24 hours, use short-term steroids, continue ventilatory support and antibiotics as needed.

❍   **Why are medications such as pilocarpine beneficial in patients with glaucoma?**

Pilocarpine cause miosis which enlarges the radius of the spaces of fontana thereby facilitating aqueous humor outflow.

❍   **How does vomiting, straining and coughing increase IOP?**

All three maneuvers increase systemic venous pressure which reduces outflow of aqueous humor, which can increase IOP 40 mm Hg or more.

❍   **What effect do CNS depressant drugs have on IOP?**

Virtually all CNS depressants, including barbiturates, neuroleptics, narcotics, tranquilizers, and hypnotics lower IOP in both normal and glaucomatous eyes.

❍   **What effect does respiratory acidosis have on IOP?**

Respiratory acidosis increases both choroidal blood volume and IOP, presumably by retinal vasodilatation occurring in conjunction with cerebral vasodilation.

❍   **What effect does hypothermia have on IOP?**

Hypothermia lowers IOP by reducing aqueous humor production and vasoconstriction.

O   Why should N_2O be avoided when sulfur hexafluoride is injected into the eye during repair of a retinal tear?

Because N_2O use can diffuse into and cause the injected intravitreal bubble to expand in size triggering a rapid and substantial increase in IOP (14 to 30 mm Hg). This may compromise retinal blood flow, causing retinal ischemia. Nitrous oxide is 117 times more soluble than sulfur hexafluoride.

O   What are potential anesthetic problems in patients taking echothiophate iodide eye drops preoperatively?

Pseudocholinesterase inhibitor and cholinergic agonist.

The prolonged action of succinylcholine and ester-linked local anesthetics owing to long-acting anticholinesterase activity, and also anticholinergic side effects such as vomiting, hypotension, and abdominal pain.

O   Describe the oculocardiac reflex arc.

Trigeminal-vagal reflex, described by Aschner and Dagnini 1908.

This reflex arc consists of a trigeminal afferent (ciliary branch of the ophthalmic division) and vagal efferent limb. It can be elicited by direct pressure on the globe and traction on all extraocular muscles (the medial rectus was initially observed to be the most potent, now questionable) as well as ocular manipulation and ocular pain. The reflex may also be triggered by a retrobulbar block, by ocular trauma, and by direct pressure on tissue remaining in the orbital apex. Sinus bradycardia is the most common manifestation, followed by a potpourri of arrhythmias.

O   What are potential maneuvers to obtund or abolish the oculocardiac reflex?

Inclusion of IM anticholinergic drug (atropine or glycopyrrolate) in the premedication regimen for oculocardiac prophylaxis is ineffective. (Near complete vagal block in the adult require 2-3 mg of atropine or 0.03-0.05 mg/kg and peak action occurs 30 minutes after administration). During pediatric strabismus surgery, current popular practice favors administration of atropine 0.02 mg/kg IV before commencing surgery.Ask the surgeon to stop ocular manipulation immediately and deepen the level of anesthesia (pain stimulus). The OCR tends to fatigue, but if the arrhythmia is malignant, the patient unstable or the reflex persists, IV atropine should be given. Atropine may cause more serious and refractory arrhythmias than the reflex itself. Local infiltration of the recti muscle may successfully block the reflex.

O   List at least 5 potential problems with retrobulbar block.

Retrobulbar hemorrhage, central retinal artery occlusion, stimulation of oculocardiac reflex, retinal detachment, puncture of the posterior globe, and intraocular injection (especially in high myopia patient), seizures secondary to intra-arterial injection, brain stem anesthesia, optic nerve penetration causing optic atrophy and permanent loss of vision, intense pain with facial nerve block, laryngospasm, dysphagia, and respiratory distress secondary to Nadbath-Rehman facial nerve block.

O   List the relative contraindications to ocular regional anesthesia.

Penetrating eye injury
Inability to lie flat
Severe tremors, chronic coughing or convulsive disorder
Claustrophobia and excessive anxiety
Inability to communicate (disoriented, mental impairment, language barrier, deafness)

Coagulation or bleeding abnormality
Patient refusal (absolute contraindication).
Age less than 15 years

○   **What are some intraoperative and postoperative problems associated with strabismus surgery?**

Oculocardiac reflex-induced dysrhythmias, postoperative nausea and vomiting, masseter spasm and malignant hyperthermia (MH-susceptible persons often have localized areas of skeletal muscle weakness or other musculoskeletal abnormalities).

○   **What are contraindications to ECT from the standpoint of the nurse anesthetist?**

Pheochromocytoma, and increased intracranial pressure must be treated prior to ECT. Unless a patient is deemed extremely suicidal, recent MI or CVA within the last 3 months are patients who are almost always postponed.

○   **What are the physiologic effects of ECT on the cardiovascular system?**

The immediate response is parasympathetic discharge potentially resulting in bradycardia, asystole, hypotension and PVCs. Sympathetic discharge then follows immediately with tachycardia, severe hypertension, dysrhythmias and increased myocardial oxygen consumption.

○   **What are the physiologic effects of ECT on the cerebrovascular system?**

Electrically induced seizures (brief tonic then clonic phase for 30 to 50 seconds) transiently result in increased cerebral oxygen consumption. Initial constriction of cerebral blood vessels is followed by an increase in cerebral blood flow, and an increase in intracranial pressure.

○   **Why should lithium be discontinued, if possible, before ECT?**

Lithium may limit the therapeutic effect of the ECT. Patients receiving lithium may show delayed awakening, memory loss, postictal confusion, acute organic brain syndrome, delirium, and other atypical neurologic findings.

○   **What effect does ECT have on the parturient?**

Anesthetic considerations include aortocaval compression, fetal hypoxia, pulmonary aspiration and specific drugs for anesthesia.

ECT may be used safely in all three trimesters. Although it appears that ECT has minimal effect on fetal heart rate, non-invasive monitoring of fetal heart rate and uterine contractions is recommended after 20 weeks gestation. Anticholinergic medications should be discontinued. The patient should be wedged to the left to avoid aortocaval compression and anticipating the increase in intragastric pressure, and lowered pH of the gastric contents, aspiration prophylaxis and tracheal intubation after the 1st trimester are mandatory. Severe respiratory alkalosis must be avoided. The patient should be observed for contractions and bleeding post-ECT.

○   **What is the muscle relaxant of choice for ECT?**

Succinylcholine.

○   **List the potential complications of laparoscopy.**

Nausea, vomiting, shoulder tip pain, hypoventilation, hypotension, subcutaneous emphysema, pneumothorax, pneumopericardium, pneumomediastinum, hemorrhage, perforated viscera, electrical burns, and neuropathy. Hypercarbia will produce hypertension and tachycardia.

O   **What is the most common complication of pelvic laparoscopy?**

Nausea and vomiting which may occur in up to 50% of patients following a general anesthetic for the procedure.

O   **How does CO_2 insufflation affect total peripheral resistance during laparoscopy?**

Total peripheral resistance is increased because of compression of the abdominal aorta directly, and an indirect sympathomimetic effect of hypercarbia increases tone of arterioles, and venous resistance.

O   **What are the potential complications of an interscalene block in a patient having outpatient shoulder surgery?**

Pneumothorax, intravascular injection into the vertebral artery (immediate CNS signs: seizures), Horner's syndrome, subarachnoid and epidural injection, 100% incidence of paralysis of the ipsilateral diaphragm (phrenic nerve blockade), and neuropathy from intraneural injection or direct needle trauma.

O   **What type of procedures would a bier block be appropriate for?**

Procedures distal to the elbow requiring an arm tourniquet time of less than 60 minutes, and surgical time not exceeding 90 minutes.

O   **What is the nerve supply of the knee joint?**

The articular nerves are branches of the obturator, femoral, tibial and common fibular (peroneal) nerves (L $_{3,4,5}$ S $_{1,2}$).

O   **How might the lung be injured during extracorporeal shock wave lithotripsy?**

The classic injury is alveolar rupture with pulmonary contusion leading to massive hemoptysis and hypoxemia. The extent of tissue injury depends on the tissue exposed and the shock wave energy at the tissue level. The lung is especially susceptible as air trapped in the alveoli creates the classic water-air interface to the shock wave.

O   **Why are kids more susceptible to shock wave induced pulmonary contusions than adults during lithotripsy?**

Children are more likely to suffer lung injury from shock waves because the lung bases are close to the upper pole of the kidney compared to the adult.

O   **How might lung injury be avoided during lithotripsy?**

By using Styrofoam boards in the back, or foam taped at the lower chest walls to shield the lungs bases from the shock waves.

O   **What are the contraindications to lithotripsy?**

Pregnancy, untreated bleeding disorders, and abdominal permanent pacemakers and AICDs.

O   **What techniques can be utilized to reduce perioperative MI in the geriatric patient?**

Preoperative beta blockade that is continued into the intraoperative and postoperative period has been shown to decrease perioperative MI in some settings. Thorough evaluation of cardiac function looking for evidence of ischemic heart disease. Continue all cardiac medications throughout the perioperative period and consider adding anti-anginal medications to preoperative medications (β-blockers and nitrates). The goal of anesthesia is to maintain the balance between myocardial O_2 supply and demand throughout the perioperative period. The most sensitive ECG lead for detecting ischemia is V_5. Transesophageal echocardiography will detect regional wall motion abnormalities and is the most sensitive monitor for myocardial ischemia, but difficult to interpret on line. The risk of perioperative MI following noncardiac surgery depends on clinical predictors (IHD: prior MI or angina, and congestive heart failure), advanced age, type of surgical procedure (major abdominal, thoracic and emergency cases) and general medical status. Hypertension alone does not place a patient at increased risk for perioperative MI.

O   **What happens to MAC (minimal alveolar concentration) in the geriatric population?**

The MAC for volatile anesthetics decreases 4 to 5% per decade after the age of 40 years.

O   **List at least 5 secondary causes of hypertension.**

Preexisting causes (excluding essential hypertension)

Renal disease: renal parenchymal diseases, renal artery stenosis, polycystic kidney disease, chronic
        pyelonephritis
Endocrine disorders: adrenocortical dysfunction, pheochromocytoma, myxedema, acromegaly, thyrotoxicosis
Coarctation of the aorta
Neurogenic: autonomic hyperreflexia, familial dysautonomia, polyneuritis, increased intracranial pressure
Obesity
Tumors (Carcinoid, Wilms' tumor, hyperthyroidism)
Preeclampsia
Drugs: cyclosporine A or FK506, amphetamines, oral contraceptives, estrogens, steroids

Perioperative-specific

Hypoxia
Hypercarbia (MH, CO_2 insufflation for laparoscopy)
Pain
Anxiety
Light anesthesia
Increased intravascular volume
shivering
Intravenous indigo carmine dye
Drugs: anesthetic agents (ketamine, cocaine), vasopressors (epinephrine, ephedrine, phenylephrine),
        withdrawal or rebound hypertension(antihypertensive medication, alcohol, narcotics)
Surgery-specific: aortic cross-clamping, tourniquet pain, drug-induced hypertension, post-carotid
        endarterectomy, trigeminal nerve stimulation
Bladder distension, hypothermia, hypoglycemia

O   **How does EKG evidence of LVH and strain affect perioperative outcome?**

Patients with EKG evidence of LVH and strain have been shown to have an eight fold increase in cardiovascular deaths.

O   **What diagnostic test is more sensitive in diagnosing LVH, EKG or echocardiography?**

Echocardiography.

O   **When in the perioperative period is myocardial ischemia most likely to occur?**

The morning of surgery when called is a time often associated with ischemia. The patient is at their greatest risk after that during the postoperative period for ischemic events, with MI's most likely to occur 2-3 days postoperatively.

Diurnal patterns in ischemia have been postulated to be the reason morning surgery patients demonstrate ischemia. Myocardial ischemia and infarction are precipitated in patients at risk for ischemic heart disease with increases in myocardial O_2 demand (tachycardia, hypertension) and decreases in O_2 supply (hypotension, hypoxemia and anemia)The intraoperative setting is a very controlled environment allowing monitoring, detection and treatment of ischemia, as well as control of the hemodynamic variables listed above.

○ **What is the ideal intraoperative blood pressure for the hypertensive patient?**

The blood pressure and heart rate should be maintained near baseline values if the patient is medically well controlled (fluctuation in a range of 20%, with a target systolic blood pressure of 150 mm Hg).

○ **What are some common causes of postoperative hypertension?**

Hypertension is due to an increase in preload, contractility, afterload, or rate. With the exception of pre-existing essential hypertension, these effects are mediated via sympathetic stimulation from a variety of causes.

Preexisting hypertensive disease: >90% have essential hypertension
Surgical procedure: CEA, CABG, aortic cross-clamping
Anesthesia-induced: hypervolemia, pain, hypoxia, hypercarbia, malignant hypertension, shivering, artifacts
Drugs: rebound hypertension from drug withdrawal, pressors
Common PACU problems: bladder distension, hypothermia, pain, hypoglycemia

○ **What is the most common type of neuropathy that develops in diabetes mellitus?**

Symmetrical peripheral polyneuropathies
Sensory changes of the lower extremities (numbness, tingling, burning)
Carpal tunnel syndrome
Segmental demyelination of nerves (cranial, median, ulnar)
Autonomic neuropathy is also common and is associated with a 50% mortality rate over a 5-year period.

○ **What are some clinical manifestations of diabetic autonomic neuropathy?**

Orthostatic hypotension, cardiac arrhythmias, loss of heart rate response to Valsalva maneuver or respirations (loss of beat-to-beat variability in heart rate), resting tachycardia, gastroparesis, bladder dysfunction, impotence, hypoglycemia, painless myocardial ischemia, unexpected cardiac arrest and impaired pupillary reflexes.

○ **What are the clinical signs and symptoms of hyperthyroidism?**

Goiter, tachycardia, anxiety, and tremor are seen in over 90% of patients. Heat intolerance, fatigue, weight loss, ocular signs (proptosis), skeletal muscle weakness, and atrial fibrillation are reported as well.

○ **How does thyroid storm manifest?**

Thyroid storm is an acute exacerbation of hyperthyroidism usually caused by a stress such as surgery or infection. Hyperthermia, extreme tachycardia, and altered mental state with severe agitation. Typically, it occurs 6 to 18 hours postoperatively.

○ **What is the best anesthetic technique for a high risk cardiac ambulatory patient undergoing non-cardiac surgery? General or Regional?**

There is no accepted randomized prospective data comparing the two types of anesthesia in the high risk cardiac patient undergoing non-cardiac surgery that has ever shown an outcome difference.

○   **How would you attenuate the hemodynamic response to intubation in a high risk cardiac ambulatory patients?**

Attenuation of this pressor response may be achieved by avoiding prolonged laryngoscopy and blunting the stimulation of airway instrumentation with ultra-short acting opiates, beta-blockers and IV or endotracheal lidocaine. 0.5mg/kg of esmolol is an excellent choice.

○   **What important actions of nitroglycerin are beneficial in treating myocardial ischemia or elevated pulmonary artery pressures?**

For ischemia; coronary vasodilation (redistributes blood flow from epicardial to subendocardial vessels and relieves abnormal coronary artery vasoconstriction) and venodilation, thereby reducing preload and subendocardial wall tension. The latter is thought most important. For increased PA pressures; decreased RV preload, and pulmonary venous dilation.

○   **What are the hallmark signs for detecting aortic stenosis in the preoperative period?**

These signs include a systolic murmur radiating to the carotids, atrial fibrillation or left ventricular hypertrophy on EKG, and calcifications (of a congenital bicuspid valve) noted on chest x-ray. The arterial pressure wave is altered with a narrowed pulse pressure (< 50 mm Hg), delayed or slow rise of the systolic pressure and a prominent anacrotic notch. Clinical presentation is often late in the course of the disease with angina, dyspnea (congestive heart failure), syncope or sudden death.

○   **Define critical aortic stenosis.**

Critical aortic stenosis occurs when the valvular cross sectional area is less than one-fifth of normal (aortic valve index < 0.5 cm^2/m^2) .

○   **What is the adverse effect of tachycardia in a patient with mitral stenosis?**

Tachycardia decreases left ventricular diastolic filling leading to increased left atrial pressure, with an increased risk of developing pulmonary edema.

○   **What are the anesthetic goals of patients with mitral regurgitation?**

Anesthetic management should aim to decrease the regurgitant fraction by promoting forward flow and decreasing stretch of the mitral valve annulus:

Maintain or increase heart rate (avoid bradycardia)
Maintain contractility – dobutamine is the choice if an inotrope required
Control atrial fibrillation – a common associated problem
Decrease SVR
Decrease pulmonary vascular resistance (avoid hypercapnia, hypoxia, nitrous oxide and pulmonary
    vasoconstrictors)
Maintain preload based on clinical response to fluid challenge but do not overfill the heart as this will stretch
    the annulus and increase regurgitation

○   **What is the most common form of valvular heart disease in ambulatory surgical patients?**

Mitral valve prolapse.

○   **When is bacterial endocarditis prophylaxis needed in patients with mitral valve prolapse?**

Prophylaxis is recommended for patients with a holosystolic murmur and/or echocardiographic evidence of regurgitation.

○ **What are some signs of Pickwickian syndrome?**

Obesity-hypoventilation syndrome.

Hypercarbia (alveolar hypoventilation), hypersomnolence and obesity. Hypoventilation causes hypoxemia, respiratory acidosis and polycythemia. Chronic hypoxemia leads to pulmonary hypertension, right ventricular hypertrophy and/or cor pulmonale. Obstructive sleep apnea may be seen.

○ **Why is the supine position potentially fatal in the morbidly obese patient?**

In the supine position, the functional residual capacity of obese patients is decreased even further, impinging on closing capacity and leading to atelectasis. Because ventilation to perfusion mismatch is exacerbated, this leads to respiratory compromise with hypoxemia and worsened pulmonary vasoconstriction and possible right-sided heart failure. There is an increased work of breathing, which in a patient at risk for cardiac disease can lead to right and left-sided heart failure, and the hypoxemia can precipitate myocardial ischemia.

○ **How can respiratory mechanics be improved postoperatively in obese patients?**

Aside from supplemental oxygen, it has been shown that positioning obese patients in a semi-recumbent position (30 degree head of bed elevation) postoperatively significantly increases the arterial oxygen tension above that seen in the supine position.

○ **What are the essential features of neuroleptic malignant syndrome?**

The essential features include:

History of psychotropic drug within the preceding 24 to 72 hours (haloperidol, fluphenazine, clozapine, perphenazine, thioridazine)
Hyperthermia, tachycardia, cyanosis
Autonomic lability
Extrapyramidal signs (akinesia and muscle rigidity)
Elevated levels of creatinine kinase
Mortality rate of 10%

○ **How do neuroleptic malignant syndrome (NMS) and malignant hyperthermia (MH) differ clinically?**

Unlike NMS, the onset of MH occurs within hours following exposure to the known triggers (volatile anesthetic agent and/or succinylcholine). NMS occurs within 24 to 72 hours of exposure to a psychotropic drug. MH also originates in skeletal muscle, whereas NMS involves dopamine receptor blockade in the hypothalamus and basal ganglia. Patients with NMS are not prone to MH. Treatment of NMS is with dantrolene or bromocriptine.

○ **What are the most common adverse effects of lithium?**

The most common adverse effects are gastric distress, weight gain, tremor, fatigue, and mild cognitive impairment. Other potential side effects include reversible T-wave EKG changes, mild leukocytosis and hypothyroidism or vasopressin-resistant diabetes insipidus-like syndrome. At toxic levels the patient may become confused, sedated, weak and develop tremor or slurred speech and then develop EKG changes include widening of the QRS complex and AV dissociation with hypotension and seizure activity.

○ **What are specific anesthetic ramifications of lithium?**

Lithium has been reported to potentiate depolarizing and non-depolarizing muscle relaxants as well as decrease MAC and prolong drowsiness following general anesthesia. Clinically these effects are minor.

O   **How might a hypertensive crisis be avoided in patients taking MAO inhibitors?**

A hypertensive crisis may be avoided by refraining from foods containing tyramine or medications that cause the presynaptic release of endogenous catecholamines (exaggerated responses to vasopressors and sympathetic stimulation). Direct-acting vasopressors are first line therapy. Sympathomimetic agents to avoid include: ketamine, pancuronium, ephedrine and epinephrine-containing solutions. Meperidine can cause hyperthemia, seizures and coma. Opioids should generally be avoided.

O   **What are the cardiovascular side effects of tricyclic antidepressants (TCAs)?**

Orthostatic hypotension is the most common cardiovascular side effect of TCAs. Quinidine-like cardiac effects include tachycardia, T-wave flattening or inversion and prolongation of the PR, QRS and QT intervals. Exaggerated responses to indirect-acting vasopressors and sympathetic stimulation should be anticipated. With chronic use and depletion of cardiac catecholamines, the patient may be at risk for the cardiodepressant action of anesthetic agents.

POSTOPERATIVE RECOVERY
AND OUTCOME

I Have Learned That Success Is To Be Measured Not So Much By The Position That One Has Reached In Life As By The Obstacles Which He Has Had To Overcome While Trying To Succeed.
Booker T. Washington

○   **What are the relative IM and p.o. potencies of the opioids?**

Drug	IM	oral
Morphine	10	30
Hydromorphone	1.5	7.5
Meperidine	75	300
Methadone	10	20
Codeine	130	200

○   **Order the hydrophilicity of opioids from most to least.**

Morphine>meperidine>methadone>alfentanil>fentanyl>sufentanil.

○   **What are the appropriate conversions from IV to epidural opioids?**

IV to epidural = 10:1.

○   **What are the appropriate conversions from IV to intrathecal opioids?**

IV to intrathecal = 100:1.

○   **What are the advantages of patient-controlled epidural analgesia?**

The ability to titrate analgesic doses in proportion to individual levels of pain intensity, lower total dose requirements compared to other systems, decreased sedation and increased patient satisfaction.

○   **What are the problems associated with the metabolites of morphine?**

Morphine is broken down to morphine-6-glucuronide and morphine-3-glucuronide. M3G is inactive, but M6G is 100 times more potent than morphine outside the CNS, and over prolonged dosing or in patients with renal impairment it may accumulate with the potential for causing respiratory depression.

○   **What are the problems associated with the metabolites of meperidine?**

Normeperidine is the first metabolite of meperidine with one-half the analgesic potency. It lowers the seizure threshold and induces CNS excitability. Normeperidine accumulation is dose-dependant and more common in patients with renal insufficiency. Seizures have been reported frequently in patients on PCA-meperidine due to the larger doses available compared to intramuscular injections.

○   **What are some of the common side effects of opiates and their treatments?**

Side effect	Treatment
Nausea	Phenothiazines, metoclopramide, scopolamine
Sedation	Naloxone, methamphetamine
Constipation	Laxatives, stool softeners
Urinary Retention	Reduction of dosage, catheterization
Pruritus	Diphenhydramine, low dose naloxone
Respiratory Depression	Naloxone

○   **What are the advantages and disadvantages of methadone administration?**

Advantages are a long drug half-life ($T_{1/2\beta} = 35$ hours), an elixir formulation, high bioavailability, and no active metabolites.
Disadvantages are accumulation and longer time to reach steady-state than other opioids. Urinary acidifiers may increase elimination and potentially precipitate an acute withdrawal syndrome.

○   **What are the differences between epidural fentanyl and morphine?**

Agent	Onset	Peak	Duration
Morphine	60 Min	30-60 Min	12-24 Hrs
Fentanyl	5-10 Min	20 Min	3-5 Hrs

○   **What is the incidence of side effects with intraspinal narcotics?**

	Spinal	Epidural
Respiratory Depression	5-7%	0.1-2%
Pruritus	60%	1-100%
Nausea	20-50%	20-30%
Urinary Retention	50%	15-25%

○   **Which epidurally administered opioid has the fewest side effects?**

Fentanyl.

○   **Why are IM injections of opioids a poor choice for postoperative analgesia?**

Variable blood levels often falling under the analgesic threshold, unpredictable absorption, delayed onset, lag to peak analgesic effect, pain and inadequate analgesia. PCA administration eliminates these problems.

○   **What are the major advantages of epidural opioid administration?**

Improved pain relief, steady pain relief, decreased postoperative morbidity, and shortened hospital stays. Improved pulmonary function has also been demonstrated.

○   **What are the signs of impending epidural opioid toxicity?**

Altered mental status, decreased level of consciousness, respiratory depression (pulse oximetry readings decrease, decreased respiratory rate, apnea and increased end tidal CO_2 levels) and miosis.

○   **What are the mechanisms of action of the nonsteroidal anti-inflammatory drugs (NSAIDs)?**

Inhibition of the cyclooxygenase and lipoxygenase pathways of prostaglandin synthesis, as well as possible CNS analgesic effects.

○   **Where are the proposed sites of action of the NSAIDs?**

They work peripherally to block the cyclooxygenase pathway and centrally to facilitate the descending neural pathways of pain modulation. There are also proposed cellular mechanisms involving release of inflammatory mediators. NSAIDs provide analgesic, anti-inflammatory and antipyretic effects.

○ **What are the major contraindications to the use of NSAIDS in the postoperative period?**

Peptic ulceration, GI bleeding, renal impairment, concurrent use of nephrotoxic drugs or prerenal acute tubular necrosis conditions (renal artery stenosis and hypovolemia) and coagulopathy or abnormal platelet function. Allergy to aspirin and aspirin-induced asthma (nasal polyps) contraindicate the use of NSAIDs. There are a host of relative contraindications to the use of NSAIDS but they must be weighed against the benefit of their use on an individual basis.

○ **What is the advantage of using NSAIDs as adjunctive analgesics in the postoperative period?**

Less overall incidence of side effects, improved overall postoperative outcomes and an additive analgesic effect.

○ **What is the recommended length of use of ketorolac tromethamine in the postoperative period?**

Ketorolac tromethamine has been extensively used in varying doses for analgesia in the postoperative setting with moderate success. A 30 mg IV dose every 6 hours for 48 hours is now recommended in patients who have a normal creatinine clearance and a 15 mg dose for the elderly or those in whom a lower dose would be more prudent. The maximum daily dose is 150 mg on the first day and 120 mg on subsequent days for a limit of 5 days.

○ **What is the estimated potency of ketorolac compared to narcotic medications?**

It has been shown that ketorolac 30 mg has a potency similar to about 5-10 mg of parenteral morphine. The oral form is limited to 10-20mg because of GI toxicity. It has 50 times the analgesic effect of naproxen and 20 times the antipyretic effect of aspirin.

○ **Are there any NSAIDs that do not affect renal blood flow?**

Sulindac (Clinoril) does not block PGE_2 or prostacyclin in the kidney and therefore does not inhibit prostaglandin-mediated autoregulation of renal blood flow.

○ **Are there any NSAIDs that have been shown to reduce the incidence of NSAID gastropathy?**

Misoprostol has been shown to reduce the incidence of peptic mucosal damage (ulceration and bleeding) when taken four times daily. Due to its cost and side effect profile (diarrhea), its clinical use is reserved for this indication.

○ **Is there an increased incidence of perioperative complications in patients taking NSAIDs?**

All NSAIDs produce reversible inhibition of platelet aggregation which potentially increases the risk of perioperative bleeding, especially if the patient has a preexisting coagulopathy or abnormal platelet function. Aspirin produces irreversible platelet dysfunction. Concurrent use of other NSAIDs, nephrotoxic drugs or acetaminophen increases the risk of nephropathy or GI side effects.

○ **What is the advantage of using acetaminophen over acetylsalicylic acid (aspirin) postoperatively?**

Although agranulocytosis and thrombocytopenia are possible, platelet dysfunction is not a side effect, as seen with aspirin. GI effects include nausea and vomiting and hepatotoxicity in overdose with fewer incidences of peptic ulceration and bleeding.

There is no significant peripheral prostaglandin synthetase inhibition with acetaminophen, although it is equipotent in inhibiting central prostaglandin synthesis. The major risk of nephropathy is administration in combination with NSAIDs.

⭕ **In what ways can local anesthetics be used for postoperative analgesia?**

Local anesthetics can be combined in the epidural space with epidural narcotics to reduce overall dose requirements and improve analgesia. Local anesthetic can also be used alone.. Pain control can be achieved with local infiltration, regional blockade, intravenous administration or topical (gel, patch) application of local anesthetics.

⭕ **What factors must be considered for the safe administration of epidural anesthesia?**

Observe contraindications to epidural anesthesia (patient refusal, sepsis with hemodynamic instability, uncorrected hypovolemia and coagulopathy), an understanding of the inherent physiologic effects (sympathetic blockade and respiratory changes) and need for maintaining preload, signs and symptoms of drug toxicity, proper epidural placement and assessment of the level of the block. It has been shown that placement of the epidural at the level of the dermatome that corresponds to the incision is associated with fewer side effects, lower drug dose requirements, and better pain control.

⭕ **What are the most common adverse reactions with local anesthetics in the postoperative period?**

Hypotension, respiratory depression, tinnitus, excessive somnolence, bradycardia, and nausea are most commonly reported.

⭕ **What are the guidelines for removing an epidural in a patient on IV or oral anticoagulants?**

Controversial. If on Coumadin, the PT and INR should be no more than 1.5 times normal. If on IV heparin, it is our policy to discontinue the heparin 2 hours prior to removal, and if the PTT is normal, remove the epidural catheter, and waited an additional 1 hour before restarting the infusion. With new low molecular weight heparin agents, there is no consensus, but current opinion is supporting the contraindication of neuraxial anesthesia. There may be a "window of opportunity" between 10 hours after the last dose and 2 hours before the next anticipated dose when it is safest to insert/withdraw a catheter. More studies are needed, and a personal institutional policy is mandatory.

⭕ **Is there any benefit to using local anesthetics for postoperative epidural analgesia versus IV PCA narcotics?**

It has been shown that patients who have postoperative epidural analgesia with local anesthetics demonstrate: improved lower extremity blood flow, better postoperative pulmonary and cardiac function, less ileus, earlier ambulation and hospital discharge, and overall better pain control, when compared to IV PCA modes of analgesia. A reduced incidence of phantom limb pain is also seen in amputations.

⭕ **When might it be advantageous to use epidural over IV PCA narcotics for postoperative analgesia?**

Upper abdominal, vascular, and thoracic surgery, especially in patients with significant lung disease.

⭕ **Is there any evidence that pre-emptive analgesia works?**

Yes. And some evidence that it does not. Many experts feel that blocking pathways involved in pain transmission before surgical stimulation reduces postoperative pain. Local infiltration along the planned surgical incision for inguinal hernia repair with general anesthesia is beneficial, if the injection is made prior to skin incision. Intravenous or epidural opiates in patients having thoracotomies and hysterectomies have shown a preemptive effect.

❍   What combination techniques have been most extensively advocated for pre-emptive analgesia?

Epidural or intrathecal continuous local anesthetics and opioids are most studied. Additionally clonidine, and NMDA antagonists have been successfully reported to reduce postoperative narcotic requirements.

❍   **What dose adjustment is required for age when administering epidural local anesthetics?**

Older patients require a smaller dose of local anesthetic to achieve the same level of block when compared with younger patients. This decrease in dose requirement is exaggerated when larger volumes of anesthetic solution are used and may be the result of narrowing of the intervertebral spaces. Elderly patient are at risk for systemic toxicity due to the diminished clearance of drugs by the liver, especially those undergoing extensive first-pass metabolism.

❍   **What surgical procedures are generally thought to warrant avoidance of ketorolac perioperatively?**

There are several case reports of bleeding following administration of a single dose of ketorolac after cosmetic surgery. It is prudent to avoid in any case where significant surgical or medical bleeding may occur, as ketorolac causes reversible inhibition of platelet aggregation. Other surgical procedures include GI bleeding or peptic ulceration and urological procedures where the risk of nephropathy (especially in patients with a creatinine greater than or equal to 1.3) is increased. If the patient has hyperactive airways disease this drug should be avoided. Despite the renal effects, urologic surgeons utilize it after nephrectomies as its use has been shown to decrease hospital stay.

❍   **A patient complains of back pain after an epidural. The surgeon suspects epidural abscess. What information is important to determine the actual etiology of this patient's pain?**

Back pain can be caused by catheter pressure on the skin, infection, hematoma, or even pre-existing back pain. Assess for leg weakness and bowel or bladder dysfunction. An abscess usually appears at least 5 days post-placement, and the incidence is rare. Epidural hematoma can occur spontaneously in clinical settings outside the operating room but when associated with regional anesthesia, there is usually a preexisting coagulopathy. If the hematoma is not surgically decompressed in 6 to 8 hours, full neurologic recovery is compromised. Confirmation is made by MRI or CT scan.

❍   **How much time do you have from the onset of symptoms related to an epidural hematoma to decompression before irreversible neurologic injury?**

Six to 8 hours is the rule.

❍   **What are the advantages of IV PCA?**

Intravenous patient controlled analgesia allows the patient to be in control of his/her pain. There is more controlled and steady analgesia, with less adverse side effects. There is less total amount of medication required for analgesia, less fluctuation in plasma opioid levels, less demand on nursing time, less delay from time of request for analgesia to delivery of the medication and less cost.

❍   **A patient requires 90 mg of IV morphine in 24 hours after surgery and you are asked to convert her/him to oral morphine for discharge home. What is the appropriate dose?**

Due to the first pass effect of agents taken orally, the conversion from IV to oral opioids is generally 1:3. Therefore this patient would require about 270 mg of oral morphine in 24 hours. Rarely is this large dose prescribed due to the high incidence of side effects.

❍   **What is the appropriate breakthrough dose of oral opioid medication in a patient taking controlled-release opioids for postoperative pain?**

Normally patients should be given 1/4 to 1/3 the dose of the scheduled controlled-release preparation every 3-4 hours for breakthrough pain. Therefore, if a patient is taking 30 mg of controlled-release morphine sulfate every 12 h, a dose of 10 mg immediate-release morphine would be sufficient.

○ **Is the anatomic location of an epidural catheter important when using *hydrophilic* opioids?**

With hydrophilic opioids (morphine) alone there is equal spread within the epidural space in a matter of several hours which avoids the need for placing the catheter in a near-dermatomal distribution of the patient's pain pattern.

○ **Is the anatomic location of an epidural catheter important when using *lipophilic* opioids?**

Using lipophilic opioids (fentanyl) it is hypothesized that there is a band-like distribution of the agent within several dermatomes. Therefore, it is generally felt that placing the catheter in the middle of the surgical dermatomal pattern affords better analgesia with the concomitant need for a reduced amount of opioid.

○ **What is the proposed mechanism of action of epidural opioids?**

The precise mechanism is not known. Most likely epidural opioids diffuse directly across the dura and bind to receptors in levels I and II of the substantia gelatinosa of the dorsal horn of the spinal cord. Other theories include uptake via the epidural vasculature promoting a systemic spread of the agent, diffusion via the CSF into rostral areas of the brain and uptake via the epidural fat and systemic absorption.

○ **What are the important terms associated with patient-controlled analgesia?**

Dose: The incremental amount of narcotic (age-dependent, renal function, body habitus) prescribed which the patient self-administers with each push.
Bolus: The loading dose of narcotic given when the patient first begins PCA, generally 2-3 times the incremental dose.
Lockout: The time between actual delivery of narcotic doses, usually a range of 6 to 10 minutes.
Basal: The continuous background infusion prescribed in addition to each dose made available to the patient.

○ **A patient receives 60 mg of IV PCA morphine in 24 hours but has intolerable nausea and vomiting and needs to be converted to hydromorphone. What is the conversion dose?**

1 mg of morphine is equal to about 0.2 mg of hydromorphone (5 times more potent than morphine), so the equivalent dose of hydromorphone in this patient would be 12 mg in 24 hours. The PCA pump would be set at basal dose 0.2 mg per hour, incremental dose 0.2 to 0.4 mg and lock-out at 6 to 10 minutes.

○ **A patient receives 300 mg of IV PCA meperidine in a 24 hour period. The internist is worried about accumulation of normeperidine and seizure activity, so he requests that you change to morphine. What would be the equivalent analgesic dose?**

This is a reasonable request as meperidine is a poor analgesic with only 1/10th the potency of morphine and has substantial risks including negative inotropic effect on the heart, allergic reactions and normeperidine-induced seizures. The appropriate 24 hour dose equivalent of morphine would be 30 mg.

○ **A patient receives a total of 60 mg of IV morphine each day in hospital. In readiness for discharge, the surgeon requests that you make recommendations for the equivalent dosing of oral hydromorphone.**

IV morphine must first be converted to the PO morphine equivalent dose. Due to the first pass effect and oral morphine's relatively poor bioavailability, the oral dose of morphine is 3 times the IV dose, or 180 mg. Hydromorphone is about 5 times more potent than morphine, therefore, the appropriate total dose in 24 hours would be 36 mg.

○   **What is the purpose of a naloxone infusion in patients receiving epidural opioids?**

Naloxone is an antagonist to opioids and can be used as a single bolus injection to reverse narcotic-induced respiratory depression. Opioid antagonists can reduce or reverse opioid-induced nausea and vomiting, pruritus, urinary retention, rigidity and biliary spasm associated with neuraxial analgesic techniques.

Naloxone 0.25μg/kg/h via continuous infusion has been reported to reduce adverse effects associated with PCA analgesia with morphine and enhance analgesia with reduced morphine requirements. The mechanism may be enhanced release of endogenous opiates and opioid receptor upregulation.

○   **What dose of IV naloxone is normally required to reverse the adverse side effects of epidural opioids?**

Generally infusions of 1-5 mcg/kg/hr are adequate to reverse side effects. At rates above 10 mcg/kg/hr analgesic effects are reversed.

○   **When is a caudal catheter better than an epidural catheter?**

Normally in very small children and infants, the placement of the caudal catheter is technically very easy and the space is better defined than the epidural space. In adult patients it may be a viable alternative to the lumbar approach in accessing the epidural space (multiple lumbar fractures, ankylosing spondylitis).

○   **What are the nonsurgical reasons to consider epidural analgesia?**

Patients with multiple rib fractures, pneumothorax, sternal fractures and chronic pain syndromes (carcinoma of the lung, chronic back pain) are very good candidates for the analgesic benefits of epidural opioid/local anesthetic mixtures. Patients with angina, claudication and severe peripheral vascular disease may benefit as well.

○   **With what procedures has epidural analgesia been shown to be particularly beneficial and why?**

Procedure	Benefit
Thoracotomy	Pulmonary function
Joint Replacement	Decreased DVT, earlier ambulation
Vascular procedures	Improved blood flow, decreased graft thrombosis
Pediatric Cardiac	Decreased ventilator time and hospital stay
Abdominal surgery	Less ileus

○   **What are alternative measures to manage postoperative upper extremity/lower extremity pain in patients intolerant to opioids?**

Central axis or peripheral nerve block with a single injection or continuous catheter technique.

Epidural catheter placement for lower extremity surgery with dilute concentrations of local anesthetics is beneficial. In upper and lower extremity surgery, an axillary or femoral/sciatic catheter with a continuous infusion of local anesthetic solution is efficacious.

○   **What is the best way to manage postoperative pain in the patient with a concurrent problem of opioid addiction (psychological dependence)?**

The risk of iatrogenic addition is less than 0.1%. The psychological dependence seen with addiction is characterized by a compulsive behavior pattern involved in acquiring opioids for nonmedical psychic effects as opposed to pain relief. Abuse potential of narcotics is related to their relative μ-receptor activity.

For addicts already withdrawn from narcotics prior to surgery, do not premedicate with a narcotic. General, regional or local anesthesia is appropriate. Narcotic antagonists butorphanol and nalbuphine are good analgesics. Adjunct analgesics such as clonidine and NSAIDs may be appropriate.

If an addict's maintenance requirements are known, simply continue them during the procedure and into recovery. Narcotic antagonists should be avoided. "PRN" injections should be avoided. After a thorough and frank discussion about the pain and expectations about pain relief the patient should receive adequate doses of either scheduled oral or IV opioids or preferably, IV PCA with a background infusion. Consideration must be made for the patient's tolerance to "usual" doses of opioids, as higher doses of opioid may be needed to produce the same pharmacologic effect.

❍ What are commonly encountered side effects of epidurally administered local anesthetic infusions?

In large quantities or high concentrations, a partial sympathetic blockade may occur precipitating hypotension, particularly orthostatic hypotension. With more dilute concentrations of, for example, 1/8 to 1/16 bupivacaine, this is avoided. Mild motor and/or sensory loss may occur. Urinary retention, particularly in the very young patient and the elderly male may occur.

❍ What are the signs and symptoms of an epidural hematoma?

Severe back pain and new onset radicular pain of the lower extremities followed quickly by weakness, paralysis, and sensory losses is an ominous sign. Loss of bowel and bladder function is a later sign. These findings all require immediate and emergent evaluation.

❍ What is the work-up for a suspected epidural hematoma?

Immediate history and thorough neurological evaluation
The catheter should be left in place
Stat consultation among the surgical, neurosurgery and anesthesia providers
MRI evaluation of the epidural space is mandatory (upper cut above the catheter tip)
Surgical evacuation (discontinue heparin and administer steroids) may be required

❍ What is clonidine and how is it used to provide analgesia?

Clonidine is a direct centrally acting alpha-2 adrenergic receptor agonist. α2-agonists are used primarily as anesthetic adjuvants for the treatment of acute and chronic pains (intractable pain, RSD and neuropathic pain). Oral clonidine can augment spinally mediated opioid analgesia whereas epidural or intrathecal clonidine can provide effective analgesia alone. Intrathecal clonidine does not provide surgical anesthesia. Clonidine decreases postoperative oxygen consumption and adrenergic stress response and only mildly potentiates opiate-induced respiratory depression. Clonidine does not cause urinary retention.

❍ What are the common side effects of epidural clonidine?

Significant hypotension, bradycardia and sedation are dose-dependent side effects of IV and epidural clonidine. A meta-analysis reported no evidence of respiratory depression by pulse oximetry.

❍ What is the role of an NMDA antagonist in post-operative pain management?

NMDA antagonists (ketamine, and dextromethorphan) have been shown to have supplemental analgesic properties when used in combination with opioids. They may decrease the amount of opioid required to achieve an analgesic response, and they may prevent tolerance to the analgesic effects which may occur with opioid use.

❍ What are non-pharmacological approaches to managing post-operative pain?

T.E.N.S. (transcutaneous electrical nerve stimulation), hypnosis and biofeedback, heat/cold therapy, acupuncture and massage are also advocated and possibly efficacious.

○ **Describe the basic physiologic processes of pain – transduction, transmission, modulation, and perception.**

Transduction the conversion at the periphery of the noxious surgical insult into an electrical action potential, precipitating the release of pain producing substances such as histamines, serotonin, bradykinin, prostaglandins, etc.
Transmission the approach of the peripheral electrical action potential to the primary sensory nerve and through the dorsal root ganglion, dorsal horn of the spinal cord, and higher central nervous system structures in an ascending, afferent pathway.
Modulation the descending, inhibitory, or efferent neurologic pathway of the pain cycle.
Perception the cortical response to pain.

○ **What medications may affect transduction?**

Peripheral local anesthetics and NSAIDs decrease transduction of pain.

○ **What medications effect transmission?**

Nerve blocks with local anesthetics decrease transmission.

○ **What medications enhance modulation of pain?**

Epidural/intrathecal opioids and alpha agonists play a role in modulation as do tricyclic anti-depressants and possibly NSAIDs.

○ **What is the primary site of action of epidural/intrathecal opioids?**

Levels I and II of the substantia gelatinosa of the dorsal horn of the spinal cord.

○ **What are the primary nerve fibers which play predominant roles in acute pain?**

The A-delta and the C fibers play the most significant role.

○ **How is acute pain assessed?**

Verbal scales (McGill Pain Questionnaire), visual analogue scale (Numerical, 10-cm line, Faces or Color Pain Intensity Scales), or verbal descriptors or functional ability are used, as pain is a subjective experience. Changes in vital signs (blood pressure, heart rate, respiratory rate) correlate poorly with the degree of pain control. Measuring pain during activity may be a better indicator of efficacy of pain control.

○ **What are the reasons to aggressively treat postoperative pain?**

Physiologic, psychologic, economic, legal reasons all exist to justify aggressive management. However, compassion and empathy are the greatest reasons.

○ **What are the major physiologic adverse effects of uncontrolled postoperative pain?**

System	Adverse Effect
Gastrointestinal	Ileus
Cardiovascular	Increased sympathetic effect (BP, Pulse), Angina
Pulmonary	Atelectasis, hypoxia, shunting, CO_2 retention
CNS	Altered mental status, stress, anxiety and depression
Immunologic	Impaired wound healing

❍   **What are the proposed mechanisms of T.E.N.S. (transcutaneous electrical nerve stimulation) therapy?**

It is proposed that T.E.N.S. therapy may work by the Gate Control Theory (closing the gate and disallowing pain transmission). Also, it is speculated that a mechanism of action occurs through the stimulation and release of endogenous opioids. T.E.N.S. works best in patients with myofascial syndromes, peripheral nerve injuries, phantom limb pain and stump pain. T.E.N.S. is unsatisfactory in patients with chronic pain that has no peripheral nociceptive cause (central pain state) and in patients with a physiologic and/or psychologic dependence on drugs.

❍   **What is postdural puncture headache (PDPH)?**

A severe headache which develops after dural puncture (often unrecognized).

❍   **When does PDPH typically present?**

It typically presents 24 to 48 hours after the puncture, sometimes earlier and rarely as late as 5 days.

❍   **What is the most common symptom?**

Intense headache in the occipital region and neck when the patient assumes the upright position and improves when the patient is recumbent.

❍   **Where is the headache usually located?**

Headache is usually in the occipital or frontal region, radiating down the posterior neck.

❍   **What is the incidence of headache?**

In a study of 10,000 spinal anesthetics the overall incidence of PDPH for all procedures and all patient types was 21%. Patients at higher risk for PDPH includes: use of large-bore spinal and cutting needles, the number of dural punctures, history of previous spinal headache, motion sickness, women, younger patients, parturients and obese patients. The use of continuous spinals and timing of ambulation are factors not increasing PDPH incidence. A meta-analysis (1994) recommended the use of noncutting needles of a gauge ≥ 26. The incidence of headache was reported as 3.9% noncutting versus 9% cutting needle and severe headache in 1.1% noncutting versus 3% cutting needle use. The incidence of headache for needle gauge less than 26 was 13.6% (5.3% for severe headache) versus 3.8% (1.2% for severe headache) using a needle gauge greater than or equal to 26. There was no difference in the incidence of backache, difficulty in insertion or failure rate for each of the groups.

❍   **What other symptoms are associated with PDPH?**

Nausea, vomiting, stiffness of the neck, diplopia, blurred vision, and hearing loss.

❍   **What complications can be associated with PDPH?**

Cranial nerve palsies, especially VI and VIII (vision and hearing disturbances due to traction on the nerves from a brain that no longer floats on a cushion of CSF). Rarely subdural hematoma and intracerebral hemorrhage occur.

❍   **What is the incidence in children?**

Headache is rare under the age of 13. One study showed no headache in children under 10 years of age following lumbar puncture.

❍   **Are any tests available for PDPH?**

No. PDPH is a diagnosis of exclusion. However, magnetic resonance imaging can visualize leaking cerebrospinal fluid in the lumbar spine. Abdominal pressure (e.g. a bear hug) will transiently relieve PDPH headache but not headaches from other sources.

○ **What is the differential diagnosis?**

Subdural hematoma, pneumocephalus, meningitis, any cause of elevated intracranial pressure, nicotine withdrawal, caffeine withdrawal, postpartum headache, and migraine.

○ **What is the proposed mechanism of the headache?**

Persistent leakage of CSF and decreased intracranial pressure causing sagging of the brain which results in traction in pain sensitive brain support structures and reflex vasodilatation of cerebral vessels.

○ **How does bevel direction of the spinal needle affect the dural hole?**

Using a paramedian approach and splitting rather than cutting the dural fibers by orienting the bevel of the needle parallel to the longitudinal axis of the dural fibers results in a lower incidence of PDPH.

○ **How are dural fibers arranged?**

They are longitudinal fibers (caudal to cephalad) arranged in a concentric ring around the spinal cord.

○ **What are the different needle types?**

There are two types: blunt pencil point (Sprotte, Whitacre, Marx and Green) and cutting diamond tip.

○ **What is the initial therapy for PDPH?**

24-hour trial of symptomatic therapy (bed rest, hydration (oral or intravenous) and analgesics) or immediate epidural blood patch, unless cranial nerve traction symptoms exist.

○ **How is caffeine thought to work in the treatment of PDPH?**

Evidence shows that the probable mechanism for caffeine's stimulatory effect on the CNS is its competitive inhibition of adenosine receptors, with results in vasoconstriction.

○ **What dose of caffeine is used to treat PDPH?**

300 mg of oral caffeine or 500 mg of intravenous caffeine sodium benzoate (which contains 250 mg of caffeine).

○ **What is the caffeine content of some common beverages?**

Freeze dried coffee 66 mg/cup; drip coffee 142 mg/cup; tea 47 mg/cup; Coke 65 mg/12oz can; Pepsi 43 mg/12oz can; Mountain Dew 55 mg/12oz can.

○ **What are the side effects of caffeine therapy?**

The most common side effects are transient flushing, palpitation and dizziness. Very rarely seizures may occur.

○ **What other cerebral vasoconstrictors are useful?**

Sumatriptan can also be used. The usual dose is 6 mg subcutaneously.

O   **What is epidural blood patching?**

This is the technique of injecting 15 to 20 ml of aseptically drawn autologous blood into the epidural space near the site of the original dural puncture. Injection is performed with the volume indicated or until mild back pressure is felt. Side effects are mild back pain and fever and occasional temporary radiculopathy from nerve pressure.

O   **What are the contraindications to EBP?**

Local infection of the back, septicemia and active neurologic disease.

O   **Can EBP be done on an HIV Patient?**

Yes.

O   **What else can be injected epidurally to help with PDPH?**

Saline and dextran has also been injected, but provides only transient relief.

O   **A nurse administers meperidine 25 mg to a patient for control of postoperative shivering. The treatment is ineffective. What are your alternate choices?**

In most patients administration of meperidine 25 mg, clonidine 150 μg, or doxapram 100 mg is efficacious in stopping shivering within 5 minutes compared to placebo. Other drugs that have been described include: ketanserin 10 mg, alfentanil 250 μg, fentanyl, morphine, nalbuphine, lidocaine, magnesium, methimazole, methylphenidate, nefopam, pentazocine and tramadol.

O   **What are the mechanisms and physiologic effects of postoperative shivering?**

The primary cause of postoperative shivering is hypothermia secondary to anesthetic agents which inhibit thermoregulation by lowering the threshold for shivering by 2-4 degrees C. The neurotransmitter pathways are complex and poorly understood. There is evidence that opioid, alpha 2 adrenergic, serotonergic and anticholinergic systems play a role. The physiologic effects include: increase in mean total-body oxygen consumption (40%), catecholamine release, cardiac output, heart rate, blood pressure and intra-ocular pressure. Oxygen consumption is directly proportional to mean body temperature. Despite similar core temperatures, men have a greater incidence of clinically significant shivering and greater total-body oxygen consumption than women. In patients following elective myocardial revascularization, shivering patients versus those paralyzed and sedated had increased VO_2, VCO_2, lower systolic blood pressure and mixed venous O_2 content and greater use of inotropic support.

O   **According to the POVL Registry of the ASA Closed Claims Study Group, what is the most common cause of postoperative blindness?**

The majority of cases are associated with spine operations (67 percent) followed by cardiac bypass procedures (10 percent). The remaining 23 percent of cases are composed of liver transplants, thoracoabdominal aneurysm resections, peripheral vascular procedures, head and neck operations, and prostatectomies. Of the 53 cases of postoperative visual loss associated with spine surgery in the registry, ophthalmologic diagnoses included ischemic optic neuropathy (n = 43, 81 percent), central retinal artery occlusion (n = 7, 13 percent) and unknown diagnosis (n = 3, 6 percent).

O   **Is there any difference in anesthetic-related mortality in patients receiving epidural or spinal anesthesia and general anesthesia?**

Meta-analysis (141 trials, 9589 patients, 2001) has reported the rate of death as 2.1 percent in patients receiving epidural or spinal anesthesia and 3.1 percent in those receiving general anesthesia. This decline of one death per 100 patients in the regional anesthesia groups resulted from reductions in pulmonary embolism, cardiac events, stroke, transfusion requirements, infections and respiratory depression. The type or location of surgery did not influence the result.

○   **T/F: Anesthesia is the cause of 15% of the 7.5 maternal deaths per 100,000 live births each year in the US.**

False. Anesthesia is the 6th most frequent cause of maternal mortality. Causes include: hemorrhage (29%), embolism (20%), PIH (18%), infection (18%), cardiomyopathy (6 %), anesthesia (3%) and others.

○   **What is the incidence of awareness following general anesthesia?**

Data published in 2004 from a multicenter trial of 19,575 patients reported that the incidence of awareness with recall after surgery under general anesthesia was 0.13% (1.3 patients per 1000).

○   **Which patients are at risk of developing postoperative pulmonary complications (atelectasis and pneumonia) following abdominal surgery?**

Six independent risk factors have been identified: age > or = 60 years; impaired preoperative cognitive function; smoking history within the past 8 weeks; body mass index > or = 27; history of cancer; and incision site-upper abdominal or both upper/lower abdominal incision.

○   **What is the treatment for corneal abrasions?**

Time heals corneal abrasions. Following general anesthesia the incidence may be as high as 44%, if the eye is left partly opened. Simple precautions, such as instilling a bland ointment (possible chemical keratitis) or taping closed the lids of the inoperative eye, may prevent surface trauma produced by the surgical drape, anesthetic mask, or exposure. Decreased tear production under general anesthesia and proptosis may worsen corneal exposure, requiring eyelid suturing in some susceptible patients. Treatment includes topical antibiotics or fluoroquinolones, ice compresses for 24 to 48 hours then warm compresses, pain management with NSAID drops to the eye or narcotics for severe pain. A soft bandage may be applied to the eye.

○   **What is the incidence of postoperative delirium in elderly patients?**

The reported incidence of postoperative delirium varies from 5.1 to 61.3%. Elderly patients usually manifest delirium following a lucid interval of one postoperative day or more, a condition known as interval delirium. Fortunately, the postoperative cognitive dysfunction is a reversible condition in the majority of elderly surgical patients. Only 1% has persistent cognitive dysfunction at 1–2 yr after the surgery. Preoperative risk factors predisposing to delirium include aging, lack of education, re-operation, polypharmacy and drug interaction, alcohol and sedative-hypnotic withdrawal, endocrine and metabolic compromise, impaired vision and hearing, sleep deficiency, anxiety, depression, and dementia.

○   **Is general anesthesia associated with a higher postoperative rate of infection?**

General anesthesia has been identified as a major "stand alone" risk factor for postoperative surgical site S. aureus infection. In a prospective case controlled study of 970 adult patients undergoing cardiovascular operation during one year follow-up; duration of general anesthesia, advanced age, urgent intervention and blood transfusion were significant risk factors for postoperative infection.

○   **What are the risk factors for postoperative nausea and vomiting?**

The incidence of nausea and vomiting in patients undergoing general anesthesia is reported as 37% and 20%, respectively. Risk factors for PONV can be divided into patient, procedural, anesthetic and postoperative risk factors. Patient: women > men; children 6 to 16 years > adults; obesity; migraine history; emergency surgery; excessive starvation, history of PONV or motion sickness; gastroparesis. Surgery: type (gynecological, gastrointestinal, laparoscopic, ear nose and throat) and longer duration. Anesthetic: choice of premedication, opioids, nitrous oxide, inhalation agents, longer procedures and greater depth of anesthesia. Postoperative: pain, opioid analgesics, dizziness, early ambulation, hypotension, premature oral intake.

○ What are the causes of hypoxemia in the PACU?

1. Even 0.1 MAC of volatile agents blunt the ventilatory response to hypoxia, and the response is abolished at 1 MAC.
2. Diffusion hypoxia: First 5-10 minutes when the patients are allowed to inhale room air at the conclusion of N_2O anesthetic
3. Opioids affect the venitlatory pattern. The ventilatory response to hypoxia is blunted and there is a dose related depression of ventilatory response to CO_2.
4. Secretions, airway obstruction
5. Atelectasis due to anesthetic and surgical effects on the respiratory system (Decreased FRC and V/Q mismatch)
6. Fluid overload

○ What are the risk factors of postoperative pulmonary complications (PPC) following a laparotomy? How can you reduce the risk o PPC?

The operative site is shown to be the single most important determinant of both the degree of pulmonary restriction and the risk of postoperative pulmonary complications.
Upper abdominal operations (nonlaparoscopic) increase the risk for PPC at least 2 fold, with rates of occurrence varying from 20-70%.
There are several strategies by which it is possible to reduce risk of PPC:
1. Use of lung-expanding therapies postoperatively: After upper abdominal operations, FRC recovers over 3-7 days. With the use of CPAP by mask, FRC will recover within 72 hours.
2. Choice of analgesia: strongly influence the risk of PPC. Use of postoperative epidural for upper abdominal operations has shown to markedly decrease the risk of PPC and decrease the overall stay in the hospital.
3. Cessation of smoking
4. Patients with obstructive disease and decreased expiratory flow may benefit from preoperative bronchodilator therapy and formal pulmonary toilet

The choice of anesthetic technique for intraoperative anesthesia does not change the risk for PPC independent of the operative site.

ASPIRATION

Most people die of a sort of creeping common sense, and discover when it is too late that the only things one never regrets are one's mistakes.
Oscar Wilde

○ **Classically, what volume and pH of aspirate is critical in causing a significant problem after gastric fluid aspiration?**

Greater than 0.4 cc/kg (25 cc) of gastric contents with a pH of 2.5 or less.

○ **What can happen to volume status and wedge pressure after a severe aspiration?**

Pulmonary capillary wedge pressure and volume status can actually decrease after severe pulmonary aspiration due to loss of fluid through pulmonary capillaries. This can cause significant hypotension.

○ **Are the chest x-ray findings of aspiration immediate or delayed in onset?**

They may be delayed up to 6-12 hours, in some cases. Look first at the right lower lobe, where findings will be most common, for evidence of infiltration, pneumonia, atelectasis, pulmonary edema and fulminant chemical pneumonitis.

○ **What is the mechanism of action of metoclopramide (Reglan)?**

It increases lower esophageal sphincter pressure, decreases pyloric pressure and speeds gastric emptying.

○ **What is the mechanism of action of ranitidine? (Zantac)?**

It is a competitive inhibitor of H_2 receptors, and thereby blocks secretion of hydrogen ions in the stomach. This effectively increases gastric pH and decreases gastric volume. The decrease in gastric volume occurs over hours.

○ **If meconium is present in the amniotic fluid or on the newborn's skin, how should you proceed?**

First, the person delivering the baby should have suctioned the oropharynx and nares with a catheter or bulb syringe before delivering the shoulders. If the baby is vigorous and has a normal respiratory effort and HR > 100, simply use a bulb syringe or suction catheter to clear secretions and any meconium from the mouth and nose. If the baby is not vigorous, has depressed respiration, muscle tone *or* HR < 100, direct suctioning of the trachea soon after delivery is indicated before many respirations have occurred.

○ **What patients are at increased risk of aspiration?**

Incidence is less than one in 35,000 - 100,000 in elective surgical patients with no specific risk factors. The majority of pulmonary aspirations occur during laryngoscopy and tracheal extubation. Risk factors include: gastric contents of increased volume or acidity; increased intragastric pressure, decreased tone of the lower esophageal sphincter, gastroesophageal reflux, ASA III or IV status, emergency surgery, inadequate muscle relaxation or difficulty during laryngoscopy, impaired laryngeal reflexes, decreased mental status, full stomach, large amounts of gas in the stomach, alcohol intoxication or ineffective cricoid pressure.

○ **How can you reduce the risk of aspiration?**

Give metoclopramide to stimulate gastric emptying (assuming no intestinal obstruction), increase gastric fluid pH with H_2 antagonists and non-particulate antacids. Consider rapid sequence intubation with effective cricoid pressure and a cuffed endotracheal tube, awake intubation or regional anesthesia avoiding heavy sedation. Delay non-emergent surgery greater than 6 hours. Nasogastric suctioning prior to extubation (when the patient is expected to have regained protective laryngeal reflexes) is prudent.

○   **What is the duration of metoclopramide? Ranitidine?**

Metoclopramide duration is 1-2 hours; ranitidine duration is 8 hours.

○   **Liquids pass from stomach to duodenum in less than 2 hours. How long does it take solids to pass from the stomach to duodenum?**

Up to 12 hours.

○   **What may delay gastric emptying?**

Idiopathic gastroparesis remains the most common cause of delayed gastric emptying. Diabetes mellitus, anorexia nervosa, gastric surgery, gastric outlet obstruction, obesity, stress from pain or anxiety, neurologic disorders, disease involving the gastric wall or nerves, drugs, such as opioids, and pregnancy. Long bone fractures are associated with incomplete gastric emptying for up to 24 hours.

○   **Where is the vomiting center located?**

Medulla.

○   **T/F: Nasogastric and gastric tubes increase the risk of aspiration.**

True.

○   **What factors characterize an aspirate?**

Particulate or liquid (secretions, blood, gastric fluid, bile), size, foodstuffs, pH, infected or non-infected aspirate.

○   **T/F: Adults are more likely to aspirate into the right mainstem bronchus.**

True, over the age of 15 years.

○   **Complete upper airway obstruction by a foreign body is treated by which maneuver?**

Heimlich – subdiaphragmatic abdominal thrusts and backslaps.

○   **What are possible complications of the Heimlich maneuver?**

Rib fractures, ruptured viscera, pneumomediastinum, regurgitation (and aspiration) and retinal detachment.

○   **What is the procedure of choice for lower airway foreign body aspiration?**

Rigid bronchoscopy. Fiberoptic bronchoscopy is an alternative procedure in adults, not in children. If bronchoscopy, postural drainage, chest physical therapy and bronchodilators fail, surgical removal may be required.

○   **What are common radiographic findings in foreign body aspiration?**

Normal film or atelectasis or infiltrates distal to the obstruction, obstructive lobar segmental overinflation in a ball-valve obstruction, and visualization of the foreign body.

○ **What are the common directly toxic (non-infected) respiratory tract aspirates?**

Gastric and small bowel contents, alcohol, hydrocarbons, mineral oil, animal and vegetable fats. All of these produce an inflammatory response and pneumonia. Gastric contents are the most common offender.

○ **What is the antibiotic choice for gastric acid aspiration?**

None.

○ **What is the role of corticosteroids in gastric acid aspiration?**

None.

○ **What is the main priority in treating gastric acid aspiration?**

Maintenance of pulmonary oxygenation. Tracheal suctioning, intubation, ventilation and PEEP (positive end expiratory pressure) may be required. Prophylactic PEEP is not effective in preventing progression of the process. Patients with clinically apparent pulmonary aspiration who do not develop symptoms within two hours are unlikely to have significant respiratory sequelae.

○ **What are the radiographic manifestations of acid aspiration?**

Varied. May be new bilateral diffuse infiltrates, irregular "patchy" bronchopneumonic pattern, or lobar infiltrates in the posterior segments of the upper lobes and the superior segment of the lower lobes.

○ **What outcomes occur in patients who do not rapidly resolve gastric acid aspiration pneumonitis?**

ARDS (adult respiratory distress syndrome), or progressive respiratory failure and death; bacterial superinfection.

○ **Under what circumstances are antibiotics used in aspiration treatment?**

Aspiration of infected material; intestinal obstruction; immune compromised host; and evidence of bacterial superinfection after a non-infected aspirate (new fever, infiltrates or purulence after the initial 2-3 days). Later findings may include necrotizing consolidation and abscess formation.

○ **What is the predominant oropharyngeal flora in outpatients?**

Anaerobes, which are responsible for nosocomial pneumonia.

○ **What is the antibiotic of choice for outpatient acquired infectious aspiration pneumonia?**

Clindamycin, high dose penicillin or Augmentin (amoxicillin and clavulanate).

○ **T/F: Aspiration of liquid gastric contents with pH greater than 2.5 produces no clinical consequences.**

False. Hypoxemia, bronchospasm and atelectasis may develop but usually resolve within 24 hours.

○ **What are the consequences of aspirating small (non-obstructing) food particles?**

Inflammation and hypoxemia, which may result in chronic bronchiolitis or granulomatosis.

O   **What is the priority treatment of near drowning?**

Correction of asphyxia and hypothermia.

O   **What are the indications for intubation and ventilation after near drowning?**

Apnea, pulselessness, altered mental status, severe hypoxemia and respiratory acidosis.

O   **What is the major complication of a double lumen tube for independent lung ventilation?**

Malpositioning. The tube may be too deep, not deep enough, or have entered the wrong side resulting in loss of lung separation and potentially hypoxemia.

O   **What are the major cardiovascular causes of hemoptysis?**

1.   Pulmonary hypertension (Eisenmenger's complex, mitral stenosis, primary recurrent pulmonary emboli).
2.   Pulmonary artery rupture.
3.   Arteriovenous malformations.
4.   Left ventricular failure with pulmonary edema.

O   **How does pulmonary artery catheterization produce hemoptysis?**

Pulmonary artery rupture, aneurysm formation or pulmonary infarction.

O   **T/F: The presence of a cuffed endotracheal tube makes aspiration pneumonia an unlikely cause of new pulmonary infiltrates.**

False. Silent aspiration previously undetected may occur prior to or after endotracheal intubation.

O   **T/F: Retrospective reviews indicate that antibiotic therapy for aspiration pneumonia will hasten the resolution of pulmonary infiltrates.**

False.

O   **With aspiration pneumonia presenting as a lobar infiltrate, which sites are the most common?**

Right lower lobe as most aspirations occur in the supine position, and the right lower lobe has the most gravity dependent position. Superior segments of lower lobes and posterior segments of the upper lobes, in general.

O   **What is the primary treatment for gastric aspiration?**

A stepwise approach using suction, analysis of arterial blood gases for pH and oxygenation, aggressive and early ventilatory support, adequate fluid resuscitation and bronchoscopy for large particulate aspiration is recommended.

O   **Are steroids and prophylactic antibiotics indicated for aspiration?**

No. Steroids can impair wound healing and antibiotics should not be given prophylactically, unless there is evidence of intestinal obstruction or fecal aspiration. Treatment is on the basis of positive culture results.

CRITICAL CARE MEDICINE

Any Idiot Can Face A Crisis – It's Day To Day Living That Wears You Out.
Anton Chekhov

○ **What are the medical indications for hyperbaric oxygen therapy?**

Air embolism; decompression sickness; poisoning with carbon monoxide, cyanide, carbon tetrachloride, or hydrogen sulfide; necrotizing soft tissue infections; clostridial myonecrosis; chronic osteomyelitis; mucormycosis; crush injury; compromised skin flaps; radiation necrosis; ischemic ulcers; central nervous system edema; acute hypoxia; burns; brown recluse spider bites.

○ **Discuss delivery of anesthesia in the hyperbaric chamber.**

Total intravenous anesthesia (TIVA) or regional anesthesia is recommended if scavenging of anesthetic gases in not available. In the chamber, nitrous oxide can be used at partial pressures exceeding its MAC which can result in supersaturation. The potential for tissue hypoxia during decompression exists and supplemental oxygen is necessary after anesthesia. The effect of volatile anesthetics is proportional to the partial pressure of the selected agent.

○ **What are the effects of hyperbaric oxygen (HBO)?**

Hyperoxia causes peripheral vasoconstriction and a decrease in tissue blood flow, while increasing tissue oxygenation.

○ **Describe the cardiovascular changes associated with sepsis?**

Clinical presentation of sepsis: hypotension with adequate fluid resuscitation and impaired end organ perfusion. Hallmarks include a high cardiac output and high mixed venous oxygen saturation. Cardiovascular changes include low systemic vascular resistance (SVR), high pulmonary vascular resistance (PVR), leaky capillaries, and a potential decrease in myocardial contractility with a reduction in oxygen extraction.

○ **What are the major causes of Adult Respiratory Distress Syndrome (ARDS)?**

Sepsis, multi-system organ failure, shock, aspiration, trauma, infection, embolism, inhalation of toxic gases, drug overdose, poisons, and numerous miscellaneous causes.

○ **What are the major effects of carbon monoxide (CO) on oxygen delivery?**

1. Decreased oxygen delivery as hemoglobin (Hb) has a 200 fold higher affinity for CO than O_2 2. Left shift of the Hb-O_2 dissociation curve which results in a decreased ability to unload O_2 at the cellular level.

○ **What is the treatment for acute hyperkalemia?**

Administration of bicarbonate, insulin, glucose and calcium. Beta agonist inhalants can also be used via nebulizer. Insulin drives potassium into cells, bicarbonate exchanges potassium for hydrogen ions, calcium stabilizes cell membranes and beta agonists increase cellular uptake of potassium.

○ **What laboratory tests will detect carbon monoxide toxicity in burn patients?**

The arterial blood gas will show lower oxygen saturation than expected, an anion gap metabolic acidosis and increased carboxyhemoglobin levels (normal < 5%).

O   **What is the frequency of sinusitis during mechanical ventilation?**

Sinusitis is most common in patients with nasotracheal intubation (2-27%), facial trauma and nasal tube feeding.

O   **In the patient with septic shock following adequate fluid status and persistent hypotension which vasopressor should be used?**

Goals: increase SVR and cardiac output. Norepinephrine and/or vasopressin are the first line drugs. If patients have a diminished cardiac output then dobutamine should be considered to augment contractility. Dopamine and epinephrine have also been successfully used to raise blood pressure in sepsis.

O   **What are the causes of hyponatremia in a patient with subarachnoid hemorrhage?**

Syndrome of inappropriate antidiuretic hormone (SIADH), volume contraction and increased concentration of atrial natriuretic factor.

O   **Describe the acute physiologic changes seen in burn patients?**

Massive intravascular fluid loss with fluid replacement calculated using the Parkland formula. Increased risk of infection compared to normal ICU patients. A systemic inflammatory response which can manifest with fever > 39° Celsius, hyperglycemia, disorientation and ileus. A hypermetabolic state starts 24-36 hours after injury which may double the patient's normal energy expenditure. Proliferation of extrajunctional acetycholine receptors, risk of hyperkalemia with succinylcholine and an increased need for nondepolarizing muscle relaxants, limited IV access, exaggerated heat loss, and hemodynamic instability are challenges for the nurse anesthetist.

O   **What is the primary goal of managing the patient with acute head trauma?**

Initial management priorities include:

Must keep sight of the ABCs of resuscitation.
1.   Immobilization of the cervical spine

2.   Early establishment of a patent airway and protection of lungs from aspiration

3.   Oxygenation and ventilation

4.   Stabilization of the circulation and adequate fluid resuscitation

To prevent secondary brain damage, avoid increases in intracranial pressure (ICP), hypotension, hypoxemia, and hypercapnia.

O   **Describe the management of acute spinal cord injury?**

Immobilization of the spinal cord and maintenance of spinal cord perfusion (mean arterial pressure (MAP) 80-85 mm Hg) with fluid and pressors, as necessary. High dose corticosteroids are given if less than 8 hours have passed since injury, with an IV bolus of 30 mg/kg, followed by an infusion of 5.4 mg/kg over the next 23 hours.

O   **What is the treatment of cerebral vasospasm?**

The goal is to improve cerebral perfusion. Nimodipine has been shown to decrease the incidence of ischemic deficits. If vasospasm occurs after an aneurysm clipping, then remember the 3H's: hypervolemia, hypertension and hemodilution.

○   **Is the use of pressure controlled ventilation necessary in ARDS?**

No. Damage to lung parenchyma can occur from overdistension due to volutrauma or barotrauma. Tidal volumes of 6 cc/kg are ideal and can be achieved through volume or pressure limited mechanical ventilation.

○   **What type of edema is caused by brain injury?**

Cytotoxic edema secondary to cellular membrane disruption which is usually trauma related. In patients with a Glasgow coma score of < 8, the risk of increased ICP is greater than 50%.

○   **Discontinuation of nitric oxide (NO) therapy requires what considerations?**

Patients may have a rebound effect with a decrease in oxygenation and an increase in pulmonary hypertension, in some cases to values worse than prior to institution of NO. Recommendations for withdrawal of NO include: low dose requirements (< 5 ppm), FiO_2 40%, PEEP < 5, and stable hemodynamics, followed by an increase in FiO_2 to 60-70%, with vasopressor support, if necessary.

○   **What are the antidotes for nerve gas poisoning?**

The specific antidotes for nerve gas (SARIN, SOMAN, TABUN, VX) counteract their anticholinesterase organophosphate properties. Toxicity is due to cholinergic overdrive at muscarinic, nicotinic and CNS sites. Antidotes include: 1. Atropine: for adults 2-5 mg IV, children 0.05 mg/kg IV with repeat doses every 10-30 minutes; 2. Pralidoxime: for adults 1-2 gm IV, children 25-50 mg/kg with repeat in 1 hour; 3. Obidoxine dichloride IV/IM injection 250 mg every 2 hours; 4. HI-6; 5. Autoinjectors – US military carry 3 atropine (2 mg) and 3 pralidoxine (600 mg); 6. Prophylactic antidote – pyridostigmine bromide.

○   **What is the classification of intraventricular hemorrhage?**

Grade I	Bleeding in just a small area of the ventricles
Grade II	Bleeding also inside the ventricles
Grade III	Ventricles are enlarged by blood
Grade IV	Beeding extends into brain parenchyma around the ventricles

○   **T/F: A recognized complication of TPN is hypophoshatemia?**

True. Unsupplemented TPN can cause severe hypophosphatemia . Symptoms include neuromuscular weakness, cardiovascular effects (CHF), and hematological effects(hemolysis, platelet dysfunction and decreased 2,3 DPG). This is most common in the severely malnourished patient and can precipitate refeeding syndrome.

○   **Why do some patients on TPN have an increased minute ventilation?**

Overfeeding of patients causes an increase in carbon dioxide production due to lipogenesis. The patient compensates by increasing their respiratory rate which can lead to hyperventilation.

○   **What are the potential complications of TPN?**

Catheter sepsis can occur as a primary or secondary infection. Metabolic complications arise from too much or too little energy source and electrolyte abnormalities. These include hyperglycemia, nonketotic hyperosmolar coma, hypoglycemia, prerenal azotemia, hypercarbia, hypertriglyceridemia, fatty acid deficiency, metabolic acidosis, hypophosphatemia, hypo/hypermagnesium, hypo/hyperkalemia, hypo/hypercalcemia and alteration in liver function tests.

○   **How should the patient on TPN scheduled for surgery be managed perioperatively?**

The patient should be changed from TPN to D10 at the same rate to maintain glucose homeostasis. Serial accuchecks for serum glucose are performed every hour to avoid hypo- or hyperglycemia and the infusion rate is titrated as indicated.

CARDIOPULMONARY RESUSCITATION

Victory Belongs To The Most Perservering.
Napoleon

O   **Which vasoactive substances are involved in the compensatory response to acute hypovolemia?**

1.   Angiotensin-renin (kidney): angiotensinogen, renin, angiotensin I, angiotensin II (lung), aldosterone (adrenal cortex)
2.   Adrenergic (adrenal medulla): norepinephrine, epinephrine
3.   AVP (pituitary): ACTH, arginine vasopressin

Blood pressure = cardiac output (contractility, sodium and water retention, capillary fluid shift) X systemic vascular resistance (vasoconstriction)

O   **What is the hormonal stress response to surgery?**

1.   Autonomic response: catecholamines, insulin and glucagon
2.   Hypothalamic-pituitary: cortisol, thyroxine, arginine vasopressin, growth hormone, ACTH, angiotensin, aldosterone, renin-angiotensin
3.   Local tissue, vascular endothelial response: cytokines and other mediators

O   **T/F: Atrial fibrillation or atrial flutter of greater than 48 hours duration should be treated with DC (direct current) cardioversion and amiodarone.**

False. First control the rate. If atrial fibrillation is > 48 hours duration, nonemergent conversion to NSR with shock or drugs may cause embolization of atrial thrombi unless the patient has been adequately anticoagulated.

O   **Explain what PATCH and 5H-5T have in common.**

Both are mnemonics for the most frequent causes of PEA (pulseless electrical activity).
5H: hypovolemia, hypoxemia, hydrogen ion (acidosis), hyper-/hypokalemia, hypothermia
5T: tablets (drug overdose, accidents), tamponade (cardiac), tension pneumothorax, thrombosis (coronary), thrombosis (pulmonary: PE)

O   **A 45-year-old male patient is scheduled for lumbar discectomy in the knee-prone position. After irrigation of the surgical wound with 25 cc 3% hydrogen peroxide the patient suddenly develops hypoxia with a decrease in end-tidal carbon dioxide and a 'mill-wheel' murmur on cardiac auscultation. What is the most likely diagnosis?**

Oxygen venous embolism. Hydrogen peroxide is degraded by catalase from human tissues into gaseous oxygen.

O   **Describe the EKG findings of venous air embolism.**

Sinus tachycardia, right axis deviation, right ventricular strain and ST depression. In healthy humans, 5 to 8 ml/kg air is needed to obstruct the right ventricle and pulmonary artery. Venous air may move paradoxically from the pulmonary artery to the systemic circulation (cardiac defects with right-to-left shunting or transpulmonary passage). As little as 0.5 ml of air may cause coronary artery occlusion with ST elevation.

O   **What is the management of acute venous air embolism?**

Prevent further air entry:
- Notify surgeon to flood or pack the field or terminate central line placement and clamp the line
- Apply jugular compression
- Lower the patient's head into the Trendelenburg position
- If feasible: rotate the patient toward the left lateral decubitus position

Remove intravascular air and treat hemodynamic consequences:
- Aspirate the right heart catheter from the distal port and attempt to remove air
- Administer 100% oxygen and intubate for respiratory distress or hypoxemia
- Discontinue nitrous oxide
- Circulatory collapse: external chest compressions and fluids/pressors/inotropes
- Hyperbaric oxygen therapy

O   **What is the treatment for acute onset Wolff-Parkinson-White syndrome?**

Synchronized DC cardioversion in the unstable patient or beta-blockers and a primary antiarrhythmic agent (one of the following: amiodarone, flecainamide, procainamide, propafenone, sotalol) followed by cardiac consultation in the hemodynamically stable patient. WPW is characterized by short PR interval, wide QRS and delta wave. WPW with atrial fibrillation often mimics ventricular tachycardia.

O   **When is it necessary to treat an intraoperative dysrhythmia?**

When it is detrimental to cardiac output (blood pressure) and tissue perfusion; a precursor of a more life threatening dysrhythmia; in the presence of myocardial ischemia. Most intraoperative dysrhythmias can be explained on the basis of an autonomic imbalance and do not need treating.

O   **Why are epinephrine, phenylephrine, vasopressin, methoxamine and dopamine thought to be equally efficacious in restoring blood pressure during CPR?**

They all cause peripheral vasoconstriction through alpha-adrenergic effects which increases aortic diastolic pressure and augments cerebral and coronary perfusion. Beta stimulation has previously been thought to facilitate defibrillation by increasing the amplitude of fine fibrillation, but actually may be detrimental by increasing myocardial oxygen consumption and decreasing the endocardial/epicardial flow ratio.

O   **What is the mechanism of sinus tachycardia?**

A heart rate of greater than 100 beats per minute originating from the sinus node (SN) which is classified as appropriate (exercise, anxiety, panic attacks, dehydration, deconditioning, hypovolemia, hyperthyroidism, pheochromocytoma, electrolyte abnormalities, hypercarbia, hypoxia, pain, inadequate anesthesia, drug effects, fever, anemia, heart failure, pulmonary embolism) or inappropriate.

Inappropriate sinus tachycardia is a diagnosis of exclusion. The proposed underlying mechanisms include: intracardiac SN abnormality (high intrinsic heart rate, depressed efferent cardiovagal reflex and beta-adrenergic hypersensitivity) and extracardiac (length-dependent autonomic neuropathy, excessive venous pooling, beta-receptor hypersensitivity, alpha-receptor hyposensitivity, altered sympathovagal balance and brainstem dysregulation).

O   **What is the treatment of a patient who develops chest pain suggestive of ischemia?**

- Immediate assessment: measure vital signs and oxygen saturation, obtain IV access, 12-lead ECG, brief targeted history and physical exam, obtain initial serum cardiac marker levels, check electrolytes, hematocrit and coagulation studies, stat portable chest x-ray
- Immediate general treatment: MONA: morphine IV, oxygen 4 L/min, nitroglycerin, aspirin 160 to 325 mg.

- 12-lead ECG shows ST depression, new T-wave inversion: patient is high risk for unstable or new-onset angina or nondiagnostic ECG but troponin positive
- start adjunctive treatments as indicated: heparin, aspirin, glycoprotein IIb/IIIa receptor inhibitors, nitroglycerin IV, beta-adrenergic receptor blocker
- cardiology consultation for monitoring or cardiac catheterization and possible revascularization

○ **Describe the ECG effects of hypokalemia.**

Progressive flattening of the T wave, increasingly prominent U wave, increased amplitude of the P wave, prolongation of the PR interval and ST-segment depression.

○ **What factors determine the treatment of ventricular tachycardia?**

- Hemodynamically stable versus unstable patient
- Monomorphic versus polymorphic
- Normal versus impaired left ventricular function

Hemodynamically stable monomorphic VT and polymorphic VT in patients with normal QT interval and *normal LV function:* procainamide, amiodarone, lidocaine and sotalol; *impaired LV function:* amiodarone or lidocaine.
Ongoing polymorphic VT and unstable patients: immediate cardioversion
Self-terminated polymorphic VT with prolonged QT interval: magnesium

○ **What is the difference between the therapeutic effect of cardioversion and defibrillation to terminate tachycardias?**

Cardioversion (*synchronized* direct current shock on the R-wave peak of the QRS complex of a stable tachycardia) terminates repetitive reentry loops, whereas, defibrillation (*unsynchronized* shock in the very unstable patient in VF and pulseless VT) depolarizes the entire myocardium. Delivery of a shock during cardiac repolarization (T wave) may precipitate VF.

○ **Successful cardioversion of atrial flutter may occur at what energy level?**

50 J.

○ **During elective repair of a right femoral hernia in a 60-yr-old woman, the patient suddenly develops profound hypotension, unresponsive to 5 mg and then 10 mg of IV ephedrine. Her heart rate increases from 72 to 150 bpm accompanied by a new intraventricular conduction delay in lead II and a decrease in end-tidal CO_2. Hypotension persists with the development of severe central cyanosis of the upper thorax and head. What is the most likely diagnosis and what are your treatment options?**

Right ventricular dysfunction from acute pulmonary embolism. Hemodynamic support (fluids, 100% oxygen, inotropic vasoactive agents:dobutamine, milrinone, norepinephrine), invasive monitoring, TEE diagnosis (acute right atrial and ventricular dilation and hypokinesis; systolic septal flattening; clot in the superior vena cava, RV and PA; altered flow through the PA; normal LV function with decreased filling; tricuspid regurgitation; changes in the right to left ventricular end-diastolic area ratio), heparin IV, centrally administered thrombolytic drugs, Greenfield filter, embolectomy by catheter or surgery.

○ **For neonatal resuscitation in the delivery room, when should you start chest compressions?**

If after 15-30 seconds of positive pressure ventilation with 100% oxygen the heart rate is below 60 bpm or between 60-80 bpm and not increasing.

BIBLIOGRAPHY/ SUGGESTED READING

BOOKS/JOURNALS

Abouleish AE. Latex Allergy and Anesthesia (Chapter 15;Lesson 10). Current Reviews in Clinical Anesthesia, Inc 1994.

Acute Pain Management Guidelines Panel Acute Pain Management: Operative or Medical Procedures and Trauma, Clinical Practice Guidelines, AHCPR Publication 92-0032, Rockville MD, US Department of Health and Human Services

Adler, JN & Plantz, SH. *Emergency Medicine Pearls of Wisdom*. 4th ed. Watertown: Mt. Auburn Press; 1997.

Advanced Cardiac Life Support. Dallas: American Heart Association; 1996.

Advanced Trauma Life Support. Chicago: American College of Surgeons; 1990.

Albert, DM. *Clinical Practice Principles and Practice of Ophthalmology*. Vol. 2. Philadelphia: W.B. Saunders Co.; 1994.

Alderson PJ, Lerman J: Oral premedication for paediatric ambulatory anaesthesia comparison of midazolam and ketamine. Can J Anaesth 41:221, 1994

Alon E, Himmelseher S: Ondansetron in the treatment of postoperative vomiting: a randomized, double-blind comparison with droperidol and metoclopramide. Anesth Analg 75:561, 1992

Ambulatory Anesthesiology, A Problem Approach, Ed: KEMcGoldrick, Williams & Wilkins (Baltimore), 1995

Ambulatory Anesthesia Handbook, Ed:RSTwersky, Mosby, 1995

Ambulatory Anesthesia and Surgery. Ed:PFWhite, Saunders (Philadelphia), Sep 1996

American College of Surgeon's Committee on Trauma. Advanced Trauma Life Support Manual. Chicago, American College of Surgeons, 1993.

Annunziato PW, Powell KR. Infections of the upper respiratory tract. In: Reese RE, BettsRF (eds.), Little, Brown, and Company, Boston

Aronchick,JM and Gefter,WB: Drug-induced pulmonary disease. J Thorac Imaging 6:19-29,1991

Ashburn M, Rice LJ, eds, The Management of Pain, Churchhill Livingstone, 1997

Avery, GB; Fletcher, MA; Macdonald, MG; Neonatology- Pathophysiology and Management of the Newborn. Fourth edition. J.B. Lippincott Company. 1994.

Badner NH, Nielson WR, Munk S, Kwiotkowska C, Gelb AW: Preoperative anxiety: detection and contributing factors. Can J Anaesth 37:444, 1990

Bakerman, S. *ABCs of Interpretive Laboratory Data*. 2nd ed. Greenville: Interpretive Laboratory Data, Inc; 1984.

Barash, Paul G., Cullen, Bruce F., and Stoelting, Robert K., eds. Clinical Anesthesia. 4th ed., Lippincott-Ravin, 2001.

Barkin, RM. Emergency Pediatrics. 3rd ed. St. Louis: CV Mosby Company; 1990.

Bates RJ, Beutler S, Resnekov L, Anagnostopoulos CE. Cardiac rupture-challenge in diagnosis and management. Am J Cardiol 1977; 40: 429-437.

Battistella F, Benfield JR. Blunt and penetrating injuries of the chest wall, pleura and lungs. In Shields TW (ed): General Thoracic Surgery, 4th ed, 1994.

Bayes de Luna A, Coumel P, Leclercq JF: Ambulatory sudden cardiac death: mechanisms of production of fatal arrhythmia on the basis of data from 157 cases. Am Heart J 117:151-159,1989.

Beasley H: Hyperthermia associated with ophthalmic surgery. Am. J. Ophthalmol 77:76-79, 1974

Beck CS. Two cardiac compression triads. JAMA 1935; 104: 714-716.

Benomof JL: Anesthesia for Thoracic Surgery (2nd ed). W.B. Saunders company, 1994

Berbari EF, Cockerill FR, Steckelberg JM: Infective endocarditis due to unusual or fastidious microorganisms. Mayo Clin Proc 72(6):532-542, 1997.

Berger PB, Ryan TJ: Inferior myocardial infarction: high-risk subgroups. Circulation 81:401-411,1990.

Berhman, RE; Vaughn, VC: Nelson Textbook of Pediatrics. 15th edition. WB Saunders Company. 1996.

Berkow, R. The Merck Manual. 15th ed. Rahway: Merck Sharp & Dohme Research Laboratories; 1987.

Bernard SL, Llull R, Nyström NA. Hand trauma. In Peitzman AB, Rhodes M, Schwab CW, Yealy DM (eds): The Trauma Manual, p. 315-330. Philadelphia: Lippincott-Raven, 1998.

Bengtston JR, Kaplan AJ, Pieper KS, et al. Prognosis in cardiogenic shock after acute myocardial infarction in the interventional area. J Am Coll Cardiol 1992; 20: 1482-1489.

Bernstein, Ralph, and Rosenberg, Andrew D. Manual of Orthopedic Anesthesia and Related Pain Syndromes. Churchill Livingstone, 1993.

Bickell WH, Wall MJ Jr, Pepe PE, Martin RR, Ginger VF, Allen MK, Mattox KL. Immediate versus delayed fluid resuscitation for hypotensive patient presenting with penetrating torso injuries. N Engl J Med 1994; 331: 1105-1109.

Blomquist IK, Bayer AS: Life-threatening deep fascial space infections of the head and neck. Infect Dis Clin N America 2 (1):237, 1988.

Bochner BS, Lichtenstein LM. Anaphylaxis. N Engl J Med 1991; 324:1785-90.

Boeke AJ, de Lange JJ, van Druenen B, Langemeijer JJ: Effect of antagonizing residual neuromuscular block by neostigmine and atropine on postoperative vomiting. Br J Anaesth 72:654-6, 1994

Bonica JJ, ed., Management of Pain 2nd Edition, Lea and Febiger, 1990

Bone LB, Johnson KD, Weigelt J, et al. Early versus delayed stabilization of femoral fractures: a prospective randomized study. J Bone Joint Surg 71:336, 1989.

Boone D, Peitzman A: Abdominal Injury, in The Trauma Manual: eds. Peitzman, Rhodes, Schwab and Yealey,. Lippincott-Raven, 1998.

Bork, K. *Diagnosis and Treatment of Common Skin Diseases*. Philadelphia: WB Saunders Company; 1988.

Bradley SF, Kauffman CA: Infections associated with vascular catheters: In Rippe JM, Irwin RS, Fink MP, Cerra FB (eds): Intensive Care Medicine, 3rd ed, 1141-1152. Boston: Little, Brown & Co., 1996.

Bradley, WG. *Neurology In Clinical Practice*. Newtown: Butterworth-Heineman; 1996.

Brant SH, Brugadu P, DeZwaan C, et al. Right and left ventricular ejection fraction in acute inferior wall infarction with or without st segment elevation in lead V_4R. J Am Coll Cardiol 1984; 4: 940-944.

Breslow MJ, Miller CF, Parker SD, Walman AT, Rogers MC: Changes in T wave morphology following anesthesia and surgery: a common recovery room phenomenon. Anesthesiology 64:398-402, 1986

Britto,J, Demling,RH: Aspiration Lung Injury. New Horizons 1:435-439, 1993

Brod, SA. *Multiple Sclerosis: clinical presentation, diagosis of treatment*. American Family Physician; 1996.

Brown CG, Werman HA, Davis EA, et al: The effect of high-dose phenylephrine versus epinephrine on regional cerebral blood flow during CPR. *Ann Emerg Med* 16:743,1987.

Brown, David L., and Factor, David A. <u>Regional Anesthesia and Analgesia</u>. W. B. Saunders Company, 1996.

Brown TM, Iannone LA, Gordon DF, et al. Percutaneous myocardial reperfusion (PMR) reduces mortality in acute myocardial infarction (MI) complicated by cardiogenic shock. Circulation 1985; 72, Suppl iii: 307.

Bryson, PD. *Comprehensive Review in Toxicology*. 2nd ed. Aspen Publishers, Inc; 1989

Buckley N: Regional vs. general anaesthesia in orthopaedics. Can J Anaesth 40:R104-R112, 1993

Buettner J, Wresch K, Klose R: Postdural puncture headache: comparison of 25-gauge Whitacre and Quincke needles. Regional Anesthesia 18:66-9, 1993

Bullock, R. *Guidelines for the Management of Severe Head Injury*. New York: Brain Trauma Foundation; 1995.

Bunker ML, McWilliams. Caffeine content of common beverages. J. Am. Diet. Assoc 74: 28-32, 1979.

Busse WW: Respiratory infections: Their role in airway responsiveness and the pathogenesis of asthma. J Allergy Clin Immunol 85:671-83, 1990

Cahill, B.C. and Ingbar, D.H., Massive hemoptysis. Clinics in Chest Medicine. 1994. 15: 147.

Capan LM, Bruce DL, Patel KP et al. Succinylcholine-induced postoperative sore throat. Anesth 59:202-6, 1983

Capone AC, Safar P, Stezoski W, Tisherman S, Peitzman, Improved outcome with fluid restriction in treatment of uncontrolled hemorrhagic shock. J Am Coll Surg 1995; 180: 49-56.

Carroll NV, Miederhoff PA, Cox FM, Hirsch JD: Costs incurred by outpatient surgery centers in managing postoperative nausea and vomiting. J Clin Anesth 6:364-9, 1994

Cepeda MS, Gonzalez F, Granados V, Cuervo R, Carr DB: Incidence of nausea and vomiting in outpatients undergoing general anesthesia in relation to selection of intraoperative opioid. J Clin Anesth 8: 324-328, 1996

Cesarini M, Torrielli R, Lahaye F, et al: Sprottte needle for intrathecal anesthesia for cacesarian section:Incidence of postdural puncture headache. Anaesthesia 45:6565, 1990.

Chernick, V; Kendig, EL: Disorders of the Respiratory Tract in Children. Sixth edition. WB Saunders Company. 1998.

Chow AW, Roser SM, Brady FA: Orofacial odotogenic infections. Ann Intern Med 88:392, 1978.

Cintron GB, Hernandez E, Linares E, Aranda JM. Bedside recognition, incidence and clinical course of right ventricular infarction. Am J Cardiol 1981; 47: 224-227.

Civetta JM, Taylor RW, Kirby RR: Critical Care (ed 3). New York, NY, Lippincott-Raven Publishers, 1997

Claxton AR, McGuire G, Chung F, Cruise C: Evaluation of morphine versus fentanyl for postoperative analgesia after ambulatory surgical procedures. Anesth Analg 84:509-514, 1997

Clements SD, Story WE, Hurst JW, et al Ruptured papillary muscle, a complication of myocardial Infarction: Clinical presentation, diagnosis and treatment. Clin Cardiol 1985; 8: 93-103.

Code WE, Yip RW, Rooney ME, Browne PM, Hertz T: Preoperative naproxen sodium reduces postoperative pain following arthroscopic knee surgery. Can J Anaesth 41:98-101, 1994

Cohen MM, Cameron CB: Should you cancel the operation when a child has an upper respiratory tract infection? Anesth Analg 72:282-288,1991

Colonna-Romano P, Shapiro BE: Unintentional dural puncture and prophylactic epidural blood patch in obstetrics, Anesth Analg 1989;69:522

Conroy, Joanne M. and Dorman, B. Hugh. Anesthesia for Orthopedic Surgery. Ravin Press, 1994.

"Controversies in Pulmonary Artery Catheterization," New Horizons vol. 5, #3, Aug 1997.

Cook, Clinical Ped 1992, Rall, The pharmac basis of therap, 1990:345-82

Cook DJ et al.: Nosocomial pneumonia and the role of gastric pH. A meta-analysis. Chest 100:7, 1991.

Cook, D.R. & Davis, P.J. Anesthetic Principles for Organ Transplantation. New York: Raven Press, Ltd., 1994.

Cooper, JAD: Drug-Related Pulmonary Diseases, in Bone,RC (ed): *Pulmonary and Critical Care Medicine*, 1993, pp 1-9,Part M, Chap 8

Cooper,JAD: Drug-Induced Lung Disease. Advances in Internal Medicine 42:231-267,1997

Cork RC, Vaughan RW, Bentley JB: General anesthesia for morbidly obese patients-An examination of postoperative outcomes. Anesthesiology 54:310-13, 1981

Cote CJ, Goudsouzian NG, Liu LMP, Dedrick DF, SzyFelbein SK. Assessment of risk factors related to acid aspiration syndrome in pediatric patients - gastric pH and residual volume. Anesthesiology 56:70-72, 1982

Cousins, Michael J., and Bridenbaugh, Phillip O. eds. Neural Blockade. 2nd ed. J. B. Lippincott, 1988.

Cranefield PF, Aronson RS: Torsade de pointes and other pause-induced ventricular tachycardias: The short-long-short sequence and early afterdepolarizations. *PACE* 11:670-677,1988.

Crawford M, Lerman J, Christensen S, Farrow-Gilespie A: Effects of duration of fasting on gastric fluid pH and volume in healthy children. Anesth Analg 71:400-03, 1990

Cullom, RD Jr. *The Wills Eye Manual: Office and Emergency Room Diagnosis and Treatment of Eye Disease.* 2nd ed. Philadelphia: JB Lippencott Co.; 1994.

Cummins RO, editor: Defibrillation. *Textbook of Advanced Cardiac Life Support* 4-1,1997.

Cummins RO: From concept to standard-of-care? Review of the clinical experience with automated external defibrillators. *Ann Emerg Med* 18:1269-1275,1989.

Cummins RO, editor: Essentials of ACLS. *Textbook of Advanced Cardiac Life Support* 1-23,1997.

Cummins RO, editor: Invasive therapeutic techniques. *Textbook of Advanced Cardiac Life Support* 14-1,1997.

Cummins RO, editor: Invasive therapeutic techniques. *Textbook of Advanced Cardiac Life Support* 14-3,1997.

Cummins RO, editor: Special resuscitation situations. *Textbook of Advanced Cardiac Life Support* 11-9,1997.

Dajani AS, Taubert KA, Wilson W, Bolger AF, et al: Prevention of bacterial endocarditis: Recommendations by the American Heart Association. JAMA 277(22):1794-1801, 1997.

David R. Goldman, Frank H. Brown and David M. Guarnieri (eds.): Perioperative Medicine. New York, McGraw-Hill Inc., 1994.

Davis PJ, McGowan FX Jr., Landsman I, Maloney K, Hoffmann P: Effect of antiemetic therapy on recovery and hospital discharge time. A double-blind assessment of ondansetron, droperidol, and placebo in pediatric patients undergoing ambulatory surgery. Anesthesiology 83:956-60, 1995

DeGowin, EL. *Bedside Diagnostic Examination.* 4th ed. New York: Macmillan Publishing Co. Inc; 1981.

Dell'llalia LJ, Starling MR, Crawford MH, et al. Right ventricular infarction: Identification by hemodynamic measurements before and after volume loading and correlation with noninvasive techniques. J Am Coll Cardiol 1984; 4: 931-939.

Dershwitz M, Randel GI, Rosow CE, Fragen RJ, Connors PM, Librojo ES, Shaw DL, Peng AW, Jamerson BD: Initial clinical experience with remifentanil, a new opioid metabolized by esterases. Anesth Analg 81: 619-623, 1995

De Wood MA, Notske RN, Hensley GR, et al. Intraaortic Balloon counterpulsation With and without reperfusion for myocardial infarction shock. Circulation 1980; 61: 1105-1112.

Dexter F, Tinker JH: Comparisons between desflurane and isoflurane or propofol on time to following commands and time to discharge. A meta-analysis. Anesthesiology 83:77-82, 1995

Ding Y, Fredman B, White PF: Use of ketorolac and fentanyl during outpatient gynecologic surgery. Anesth Analg 77:205-10, 1993

Duke, J. Anesthesia Secrets (Second Edition). Philadelphia: Hanley & Belfus, Inc., 2000.

Ebert TJ, Muzi M: Sympathetic hyperactivity during desflurane anesthesia in healthy volunteers: a comparison with isoflurane. Anesth 79:444-53, 1993

Edelstein PH: Legionnaire's disease. Clin Infect Dis 16:741, 1993.

Escolano F, Sierra P, Ortiz JC, Cabrera JC, Castano J: The efficacy and optimum time of administration of ranitidine in the prevention of acid aspiration syndrome. Anaesthesia 51:182, 1996

Fabian T, Croce M: Abdominal Trauma, including indications for celiotomy. In Feliciano, Moore, Mattox (eds): Trauma, 3rd ed. Stamford, CT: Appleton and Lange, 1996.

Farley MM et al.: Invasive Haemophilus influenzae disease in adults. Ann Intern Med 116:806, 1992.

Farraj RS, McCully RB, Oh JK, Smith TF. Mycoplasma-associated pericarditis. Mayo Clin Proc 72(1):33-36, 1997.

Faust, R.J., Cucchiara, R.F., Rose, S.H., Spackman, T.N., Wedel, D.J. & Wass, C.T. Anesthesiology Review (3rd ed.). New York: Churchill Livingstone, Inc., 2002.

Feliciano DV, Moore EE, Mattox KL (eds): Trauma, 3rd ed, 345-440. Stamford: Appleton & Lange, 1996.

Ferrante FM, Ostheimer GW, Covino BG, eds. Patient Controlled Analgesia, Blackwell Scientific Publications, 1990

Fishman, AP, editor. Pulmonary Diseases and Disorders, 3rd Edition. New York: McGraw-Hill, 1998.

Fitzpatrick, TB. Color Atlas and Synopsis of Clinical Dermatology. New York: McGraw-Hill Publishing Company; 1990.

Fleisher LA, Barash PG: Preoperative cardiac evaluation for noncardiac surgery: A functional approach. Anesth Analg 74:586-598,1992

Fleming DW, Cochi SL, Hightower AW, et al: Childhood upper respiratory tract infections. To what degree is incidence affected by day care attendance? Pediatrics 79:56-60, 1987

Flomenbaum, Neal. Emergency Diagnostic Testing. 2nd ed. St. Louis: Mosby-Year Book, Inc.; 1995.

Fonda J, et al. The medical and economic impact of severely injured lower extremities. J Trauma 28: 1270-2, 1988.

Forrester JS, Diamond G, Chatterjee K, Swan JC. Medical therapy of acute myocardial infarction by application of hemodynamic subsets (parts 1 and 2). N Engl J Med 1976; 295; 1356-1362 and 1204-1213.

Galford, R.E. Problems in Anesthesiology: Approach to Diagnosis. Boston: Little, Brown and Company, 1992.

Gambling, D.R. & Douglas, M.J. Obstetric Anesthesia and Uncommon Disorders. Philadelphia: W.B. Saunders Company, 1998.

George, RB, Light, RW, Matthay, MA, Matthay, RA. Chest Medicine: Essentials of Pulmonary and Critical Care Medicine, 3rd Edition. Baltimore: Williams & Wilkins, 1995.

Gibbon JH, Hopkinson M, Churchill ED. Changes in circulation produced by gradual occlusion of pulmonary artery. J Clin Invest 1932; 11: 543-553.

Gilbert SS, Easy WR, Fitch WW: The effect of pre-operative oral fluids on morbidity following anesthesia for minor surgery. Anaesthesia 50:79-81, 1995

Gooch, CL. Neuroimmunology for Clinicians. Rolak & Harati; 1996.

Goodman AG, Rall TW, Nies AS, Taylor P. ìGoodman and Gilmanís the Pharmacological Basis of Therapeutics,î 8th ed. Pergamon Press: New York, 1990.

Green G, Jonsson L: Nausea: the most important factor determining length of stay after ambulatory anaesthesia. A comparative study of isoflurane and/or propofol techniques. Acta Anaesthesiol Scand 37:742-6, 1993

Greenfield Lj. Surgery Scientific Principles and Practice. J.B. Lippincott Company, Philadelphia, 1993. Chps 2, 20.,pp. 38-62 and 692.

Gregory R, et al. The mangled extremity (M.E.S.): A severity grading system for multisystem injury of the extremity. *J Trauma* 25: 1147-50, 1985.

Grippi, MA. Pulmonary Pathophysiology. Philadelphia, J. B. Linpincott Company, 1995.

Guberman BA, Fowler NO, Engel PJ, et al. Cardiac tamponade in medical patients Circulation 1981; 64: 633-640.

Guerci AD, Gerstenblith G, Brinker JA, et al. A randomized trail of intravenous tissue plasminogen activator for acute myocardial infarction with subsequent randomization to elective coronary angioplasty. N Engl J Med 1987; 317; 1613-1618.

Guyton AC. Textbook of Medical Physiology. 10th ed. W.B. Saunders Co., Philadelphia, 2000.

Hands ME, Rutherford JD, Muller JE, et al. The in-hospital development of cardiogenic shock after myocardial infarction: Incidence, predictors of occurrence, outcome and prognostic factors. J Am Coll Cardiol 1989; 14: 40-46.

Hannallah RS, Patel RI: Low-dose intramuscular ketamine for anesthesia pre-induction in young children undergoing brief outpatient procedures. Anesthesiology 70:598-600, 1989

Hannalah RS, Britton JT, Schafer PG, Patel RI, Norden JM: Propofol anaesthesia in paediatric ambulatory patients: a comparison with thiopentone and halothane. Can J Anaesth 41:12-8, 1994

Harnarayan C, Bennett MA, Pentecost BL, Brewer DB. Quantitative study of infarcted myocardium in cardiogenic shock. Br Heart J 1970; 32: 728-32.

Haynes SR, Morton NS: The laryngeal mask airway: A review of its use in paediatric anaesthesia. Ped Anes 3:65-73, 1993

Healy TEJ, Cohn PJ, *Wyllie and Churchill Davidsons, A Practice of Anesthesia*, Sixth Edition, Edward Arnold, London 1995.

Heath PJ, Kennedy DJ, Ogg TW, et al: Which intravenous induction agent for day surgery? A comparison of propofol, thiopentone, methohexitone and etomidate. Anaesthesia 43:365-368, 1988

Helman JD, Leung JM, Bellows WH, et al: The risk of myocardial ischemia in patients receiving desflurane versus sufentanil anesthesia in patients undergoing coronary artery bypass graft surgery. The S.P.I. Research Group. Anesthesiology 77:47-62 , 1992

Hermens JM, Bennet MJ, Hirshman C Anesthesia for laser surgery. Anesth Analg 62:218, 1983

Hensley, F.A. Jr. & Martin, D.E. A Practical Approach to Cardiac Anesthesia (Second Edition). New York: Little, Brown and Company, 1995.

Hensley, F.A. Jr. & Martin, D.E. The Practice of Cardiac Anesthesia. Boston: Little, Brown and Company, 1990.

Hoerster, W., Kreuscher, H., Niesel, H.Chr. & Zenz, M. Regional Anesthesia (Second Edition). St. Louis: Mosby-Year Book, Inc., 1990.

Holesha W, Dziura-Murauski J: Extrapyramidal side effects of metoclopramide in outpatient surgery patients. J Post Anesth Nurs 9:107-10, 1994

Holland, JF. *Cancer Medicine*. 4th ed. Baltimore: Williams & Wilkins; 1997.

Hughes CW: Anesthesia for Remote Locations. In: Bell C, Hughes Cw, Oh TH, eds. The Pediatric Anes Handbook. St Louis:Mosby Year Book, Inc.:485-96, 1991

Idris A, Staples E, O'Brien D, et al: End-tidal carbon dioxide during extremely low cardiac output. *Ann Emerg Med* 23:568-572,1994.

Isner JM, Roberts WC. Right Venticular infarction comoplicating left ventricular infarction secondary to coronary heart disease. Am J Cardiol 1978; 42: 885-894.

Johannsen G, Andersen M, Juhl B: The effect of general anesthesia on the haemodynamic events during laparoscopy with CO2-insufflation. Acta Anaesthesiol Scand 33:132-36, 1989

Johansen K, et al. Objective criteria accurately predict amputation following lower extremity trauma. *J Trauma* 30: 568-71, 1990.

Johnson SA, Scanlon PJ, Loeb HS, et al. Treatment of cardiogenic shock in myocardial infarction by intraaortic balloon counterpulsation and surgery. Am J Med 1977; 93: 687-692.

Jones T, Isaacson JH:Preoperative screening: What tests are necessary? Cliv Clin J of Med 62(6):374-8, 1995

Kalenda Z: The capnogram as a guide to the efficacy of cardiac massage. *Resuscitation* 6:259-263,1978.

Kane JM. Compartment syndrome. In Peitzman AB, Rhodes M, Schwab CW, Yealy DM (eds): The Trauma Manual, p. 315-330. Philadelphia: Lippincott-Raven, 1998.

Kannel WB: Prevalence and natural history of electrocardiographic left ventricular hypertrophy. Am J Med 26:4-11, 1983

Kaplan, HI. *Comprehensive Textbook pf Psychiatry/VI*. 6th ed. Vol. 1.

Katz J, Benumof J, Kadis LB, *Anesthesia and Uncommon Diseases*, Third Edition, Saunders Company, Philadelphia 1990.

Kearney RA, Eisen HJ, Wolf JE: Nonvalvular infections of the Cardiovascular system. Ann Intern Med 121(3):219-230, 1994.

Keenan RL, Boyan CP: Cardiac arrest due to anesthesia: A study of incidence and causes. *JAMA* 253:2373,1985.

Keeter S, Benator RM, Weinberg SM, Hartenberg M: Sedation in pediatric CT: National survey of current pratice. Radiology 175:745-52, 1990

Kennedy JW, Gensini GG, Timmis GC, Maynard C. Acute myocardial infarction Treated with intracoronary streptokinase: A report of the Society for Cardiac Angiography. Am J Cardiol 1985; 55: 871-877.

Khambatta HJ, Sonntag H, Larsen R et al. Global and regional myocardial blood flow and metabolism during equipotent halothane and isoflurane anesthesia in patients with coronary artery disease. Anesth Analg 67: 936-42, 1988

Killenberg, P.G. & Clavien, P. Medical Care of the Liver Transplant Patient (Second Edition). Malden: Blackwell Science, Inc., 2001.

Killip T., Kimball JT. Treatment of myocardial infarction in a coronary care unit. Am J Cardiol 1967; 20 457-464.

Kinch JW, Ryan TJ: Right ventricular infarction. *N Engl J Med* 330:1211-1217,1994.

Kirkland LL, Taylor RW. Pericardiocentesis. Critical Care Clinics 1992; 8:699-712.

Koenig, K. *Clinical Emergency Medicine*. New York: McGraw-Hill; 1996.

Klug D, Lacroix D, Savoye C, Goullard L, et al: Systemic infection related to endocarditis on pacemaker leads: Clinical presentation and management. Circulation 95(8):2098-2107, 1997.

Lampotang S, Nyland ME, Gravenstein N: The cost of wasted anesthetic gases [Abstract]. Anesth Analg 71:s151, 1991

Langer JC, Shandling B, Rosenberg M: Intraoperative Bupivacaine during outpatient hernia repair in children: A randomized double blind trial. J Pediatr Surg 22:267-270, 1987

L, Bates ER, Pitt B, et al. Percutaneous transluminal coronary angioplasty improves survival in acute myocardial infarction complicated by cardiogenic shock. Circulation 1988; 78:1345-1351.

Leaverton, PE. *A Review of Biostatistics*. 3rd ed. Boston: Little Brown and Company; 1986.

Lerman J, David PJ, Welborn LG, Orr RJ, Rabb M, Carpenter R, Motoyama E, Hannallah R, Haberkem CM: Induction , recovery, and safety characteristics of sevoflurane in children undergoing ambulatory surgery. A comparison with halothane. Anesthesiology 84:1332-1340, 1996

Levin, DL; Morris, FC: Essentials of Pediatric Intensive Care. Quality Medical Publishing, Inc. 1990.

Levine MF, Spahr-Schopfer LA, Hartley E, Lerman J, MacPherson B: Oral midazolam premedication in children: the minimum time interval for separation from parents. Can J Anaesth 40:726, 1993

Levy JH. Anaphylactic Reactions in Anesthesia and Intensive Care. Second Edition. Butterworth-Heinemann Publishers, 1992.

Lineberger CF, Ginsberge B, Franiak RJ, Glass PS: Narcotic agonist and antagonists. Anesthesiology Clinics North Am 12:65-89, 1994

Loach, Alan. Orthopedic Anesthesia. 2nd ed. Hodder and Stoughton, 1994.

London MJ, Hollenberg M, Wong MG, et al: Intraoperative myocardial ischemi localization by continuous 12-lead electrocardiography. Anesthesiology 69:232-41, 1988

Lorenz W, Ennis M, Doenicke A, Dick W. Perioperative Uses of Histamine Antagonists. J Clin Anesth 1990; 2:345-360.

Lorh DG, Sahn S Postextubation pulmonary edema following anesthesia induced by upper airway obstruction: Are certain patients at increased risk? Chest 90:802-5, 1986

Ly B, Arnesen H, Eie H, Hol R. A controlled clinical trail of streptokinase and heparin in the treatment of major pulmonary embolism. Acta Med Scand 1978; 203: 465-470.

Lyn DJ, Woda RP, Mendell JR. Respiratory dysfunction in muscular dystrophy and other myopathies. Clin Chest Med 1994; 15:661-74.

Lysak SZ, Anderson PT, Carithers RA, DeVane GG, Smith ML, Bates GW: Postoperative effects of fentanyl, ketorolac, and piroxicam as analgesics for outpatient laparoscopic procedures. Obstet Gynecol 83(2):270-5, 1994

Magahon JP, Rob GT, Dublin A. Fractures of the Scapula. J Trauma 20, 1980.

Malviya S, Swartz J, Lerman J: Are all preterm infants younger than 60 weeks postconceptual age at risk for postanesthetic apnea? Anesthesiology 78:1076-81, 1993

Marrie TJ: Community-acquired pneumonia. Clin Infect Dis 18:501, 1994.

Marriott, HJL. *Practical Electrocardiography*. 7th ed. Baltimore: Williams and Wilkins; 1983.

Martin C, Boisson C, Haccoun M, Mege JL. Patterns of cytokine evolution (tumor necrosis factor-alpha and interieukin-6) after septic shock, hemorrhagic shock, and severe trauma. Crit Care Med 1997; 25: 1813-1819.

Martin LD, Pasternak LR, Pudimat M Total intravenous anesthesia with propofol in pediatric patients outside the operating room. Anesth Analg 74:609-612, 1992

Martin TM, Nicolson SC, Bargas MS: Propofol anesthesia reduces emesis and airway obstruction in pediatric outpatients. Anesth Analg 76:144-8, 1993

Maynard N, Bihari D, Beale R, Smithies M, Baldock G, Mason R, McColl I. Assessment of splanchinic oxygenation by gastric tonometry in patients with acute circulatory failure. JAMA 1993; 270: 1203-1210.

MayoSmith MF, Hirsch PJ, Wodzinski SF, Schiffman FP: Acute epiglottitis in adults. An eight-hyear experience in the state of Rhode Island. N Engl J Med 314(18): 1133, 1986

McDowall RH: Anesthesia considerations for pediatric cancer. Sem Surg Oncol 9:478-488, 1993

Mcintyre KM, Sashara AA. The hemodynamic response to pulmonary embolism in patients without prior cardiopulmonary disease. Am J Cardiol 1971; 28: 288-294.

McNally, P.R. GI/Liver Secrets. Philadelphia: Hanley & Belfus, Inc., 1996.

Meduri GU: Diagnosis of ventilator-associated pneumonia. Infect Dis clin North AM 7:295, 1993.

Meinertz T, Kasper W, Schumacher M, et al. The German multicenter trial of anisoylated plasminogen streptokinase activator Complex versus heparin for acute myocardial infarction. Am J Cardiol 1988; 62: 347-352.

Melnick BM: Extrapyramidal reactions to low-dose droperidol. Anesthesiology 69:424-426, 1988

Mendel HG, Guarnieri KM, Sundt LM, Torjman MC: The effects of ketorolac and fentanyl on postoperative vomiting and analgesic requirements in children undergoing strabismus surgery. Anesth Analg 80: 1129-1133, 1995

Miller, R.D. Anesthesia (Fifth Edition), Volume 1. Philadelphia: Churchill Livingstone, 2000.

Miller J, Tresch D, Horwitz L, et al: The precordial thump. *Ann Emerg Med* 13:791-794,1984.

Minami H, McCallum RW: The physiology and pathophysiology of gastric emptying in humans. Gastroenterology 86:1592-610, 1984

Mitchell AA, Louik C, Lacouture P, Slone D, Goldman P, Shapiro S: Risks to children from computed tomographic scan premedication. JAMA 247:2385-88, 1982

Moore DC, Batra MS: The components of an effective test dose prior to epidural block. Anesthesiology 55:643-6, 1981

Moore, K.L. Clinically Oriented Anatomy (Third Edition). Baltimore: Williams & Wilkins, 1992.

Moore RA, McNicholas KW, Warran SP: Atlantoaxial subluxation with symptomatic spinal cord compression in a child with Down's syndrome. Anesth Analg 66:89-90, 1987

Mordis CJ: Anesthesia for magnetic resonance imaging. Anesth Review 18:15-20, 1991

Morgan, G.E. Jr., Mikhail, M.S. & Murray, M.J. Clinical Anesthesiology (Second Edition). Stamford: Appleton & Lange, 2002.

Motoyama, E.K. & Davis, P.J. Smith's Anesthesia for Infants and Children (Sixth Edition). New York: Mosby, 1996.

Mulroy, Michael F. Regional Anesthesia: An illustrated Procedural Guide. Little, Brown and Company, 1996

Nagelhout, J., Zaglaniczny, K. Nurse Anesthesia. 3rd ed., 2004

Narayan, RK. Neurotrauma. New York: McGraw-Hill; 1996.

Neal JM: Management of Postdural Puncture Headaches. Anesthesiology Clinics of North America 10(1): 163-178, 1992.

Nelson, W.E. Textbook of Pediatrics. Philadelphia W.B. Saunders Company, 1984.

Niederman MS et al.: Guidelines for the initial management of adults with community-acquired pneumonia: Diagnosis, assessment of severity, and initial antimicrobial therapy. Am Rev Respir Dis 148:1418, 1993.

Niemann JT, Rosborough JP, Ung S, et al: Coronary perfusion pressure during experimental cardiopulmonary resuscitation. Ann Emerg Med 11:127-131,1982.

Olsson GL, Hallen B: Cardiac arrest during anaesthesia. A computer-aided study in 250543 anaesthetics. Acta Anaesthesiol Scand 31:653,1988.

O'Neill W, Erbel R, Laufer N, et al. Coronary angioplasty therapy of cardiogenic shock complicating acute myocardial infarction. Circulation 1985; 72, Suppl III; 307.

Orkin FK: Economic and regulatory issues. In: White PF, ed. Outpatient anesthesia. New York: Churchill & Livingstone, 87-105, 1990

O'Rourke PP: Out-of-hospital cardiac arrest in pediatric patients: Outcome. Crit Care Med 12:283,1984.

Otto CW, Yakaitis RW, Ewy GA, et al: Comparison of dopamine, dobutamine, and epinephrine in CPR. Crit Care Med 9:640,1981.

Owens TM, Watson WC, Prough DS, Uchida T, Kramer GC. Limiting initial resuscitation of uncontrolled hemorrhage reduces internal bleeding and subsequent volume requirements. J Trauma 1995; 39: 200-207.

Owings JT, Kennedy JP, Blaisdell. FW. Injuries to the extremities. Surgery, Scientific American, 1997.

Paradis NA, Martin GB, Rivers EP, et al: Coronary perfusion pressure and return of spontaneous circulation in human cardiopulmonary resuscitation. JAMA 263:1106,1990.

Patel RI, Hannallah RS: Preoperative screening for pediatric ambulatory surgery: evaluation of a telephone questionnaire method. Anesth Analg 75:258,1992

Patel RI, Hannallah RS: Anesthetic complications following pediatric ambulatory surgery: A 3-year study. Anesth 69:1009-12, 1988

Pedersen T, Eliasen K, Hendriksen E: A prospective study of mortality associated with anaesthesia and surgery: risk indicators of mortality in hospital. Acta Anaesth Scand 37:176,1990

Penn RL and Betts RF: Lower respiratory tract infections (including tuberculosis) In: Reese Re and Betts RF (eds). A Practical Approach to Infectious Diseases, fourth edition. Little, Brown and Company, Boston, New York, Toronto, London.

Petros AJ: Oral ketamine: Its use for mentally retarded adults requiring day care dental treatment. Anaesthesia 46:646-647, 1991

Phillip BK: Drug reversal: benzodiazepine receptors and antagonists. J Clin Anesth 5:46s-51s, 1993

Phillip BK, Kallar SK, Bogetz MS, Scheller MS, Wetchler BV: A multicenter comparison of maintenance and recovery sevoflurane or isoflurane for adult ambulatory anesthesia. The Sevoflurane Multicenter Ambulatory Group. Anesth Analg 83: 314-319, 1996

Philip BK: Patients assessment of ambulatory anesthesia and surgery. J Clin Anesth 4:355-8, 1992

Phillips S, Hutchinson S, Davidson T: Preoperative drinking does not affect gastric contents. Br J Anesth 70:6-9,1993

Phillips T. Extremities. In Ivatury RR, Cayten CG (eds): The Textbook of Penetrating Trauma, p. 319-332. Philadelphia: Williams & Wilkins, 1996.

Physicians' Desk Reference. 50th ed. Oradell: Medical Economics Company Inc; 1996.

Pirolo JS, Hutchins GM, Moore GW. Infarct Expansion: Pathological analysis of 204 patients with a single myocardial infarct. J Am Coll Cardiol 1986; 7: 349-354.

Plantz, SH. *Emergency Medicine*. Baltimore: Wiiliams & Wilkins; 1998.

Powell MA, McMahon D, Peitzman AB: Thoracic injury: In Peitzman AB, Rhodes M, Schwab CW, Yealy DM (eds): The Trauma Manual, 199-225. Philadelphia: Lippincott-Raven, 1998.

Preoperative fasting time: Is the traditional policy changing? Results of a national survey. Anesth & Analg 83:123-8, 1996

Prewitt RM, Downers AM, Gu S, et al. Effects of hydralazine and increased cardiac output on recombinant tissue plaminogen activator induced thrombolysis in canine pulmonary embolism. Chest 1991; 99: 708-714.

Pugsley WB, Baldwin T, Trasure T, et al: Low energy level internal defibrillation during cardiopulmonary bypass. *Eur J Cardiothorac Surg* 3:278,1989.

Puhringer FK, Khuenl-Brady KS, Koller J, Mitterschiffthaler G: Evaluation of the endotracheal intubating conditions of rocuronium and succinylcholine in outpatient surgery. Anesth Analg 75:37, 1992

Radford MJ, Johnson RA, Daggett WM. Ventricular septal rupture: A review of clinical and physiologic features and an analysis of survival. Circulation 1981; 64: 545-553.

Raj, P. Prithvi. <u>Clinical Practice of Regional Anesthesia</u>. Churchill Livingstone, 1991.

Raj PP, Practical Management of Pain, 2nd Ed, Mosby-YearBook, Inc. 1992

Ramoska E, Sacchetti AD: Propanolol-induced hypertension in treatment of cocaine intoxication. Ann Emerg Med 14:112-13, 1985

Rasmussen S, Leth A, Kjoller E, Pedersen A. Cardiac rupture in acute myocardial infarction. Acta Med Scand 1979; 205: 11-16.

Ratliff NB, Hackel DB. Combined right and left ventricular infarction: pathogenesis and clinicopathologic correlations. Am J Cardiol 1980; 4:: 217-221.

Robert K. Stoelting and Stephen F. Dierdorf: Anesthesia and Co-Existing Disease. 4th ed. New York, Churchill Livingstone Inc., 2002.

Robbins, SL. *Pathologic Basis of Disease*. 3rd ed. Philadelphia: WB Saunders Company; 1984.

Rogers MC, Tinker JH, Covino BG, and Longnecker DE, *Principles and Practices of Anesthesiology*, Mosby Year Book, Inc., St Louis, Missouri 1993.

Roland, L. *Merritt's Textbook of Neurology*. Williams & Wilkins; 1995.

Rosenblum M, Weller RS, Conard PL, Falvey EA, Gross JB: Ibuprofen provides longer lasting analgesia than fentanyl after laparoscopic surgery. Anesth Analg 73:255-259, 1991

Rosenow,EC: Drug-Induced Pulmonary Disease, in Murray,JF and Nadel,JA (ed): *Textbook of Respiratory Medicine*, 2nd Edition, 1994, pp 2117-2144

Rothenberg DM: Ethical considerations for cardiopulmonary resuscitation. *Anesthesiology Clinics of North America* 13:4,999-1012,1995.

Rothenberg DM, Parnass SM, Litwack K, McCarthy RJ, Newman LM: Efficacy of ephedrine in the prevention of postoperative nausea and vomiting. Anesth Analg 72:58-61, 1991

Rowe, RC. *The Harriet Lane Handbook*. 11th ed. Chicago: Year Book Medical Publishers, Inc; 1987.

Rutherford BD, Hartier GO, McConahay DR, Johnson WL. Direct balloon angioplasty during acute myocardial infarction in patients. Circulation 1985; 72, Suppl III; 308.

Ryan, SJ. *Retina: Medical Retina*. 2nd ed. St. Louis: Mosby-Year Book, Inc.; 1994.

Salvo I, Columbo S, Capocasa T, et al: Pulseoximetry in MRI units. J Clin Anesth 2:65-66, 1990

Sanders AB, Kern KB, Otto CW, et al: End-tidal carbon dioxide monitoring during cardiopulmonary resuscitation: a prognostic indicator for survival. *JAMA* 262:1347-1351,1989.

Sanders AB, Atlas M, Ewy GA, et al: Expired CO_2 as an index of coronary perfusion pressure. *Am J Emerg Med* 3:147-149,1985.

Sanders AB, Kern KB, Ewy GA, et al: Improved resuscitation from cardiac arrest with open-chest massage. *Ann Emerg Med* 13:672-675,1984.

Sanders AB, Kern KB, Atlas M, et al: Importance of the duration of inadequate coronary perfusion pressure on resuscitation from cardiac arrest. *J Am Coll Cardiol* 6:113-118,1985.

Santos DJ, Barrett J, Lachia R, et al: Efficacy of epidural saline patch in preventing post dural puncture headache, Reg Anesth 1986; 11;42(abstract).

Sasyniuk BI: Symposium on the management of ventricular dysrhythmias: concept of reentry versus automaticity. *Am J Cardiol* 54:1A-6A,1984.

Schleien CL, Gelman B, Kuluz JW: Pediatric Cardiopulmonary Resuscitation. *Anesthesiology Clinics of North America* 13:4,943-979,1995.

Sears DH, Leeman MI, O'Donnell RH, et al: Incidence of postdural puncture headache in cesarean section patients using the 24G Sprotte needle. Anesthesiology 73:A1003, 1990

Selvin B: Electroconvulsive therapy-1987. Anesthesiology 67:367-85, 1987

Sloan MH, Conard PF, Karsunky PK, Gross JB: Sevoflurane versus isoflurane: Induction and recovery characteristics with single-breath inhaled inductions of anesthesia. Anesth Analg 82:528-532, 1996

Shapiro M. Abdominal Vascular Injury, in The Trauma Manual: eds. Peitzman, Rhodes, Schwab and Yealey, Lippincott-Raven, 1998.

Sharpe, M.D. & Gelb, A.W. Anesthesia and Transplantation. Boston: Butterworth-Heinemann, 1999.

Sheehan DV, Caycomb JB, Kouretas N: The monoamine oxidase inhibitors: Prescription and patient management. Int J Psychiatric Med 10:99-121, 1980-1981

Sinatra RS, et al, Acute Pain: Mechanisms and Management, Mosby Year Book, 1992

Slaby, F. *Radiographic Anatomy*. New York: John Wiley & Sons; 1990.

Smith I, Van Hemelrijck J, White PF, Shively R: Effects of local anesthesia on recovery after outpatient arthroscopy. Anesth Analg 73:536-539, 1991

Smith RM: Pediatric anesthesia in perspective. Anesthesiology 57:634-46, 1978

Spelina KR, Contes DP, Monk CR, Prys-Roberts C, Norley I, Turtle MJ: Dose requirements of propofol by infusion during nitrous oxide anaesthesia in man. Br J Anaesth 58:1080-84, 1986

Stalker R, Ward RL: Hazards of fiberoptic bronchoscopy. *BMJ* 1:553,1979.

Stevens RA, Urmey WF, Urquhart BL, Kao TC: Back pain after epidural anesthesia with chloroprocaine. Anesthesiology 78:492, 1993

Tetzlaff, J.E. Clinical Orthopedic Anesthesia. Boston: Butterworth-Heinemann, 1995.

Textbook of Neonatal Resuscitation. American Heart Association. 1994.

Textbook of Pediatric Advanced Life Support. Dallas: American Heart Association; 1988.

The child with a runny nose. In: Berry FA, ed. Anesthetic management of difficult and routine pediatric patients. New York: Churchill Livingstone, 1986:349-68

The Hand Examination and Diagnosis. 2nd ed. London: Churchill Livingstone; 1983.

The Hand Primary Care of Common Problems. 2nd ed. London: Churchill Livingstone; 1990.

The International Study Group. In-hospital mortality and clinical course of 20,891 patients with suspected acute myocardial infarction randomized between alteplase and streptokinase with and without heparin. Lancet 1990; 336; 71-75.

Thomas, S.J. & Kramer, J.L. Manual of Cardiac Anesthesia (Second Edition). New York: Churchill Livingstone, 1993.

Weiskopf RB, Moore MA, Eger EI II, et al: Rapid increase in desflurane concentration is associated with greater transient cardiovascular stimulation than with rapid increase in isoflurane concentration in humans. Anesthesiology 80:1035-1045, 1994

Welborn LG, Hannallah RS, Norden JM, Ruttimann UE, Callan CM: Comparison of emergence and recovery characteristics of sevoflurane, desflurane, and halothane in pediatric ambulatory patients. Anesth Analg 83:917-920, 1996

Welborn LG, McGill WA, Hannallah RS, Nisselson CL, Ruttiman UE, Hicks JM: Perioperative blood glucose concentrations in pediatric outpatients. Anesthesiology 65:543-47, 1986

West JB: Respiratory Physiology--the essentials (ed 4). Baltimore, MD, Williams & Wilkins, 1990

White PF: Studies of desflurane in outpatient anesthesia. Anesth Analg 75: 4 Suppl, S47-53;1992

White, PF: Anesthesia: Drug Manual. Philadelphia: W.B. Saunders Company, 1996.

Winnie, Alon P. Plexus Anesthesia. Vol. 1. W. B. Saunders, 1983.

Yacoub OF, Cardona I, Coveler LA, Dodson MG: Carbon dioxide embolism during laparoscopy. Anesthesiolog 57:533-35, 1982

Yoshikawa TT and Quinn W: The aching head: intracranial suppuration due to head and neck infections. Infect Dis Clin N America 2 (1):265, 1988

Zaloga GP, Sager A, Black KW, Prielipp R. Low dose calcium administration increases mortality during septic peritonitis in rats. Circ Shock 1992 37: 226-229.

Zaidan, JR: Initiating electrical therapy for acute intraoperative arrhythmias. *Anesthesiology Clinics of North America* 13:4,817-833,1995.

Zehender M, Kasper W, Kauder E, et al: Right ventricular infarction as an independent predictor of prognosis after acute inferior myocardial infarction. *N Engl J Med* 328:981-988,1993.

Zeni F, Freeman B, Natanson C. Anti-inflammatory theraples to treat sepsis and septic shock: a reassment. Crit Care Med 1997; 25: 1095-1100.

ADDITIONAL REFERENCES:

Woodcock B, Tremper K. Red Blood Cell Substitutes. In evers AS, Maze M (Eds) Anesthetic Pharmacology. Churchill Livingstone. Philadelphia, PA. 2004:913-4.

Norman GR, Streiner DL. PDQ Statistics. 2nd edition. B.C Decker Inc. Hamilton, London, St. Louis. 1999:25.

Rosenthal JA. Statistics and Data Interpretation for the Helping Profession. Wadswarth/ Thomas LearningBelmont, CA 2000: 4-49.

Atlee JL. Arrhythmia, Rhythm Management Devices, and Catheter and Surgical Ablation. In Hensley, Jr. FA, Martin DE, Gravlee GP.(eds): A Practical Approach to Cardiac Anesthesia. 3rd edition. Lippincott Williams & Wilkins, Philadelphia, PA. 2003:80-81.

Spies CD, Rommelspacher H. Alcohol withdrawal in the surgical patient: prevention and treatment. Anesthesia & Analgesia. 1999;88:946-54.

Dobrydnjov I, Axelsson K, Berggren L et al. Intrathecal and oral clonidine as prophylaxis for postoperative alcohol withdrawal syndrome: a randomized double-blinded study. Anesthesia & Analgesia. 2004;98:738-44, table of contents.

Chobanian AV, Bakris GL, Black HR et al. The Seventh Report of the Joint National Committee on Prevention, Detection, Evaluation, and Treatment of High Blood Pressure: the JNC 7 report.[see comment][erratum appears in JAMA. 2003 Jul 9;290(2):197]. Jama. 2003;289:2560-72.

Prys-Roberts C. Isolated systolic hypertension: pressure on the anaesthetist?[see comment]. Anaesthesia. 2001;56:505-10.

Stone JG, Foex P, Sear JW et al. Risk of myocardial ischaemia during anaesthesia in treated and untreated hypertensive patients. British Journal of Anaesthesia. 1988;61:675-9.

Eagle KA, Berger PB, Calkins H et al. ACC/AHA guideline update for perioperative cardiovascular evaluation for noncardiac surgery---executive summary a report of the American College of Cardiology/American Heart Association Task Force on Practice Guidelines (Committee to Update the 1996 Guidelines on Perioperative Cardiovascular Evaluation for Noncardiac Surgery). Circulation. 2002;105:1257-67.

Nicholson G, Pereira AC, Hall GM. Parkinson's disease and anaesthesia.[see comment]. British Journal of Anaesthesia. 2002;89:904-16.

Michelakis ED, Tymchak W, Noga M et al. Long-term treatment with oral sildenafil is safe and improves functional capacity and hemodynamics in patients with pulmonary arterial hypertension. Circulation. 2003;108:2066-9.

Leuchte HH, Schwaiblmair M, Baumgartner RA et al. Hemodynamic response to sildenafil, nitric oxide, and iloprost in primary pulmonary hypertension. Chest. 2004;125:580-6.

Apfel CC, Laara E, Koivuranta M et al. A simplified risk score for predicting postoperative nausea and vomiting: conclusions from cross-validations between two centers. Anesthesiology. 1999;91:693-700.

Salpeter SR, Ormiston TM, Salpeter EE et al. Cardioselective beta-blockers for chronic obstructive pulmonary disease: a meta-analysis. Respiratory Medicine. 2003;97:1094-101.

Pauwels RA, Buist AS, Ma P et al. Global strategy for the diagnosis, management, and prevention of chronic obstructive pulmonary disease: National Heart, Lung, and Blood Institute and World Health Organization Global Initiative for Chronic Obstructive Lung Disease (GOLD): executive summary. Respiratory Care. 2001;46:798-825.

Salpeter SS, Ormiston T, Salpeter E et al. Cardioselective beta-blockers for chronic obstructive pulmonary disease.[see comment]. Cochrane Database of Systematic Reviews. 2002:CD003566.

Poldermans D, Boersma E, Bax JJ et al. The effect of bisoprolol on perioperative mortality and myocardial infarction in high-risk patients undergoing vascular surgery. Dutch Echocardiographic Cardiac Risk Evaluation Applying Stress Echocardiography Study Group.[comment]. New England Journal of Medicine. 1999;341:1789-94.

Mangano DT, Layug EL, Wallace A, Tateo I. Effect of atenolol on mortality and cardiovascular morbidity after noncardiac surgery. Multicenter Study of Perioperative Ischemia Research Group.[comment][erratum appears in N Engl J Med 1997 Apr 3;336(14):1039]. New England Journal of Medicine. 1996;335:1713-20.

Raby KE, Brull SJ, Timimi F et al. The effect of heart rate control on myocardial ischemia among high-risk patients after vascular surgery.[comment]. Anesthesia & Analgesia. 1999;88:477-82.

Urban MK, Markowitz SM, Gordon MA et al. Postoperative prophylactic administration of beta-adrenergic blockers in patients at risk for myocardial ischemia. Anesthesia & Analgesia. 2000;90:1257-61.

Salpeter S, Greyber E, Pasternak G, Salpeter E. Risk of fatal and nonfatal lactic acidosis with metformin use in type 2 diabetes mellitus.[update of Cochrane Database Syst Rev. 2002;(2):CD002967; PMID: 12076461]. Cochrane Database of Systematic Reviews. 2003:CD002967.

Boersma E, Poldermans D, Bax JJ et al. Predictors of cardiac events after major vascular surgery: Role of clinical characteristics, dobutamine echocardiography, and beta-blocker therapy. Jama. 2001;285:1865-73.

Bluman LG, Mosca L, Newman N, Simon DG. Preoperative smoking habits and postoperative pulmonary complications.[see comment]. Chest. 1998;113:883-9.

Egan TD, Wong KC. Perioperative smoking cessation and anesthesia: a review. Journal of Clinical Anesthesia. 1992;4:63-72.

Sorensen LT, Karlsmark T, Gottrup F. Abstinence from smoking reduces incisional wound infection: a randomized controlled trial. Annals of Surgery. 2003;238:1-5.

Gottlieb SO. Cardiovascular benefits of smoking cessation. Heart Disease & Stroke. 1992;1:173-5.

Warner MA, Offord KP, Warner ME et al. Role of preoperative cessation of smoking and other factors in postoperative pulmonary complications: a blinded prospective study of coronary artery bypass patients. Mayo Clinic Proceedings. 1989;64:609-16.

Moller AM, Villebro N, Pedersen T, Tonnesen H. Effect of preoperative smoking intervention on postoperative complications: a randomised clinical trial.[see comment]. Lancet. 2002;359:114-7.

Schwartz KA, Schwartz DE, Pittsley RA et al. A new method for measuring inhibition of platelet function by nonsteroidal antiinflammatory drugs. Journal of Laboratory & Clinical Medicine. 2002;139:227-33.

Horlocker TT, Wedel DJ, Benzon H et al. Regional anesthesia in the anticoagulated patient: defining the risks (the second ASRA Consensus Conference on Neuraxial Anesthesia and Anticoagulation).[see comment]. Regional Anesthesia & Pain Medicine. 2003;28:172-97.

Wilson SH, Fasseas P, Orford JL et al. Clinical outcome of patients undergoing non-cardiac surgery in the two months following coronary stenting.[see comment]. Journal of the American College of Cardiology. 2003;42:234-40.

Smetana G. Preoperative pulmonary assessment of the older adult. Clinics in Geriatric Medicine 2003;19:35-55.

Smetana GW. Preoperative pulmonary evaluation.[see comment]. New England Journal of Medicine. 1999;340:937-44.

Lawrence VA, Dhanda R, Hilsenbeck SG, Page CP. Risk of pulmonary complications after elective abdominal surgery.[see comment]. Chest. 1996;110:744-50.

National Asthma E, Prevention P. National Asthma Education and Prevention Program. Expert Panel Report: Guidelines for the Diagnosis and Management of Asthma Update on Selected Topics--2002.[erratum appears in J Allergy Clin Immunol. 2003 Mar;111(3):466]. Journal of Allergy & Clinical Immunology. 2002;110:S141-219.

ACLS:Principles and Practice Dallas: American Heart Assoc, 2003.

AS Dajani KT, W Wilson, AF Bolger, A Bayer, P Ferrieri, MH Gewitz, and G Zuccaro. Prevention of Bacterial Endocarditis : Recommendations by the American Heart Association. Circulation 1997;96:358-66.

Tiao JY, Semmens JB, Masarei JR, Lawrence-Brown MM. The effect of age on serum creatinine levels in an aging population: relevance to vascular surgery. Cardiovascular Surgery. 2002;10:445-51.

S. Moncada, R.M.J. Palmer, E.A. Higgs, "Nitric oxide-physiology, pathophysiology and pharmacology," Pharmacological Reviews, 43:109-42, 1992

Dorsch and Dorsch: Understanding Anesthesia Equipment, 2nd ed., Copyright 1984 Williams and Wilkens pp.83

Fliser D, Zeier M, Nowack R and Ritz E. Renal functional reserve in healthy elderly people. Journal of the American Society of Nephrology 1993; 3: 1371-1377

Muhleberg W, Platt D. Age dependent changes in the kidneys: pharmacological implications. Gerontology 1999; 45: 243-253
Amar D, Hao Z, Leung DHY et al. Older age is the strongest predictor of postoperative atrial fibrillation. Anesthesiology 2002; 96: 352-356

Lakatta EG. Changes in cardiovascular function with aging. European Heart Journal 1990; II (supplement C): 22-29

Lakatta EG. Cardiovascular aging research: the next horizons. Journal of the American Geriatric Society 1999; 47: 613-625

Klein AL, Leung DY, Murray RD et al. Effects of age and physiologic variables on right ventricular dynamics in normal subjects. American Journal of Cardiology 1999; 84: 440-448

Amar D, Hao Z, Leung DHY et al. Older age is the strongest predictor of postoperative atrial fibrillation. Anesthesiology 2002; 96: 352-356

Priebe HJ. The aged cardiovascular risk patient. British Journal of Anaesthesia 2001; 86: 897-898
Lakatta EG. Changes in cardiovascular function with aging. European Heart Journal 1990; II (supplement C): 22-29

Olivetti G, Melissari M, Capasso JM, Anversa P. Cardiomyopathy of the aging human heart. Myocyte loss and relative cellular hypertrophy. Circulation Research 1991; 68: 1560-1568

Janssen JP, Pace JC and Nice LP. Physiological changes in respiratory function associated with ageing. European Respiration Journal 1999; 13:197-205

Zeeh J and Platt D. The aging liver: structure and functional changes and their consequences for drug treatment in old age. Gerontology 2002; 48: 121-127

Seaman DS. Adult living donor transplantation: current status. Journal of Clinical Gastroenterology 2001; 33: 97-106

Fielding RA. The role of progressive resistance training and nutrition in the preservation of lean body mass in the elderly. Journal of the American College of Nutrition 1995; 14: 587-594

Wilmore DW. The metabolic management of the critically ill., pp28. New York: Plenum 1977

Schwartz RS, Jaeger LF and Veith RC. The importance of body composition to the increase in plasma norepinephrine appearance in elderly men. Journal of Gerontology 1987; 42: 546-551

Feldmann RD, Limbird LE, Nadeau J et al. Alterations in leukocyte beta-receptor affinity with aging: a potential explanation for altered beta-adrenergic sensitivity in the elderly. New England Journal of Medicine 1984; 310: 815-819

Schwartz RS, Jaeger LF and Veith RC. The thermic effect of feeding in older men: the importance of the sympathetic nervous system. Metabolism 1990;39:
733-737
Kerckoffs DAJM, Blaak EE, van Baak M and Saris WHM, Effect of aging on beta-adrenergically mediated thermogenesis in men. Journal of Applied Physiology 1998; 274: E1075-1079

Vaughan MS, Vaughan RW, Cork RC. Postoperative hypothermia in adults: relationship of age, anesthesia, and shivering to rewarming. Anesth Analg 1981; 60:746-751.

Rooke GA, Robinson BJ. Cardiovascular and autonomic nervous system aging. Problems in Anesthesia. 1997; 9(4):482-497.

White PF. Anesthetic techniques for the elderly outpatient. Int Anesthesiol Clin. 1988; 26(2):105-111.

Schnider TW, Minto CF, Shafer SL, et al. The influence of age on propofol pharmacodynamics. Anesthesiology. 1999; 90:1502-1516.

Dundee JW, Robinson FP, McCollum JSC, Patterson CC. Sensitivity to propofol in the elderly. Anaesthesia. 1986; 41:482-485.

Hilgenberg JC. Inhalation and intravenous drugs in the elderly patient. Seminars in Anesthesia 1986; 5:44-53.

Rampil IJ, Lockhart SH, Zwass MS, et al. Clinical characteristics of desflurane in surgical patients: Minimum alveolar concentration. *Anesthesiology.* 1991; 74:429-433

Wollner L, McCarthy ST, Soper NDW, et al. Failure of cerebral autoregulation as a cause of brain dysfunction in the elderly. Br Med J. 1979; 1:1117-1118.

Kobayashi H, Okada K, Yamashita K. Incidence of silent lacunar lesion in normal adults and its relation to cerebral blood flow and risk factors. Stroke. 1991; 22:1379-1383.

Kario K, Matsuo T, Kobayashi H, et al. Nocturnal fall of blood pressure and silent cerebrovascular damage in elderly hypertensive patients. Hypertension. 1996; 27:130-135.

Kohara K, Jiang Y, Igase M, et al. Post-prandial hypotension is associated with asymptomatic cerebrovascular damage in essential hypertensive patients. Hypertension. 1999; 33:565-568

Kohara K, Igase M, Yinong J, et al. Asymptomatic cerebrovascular damage in essential hypertension in the elderly. Am J Hypertens. 1997; 10:829-835.

Karemaker JM, Wieling W, Dunning AJ. Aging and the baroreflex. In: Amery A, Staessen, Eds. Hypertension in the Elderly. Amsterdam, The Netherlands: Elsevier Science Publishers BV; 1989:24-38.

Finucane BT, Hammonds WD and Welch MB. **Influence** of age on vascular absorption of lidocaine from the epidural space . Anesth Analg 1988 Feb; 67(2): 204

White PF. Anesthetic techniques for the elderly outpatient. Int Anesthesiol Clin. 1988; 26(2):105-111.

White PF. Clinical pharmacology of intravenous induction drugs. Int Anesthesiol Clin. 1988; 26(2):98-104.

Kanto J, Aaltone L, Himbrerg JJ et al: Midazolam as an intravenous induction agent in the elderly> A clinical and pharmacokinetic study. Anesth Analg 1986; 65: 15.

Klotz U, Avant GR, Hoyumpa A et al: The effects of age and liver disease on the disposition and elimination of diazepam in adult man. J Clin Invest 1975; 55: 347

Schnider TW, Minto CF, Shafer SL, et al. The influence of age on propofol pharmacodynamics. *Anesthesiology*. 1999; 90:1502-1516.

Dundee JW, Robinson FP, McCollum JSC, Patterson CC. Sensitivity to propofol in the elderly. *Anaesthesia*. 1986; 41:482-485.

Frolkis VV, Martynenko OA, Zamostyan VP. Aging of the neuromuscular apparatus. Gerontology. 1976; 22(4):244-279.Matteo RS, Backus WW, McDaniel DD, et al.

Pharmacokinetics and pharmacodynamics of d-tubocurarine and metocurine in the elderly. Anesth Analg. 1985; 64(1):23-29.

Tasch MD, Stoelting RK. Autonomic nervous system. In: McLeskey CH, ed. Geriatric Anesthesiology. Baltimore: Williams & Wilkins; 1997:57-70.

Muravchic S: Current concepts: Anesthetic pharmacology in geriatric patients. Prog Anesthesiol 1987; 1:2

Clinical pharmacology of intravenous induction drugs. Int Anesthesiol Clin. 1988; 26(2):98-104.

Aronow WS, Ahn C, Mercando A et al. Prevalence and association of ventricular tachycardia and complex ventricular arrhythmias and new coronary events in older men and women with and without cardiovascular disease. J Gerontol a Biol Sci Med Sci 2002; 57: 333-5

Lee KH, Kerwin BA, Miro AM. Respiratory Function. In Shoemaker (ed): Pocket Companion to Textbook of Critical Care. Philadelphia, W.B. Saunders, 1996, p. 232-4.

Terris DJ, Arnstein DP, Nguyen HH. Contemporary evaluation of unilateral vocal cord paralysis. Otolaryngol Head Neck Surg1992; 107:84.

Yentis SM, Hirsch NP, Smith GB. Anaesthesia and Intensive Care A-Z An Encyclopaedia of Principles and Practice. 2nd Edition, Oxford, Butterworth Heinemann, 2000, p. 332.

Lindeman RD, Roche RJ. Minerals. In Zaloga (ed): Nutrition in Critical Care. St. Louis, Mosby, 1994, p. 257-258.

Nussbaum MS, Fischer JE. Parenteral Nutrition. In Zaloga (ed): Nutrition in Critical Care. St. Louis, Mosby, 1994, p. 374-78.

Kudsk KA, Jacobs DO. Nutrition. In Norton (ed): Surgery: Basic Science and Clinical Evidence. New York, Springer-Verlag, 2001, p. 144-46.

Moon RE, Dear GdL, Stolp BW. Hyperbaric Oxygen in Critical Care. In Shoemaker (ed): Textbook of Critical Care. 4th Edition. Philadelphia, WB Saunders, 2000, p.1524.

Lew TWK, Darby JM. Central Nervous System. In Shoemaker (ed): Pocket Companion to Textbook of Critical Care. Philadelphia, W.B. Saunders, 1996, p. 589.

Yurn R. Burns. In Norton (ed): Surgery: Basic Science and Clinical Evidence. New York, Springer, 2001, p. 327-336.

Morris GF, Taylor WR. Modern Management of Acute Spinal Cord Injury. In Shoemaker (ed): Textbook of Critical Care. 4th Edition. Philadelphia, WB Saunders, 2000, p.328.

Lew TWK, Darby JM. Central Nervous System. In Shoemaker (ed): Pocket Companion to Textbook of Critical Care. Philadelphia, W.B. Saunders, 1996, p. 587-588.

Knudsen NW, Fulkerson WJ. Lung Injury from Mechanical Ventilation. In MacIntyre (ed): Mechanical Ventilation. Philadelphia, WB Saunders, 2001, p.212-219.

Chandler CF, Waxman K. Monitoring. In Shoemaker (ed): Pocket Companion to Textbook of Critical Care. Philadelphia, W.B. Saunders, 1996, p. 115.

Hess D. Heliox and Inhaled Nitric Oxide. In MacIntyre (ed): Mechanical Ventilation. Philadelphia, WB Saunders, 2001, p.465-466.

Warfare Agents (Accessed on March 25, 2004 at http://micromedex.duhs.duke.edu/mdxcgi/display.exe?CTL=D%3A%5Cmdx%5Cmdxc).

Intraventricular Hemorrhage (Accessed March 27, 2004 at http://web1.tch.harvard.edu/cfapps/A2ZtopicDisplay.cfm?Topic=Intraventricular%20Hemorrha).

Matteo RS, Ornstein E, Schwartz AE, et al. Pharmacokinetics and pharmacodynamics of rocuronium (ORG 9426) in elderly surgical patients. Anesth Analg 1993; 77: 1193-1197.

Buckley FP, Martay K: Anesthesia and Obesity and Gastrointestinal Disorders. In Barash PG, Cullen BF, and Stoelting RK (eds): Clinical Anesthesia, 4th edition. Philadelphia, Lippincott Williams and Wilkins, 2001, pp. 1037-1038.

Fleming NW. Macres S. Antognini JF. Vengco J. Neuromuscular blocking action of suxamethonium after antagonism of vecuronium by edrophonium, pyridostigmine or neostigmine. British Journal of Anaesthesia. 77(4):492-5, 1996 Oct.

McCoy EP. Mirakhur RK. Comparison of the effects of neostigmine and edrophonium on the duration of action of suxamethonium. Acta Anaesthesiologica Scandinavica. 39(6):744-7, 1995 Aug.

Atherton DP. Hunter JM. Clinical pharmacokinetics of the newer neuromuscular blocking drugs. Clinical Pharmacokinetics. 36(3):169-89, 1999 Mar.

Szenohradszky J. Fogarty D. Kirkegaard-Nielsen H. Brown R. Sharma ML. Fisher DM. Effect of edrophonium and neostigmine on the pharmacokinetics and neuromuscular effects of mivacurium. Anesthesiology. 92(3):708-14, 2000 Mar.

Motamed C. Kirov K. Combes X. Dhonneur G. Duvaldestin P. Effect of metoclopramide on mivacurium-induced neuromuscular block. Acta Anaesthesiologica Scandinavica. 46(2):214-6, 2002 Feb.

Gruber M. Lindner R. Prasser C. Wiesner G. The effect of fluoride and hypothermia on the in vitro metabolism of mivacurium. Anesthesia & Analgesia. 95(2):397-9, table of contents, 2002 Aug.

McGehee DS. Krasowski MD. Fung DL. Wilson B. Gronert GA. Moss J. Cholinesterase inhibition by potato glycoalkaloids slows mivacurium metabolism. Anesthesiology. 93(2):510-9, 2000 Aug.

Stoelting RK, Miller RD (eds): Basics of Anesthesia, 4th edition. Philadelphia, Churchill Livingston, 2000, pp.101.

Wight WJ. Wright PM. Pharmacokinetics and pharmacodynamics of rapacuronium bromide. Clinical Pharmacokinetics. 41(13):1059-76, 2002.

Stoelting RK, Miller RD (eds): Basics of Anesthesia, 4th edition. Philadelphia, Churchill Livingston, 2000, pp.101.

Jooste E. Klafter F. Hirshman CA. Emala CW. A mechanism for rapacuronium-induced bronchospasm: M2 muscarinic receptor antagonism. Anesthesiology. 98(4):906-11, 2003 Apr.

Wight WJ. Wright PM. Pharmacokinetics and pharmacodynamics of rapacuronium bromide. Clinical Pharmacokinetics. 41(13):1059-76, 2002.

Bevan DR, Donati F: Muscle Relaxants. In Barash PG, Cullen BF, and Stoelting RK (eds): Clinical Anesthesia, 4th edition. Philadelphia, Lippincott Williams and Wilkins, 2001, pp. 437-438.

Sokoll MD. Gergis SD. Antibiotics and neuromuscular function. Anesthesiology. 55(2):148-59, 1981 Aug

Stoelting RK. Pharmacology and Physiology in Anesthetic Practice. 3rd edition, Philadelphia, Lippincott Williams and Wilkins, 1999, pp. 196-199.

Ghoneim MM. Long JP. The interaction between magnesium and other neuromuscular blocking agents. Anesthesiology. 32(1):23-7, 1970 Jan.

Dailey PA. Fisher DM. Shnider SM. Baysinger CL. Shinohara Y. Miller RD. Abboud TK. Kim KC. Pharmacokinetics, placental transfer, and neonatal effects of vecuronium and pancuronium administered during cesarean section. Anesthesiology. 60(6):569-74, 1984 Jun.

Herman NL: The Placenta: Anatomy, Physiology, and Transfer of Drugs. In Chestnut DH (ed): Obstetric Anesthesia: Principles and Practice, 2nd edition. St. Louis, Missouri, Mosby, 1999, p. 69.

Wang K. Asinger RW. Marriott HJ. ST-segment elevation in conditions other than acute myocardial infarction. New England Journal of Medicine. 349(22):2128-35, 2003 Nov 27.

Prough DS, Mathru M: Acid-Base, Fluids, and Electrolytes. In Barash PG, Cullen BF, and Stoelting RK (eds): Clinical Anesthesia, 4th edition. Philadelphia, Lippincott Williams and Wilkins, 2001, pp. 187-189.

Bevan DR, Donati F: Muscle Relaxants. In Barash PG, Cullen BF, and Stoelting RK (eds): Clinical Anesthesia, 4th edition. Philadelphia, Lippincott Williams and Wilkins, 2001, pp. 421.

Stoelting RK, Miller RD (eds): Basics of Anesthesia, 4th edition. Philadelphia, Churchill Livingston, 2000, pp.91-93.

Stoelting RK, Miller RD (eds): Basics of Anesthesia, 4th edition. Philadelphia, Churchill Livingston, 2000, pp.94-95.

Hayes AH. Breslin DS. Mirakhur RK. Reid JE. O'Hare RA. Frequency of haemoglobin desaturations with the use of succinylcholine during rapid sequence induction of anesthesia. Acta Anaesthesiologica Scandinavica. 45(6):746-9, 2001 Jul.

Heier T. Feiner JR. Lin J. Brown R. Caldwell JE. Hemoglobin desaturations after succinylcholine-induced apnea: a study of the recovery of spontaneous ventilation in healthy volunteers. Anesthesiology. 94(5):754-9, 2001 May.

Ding Z. White PF. Anesthesia for electroconvulsive therapy. Anesthesia & Analgesia. 94(5):1351-64, 2002 May.

Stoelting RK, Miller RD (eds): Basics of Anesthesia, 4th edition. Philadelphia, Churchill Livingston, 2000, pp.89-90.

Cantineau JP, Porte F, Dhonneur G, Duvaldestin P: Neuromuscular effects of rocuronium on the diaphragm and adductor pollicis muscles in anesthetized patients. Anesthesiology 1994; 81: 585–90

Laycock JR, Donati F, Smith CE, Bevan DR: Potency of atracurium and vecuronium at the diaphragm and the adductor pollicis muscle. Br J Anaesth 1988; 61: 286–91

Hemmerling TM, Schmidt J, Hanusa C, Wolf T, Schmidt H: Simultaneous determination of neuromuscular block at the larynx, diaphragm, adductor pollicis, orbicularis oculi and corrugator supercilii muscles. Br J Anaesth 2000; 85: 856–60.

Hemmerling TM. Donati F. Neuromuscular blockade at the larynx, the diaphragm and the corrugator supercilii muscle: a review. Canadian Journal of Anaesthesia. 50(8):779-94, 2003 Oct.

Bevan DR, Donati F: Muscle Relaxants. In Barash PG, Cullen BF, and Stoelting RK (eds): Clinical Anesthesia, 4th edition. Philadelphia, Lippincott Williams and Wilkins, 2001, pp. 424-430.

Monk TG, Weldon BC: The Renal System and Anesthesia for Urologic Surgery. In Barash PG, Cullen BF, and Stoelting RK (eds): Clinical Anesthesia, 4th edition. Philadelphia, Lippincott Williams and Wilkins, 2001, pp. 1013-1014.

Powell DR. Miller R. The effect of repeated doses of succinylcholine on serum potsssium in patients with renal failure. Anesthesia & Analgesia. 54(6):746-8, 1975 Nov-Dec.

Koide M. Waud BE. Serum potassium concentrations after succinylcholine in patients with renal failure. Anesthesiology. 36(2):142-5, 1972 Feb.

Bevan DR, Donati F: Muscle Relaxants. In Barash PG, Cullen BF, and Stoelting RK (eds): Clinical Anesthesia, 4th edition. Philadelphia, Lippincott Williams and Wilkins, 2001, pp. 433.

Berry FA, Castro BA: Neonatal Anesthesia. In Barash PG, Cullen BF, and Stoelting RK (eds): Clinical Anesthesia, 4th edition. Philadelphia, Lippincott Williams and Wilkins, 2001, pp. 1179

Airways. In: Murray & Nadel: Textbook of Respiratory Medicine, 3rd Ed, 2000, WB Saunders Company, p 6, 823

Respiratory Physiology. In: Miller: Anesthesia, 5th Ed, 2000, Churchill Livingstone Inc, p 594

Respiratory Care. In: Miller: Anesthesia, 5th Ed, 2000, Churchill Livingstone Inc, p 1281

Respiratory Care. In: Miller: Anesthesia, 5th Ed, 2000, Churchill Livingstone Inc, p 2436

Gotta AW, Ray C, Sullivan CA, Goldiner PL: Anatomical dead space and airway resistance after glycopyrrolate or atropine premedication. Can An Soc J 28(1)1981:51-4

Ashutosh K, Dev G, Steele D: Nonbronchodilator effects of pirbuterol and ipratropium in chronic obstructive pulmonary disease. Chest 107(1) 1995: 173-8

Hansen D, Syben R, Vargas O, Spies C, Welte M: The alveoloar-arterial difference in oxygen tension increases with temperature-corrected determination during moderate hypothermia. Anesth Analg 88(3)1999:538-41

Mummery HJ, Stolp BW, Dear GdL, Doar PO, et al: Effects of age and exercise on physiological dead space during simulated dives at 2.8 ATA. J Appl Physiol 94(2)2003:507-17

Respiratory Physiology. In: Miller: Anesthesia, 5th Ed, 2000, Churchill Livingstone Inc, p 594

Chronic obstructive pulmonary desease. In: Murray & Nadel: Textbook of Respiratory Medicine, 3rd Ed, 2000, WB Saunders Company, p 1207

Respiratory Physiology. In: Miller: Anesthesia, 5th Ed, 2000, Churchill Livingstone Inc, p 584

Respiratory Physiology. In: Miller: Anesthesia, 5th Ed, 2000, Churchill Livingstone Inc, p 594

The post anesthesia care unit. In: Miller: Anesthesia, 5th Ed, 2000, Churchill Livingstone Inc, p 2312

Respiratory Physiology. In: Miller: Anesthesia, 5th Ed, 2000, Churchill Livingstone Inc, p 93

Fink BR. Diffusion anoxia. Anesthesiology 16.1955:511-19

Rackow H, Salanitre E, Frumin MH: Dilution of alveolar gases during nitrous oxide excretion in man. J Appl Physiol 16. 1961:723-8

Respiratory Care. In: Miller: Anesthesia, 5th Ed, 2000, Churchill Livingstone Inc, p 2422

Bluman LG, Mosca L, Newman N, Simon DG: Preoperative smoking habits and postoperative pulmonary complications. Chest 113, 1998:883-9

Kotani N, Kushikata T, Hashimoto H, Sessler DI, et al: Recovery of intraoperative microbicidal and inflammatory functions of alveolar immune cells after a tobacco free period. Anesthesiology 94(6)2001:999-1006

Pulmonary function testing . In: Miller: Anesthesia, 5th Ed, 2000, Churchill Livingstone Inc, p 894

Nelson NM: Neonatal pulmonary function. Pediatr Clin North Am 13.1966:769

Camporesi EM, Bosco G: Ventilation, gas exchange and exercise under pressure. In: Bennett and Elliott's Physiology and Medicine of Diving, 5th Ed. Saunders 2004, p 86

In: Murray & Nadel: Textbook of Respiratory Medicine, 3rd Ed, 2000, WB Saunders Company, p 1582

Mellemgaard K: The alveolar-arterial oxygen difference: Its size and components in normal man. Acta Physiol Scand 67. 1966:10

Respiratory Pathophysiology. In: Behrman: Nelson Textbool of Pediatrics. 17th Ed. 2004 Elsevier, p 1369

Respiratory Care. In: Miller: Anesthesia, 5th Ed, 2000, Churchill Livingstone Inc, p 2422

Ventilation - Perfusion Relationships. In: Murray & Nadel: Textbook of Respiratory Medicine, 3rd Ed, 2000, WB Saunders Company, p 826

Respiratory Care. In: Miller: Anesthesia, 5th Ed, 2000, Churchill Livingstone Inc, p 894

Pulmonary function testing . In: Miller: Anesthesia, 5th Ed, 2000, Churchill Livingstone Inc, p 894

Ventilation - Perfusion Relationships. In: Murray & Nadel: Textbook of Respiratory Medicine, 3rd Ed, 2000, WB Saunders Company, p 823

Respiratory Care. In: Miller: Anesthesia, 5th Ed, 2000, Churchill Livingstone Inc, p 2417

Respiratory Care. In: Miller: Anesthesia, 5th Ed, 2000, Churchill Livingstone Inc, p 2436

Surfactant. In: Murray & Nadel: Textbook of Respiratory Medicine, 3rd Ed, 2000, WB Saunders Company, p 307-325

Respiratory Care. In: Miller: Anesthesia, 5th Ed, 2000, Churchill Livingstone Inc, p 2416

Eger EII, Severinghaus JW: Effect of uneven pulmonary distribution of blood and gas on induction with inhalatin anesthetics. Anesthesiology 25.1964:620-6

Respiratory Care. In: Miller: Anesthesia, 5th Ed, 2000, Churchill Livingstone Inc, p 2436

Pulmonary Pharmacology. In: Miller: Anesthesia, 5th Ed, 2000, Churchill Livingstone Inc, p 134

Respiratory Physiology and Respiratory Function during Anesthesia. In: Miller: Anesthesia, 5th Ed, 2000, Churchill Livingstone Inc, p 609

Anesthesia for Thoracic Surgery. In: Miller: Anesthesia, 5th Ed, 2000, Churchill Livingstone Inc, p 1710

Respiratory Physiology and Respiratory Function during Anesthesia. In: Miller: Anesthesia, 5th Ed, 2000, Churchill Livingstone Inc, p 610

Respiratory Care. In: Miller: Anesthesia, 5th Ed, 2000, Churchill Livingstone Inc, p 2436

Luft UC, Mostyn EM, Loeppky JA, Venters MD: Contribution of the Haldane effect to the rise of arterial PCO_2 in hypoxic patients breathing oxygen. Critical Care Medicine1981:9(1)32-7

Respiratory Physiology and Respiratory Function during Anesthesia. In: Miller: Anesthesia, 5th Ed, 2000, Churchill Livingstone Inc, p 581

Respiratory Physiology and Respiratory Function during Anesthesia. In: Miller: Anesthesia, 5th Ed, 2000, Churchill Livingstone Inc, p 581

Gronkvist M, Bergsten E, Eiken O, Gustafsson PM: Inter- and intraregional venilation inhomogeneity in hypergravity and after pressurization of an anti-G suit. J Appl Physiol 2003.94(4):1353-64

Elliott AR, et al: Microgravity reduces sleep-disordered breathing in humans. Am J Respir Crit Care Med 2001.164(3):478-85

Frerichs I, et al: Gravity effects on regional lung ventilation determined by functional EIT during parabolic flights. J Appl Physiol 2001.91(1):39-50

Rehder K: Postural Changes in respiratory function, Acta Anaesth Scand 1998.113:13-6

Prisk GK, Guy HJ, Elliott AR, West JB: Cardiopulmonary adaptation to weightlessness.

Journal of Gravitational Physiology 1994.1(1)118-21

Respiratory Physiology and Respiratory Function during Anesthesia. In:
Miller: Anesthesia, 5th Ed, 2000, Churchill Livingstone Inc, p 581

Acid - Base Balance. In: Miller: Anesthesia, 5th Ed, 2000, Churchill
Livingstone Inc, p 1404

Lanzinger MJT, Mark JB. The pulmonary artery catheter. In: Mackay JH,
Arrowsmith JE (Eds). Core Topics in Cardiac Anaesthesia. London: Green Medical
Media. 2004. pp 125-8.

Respiratory Physiology and Respiratory Function during Anesthesia. In:
Miller: Anesthesia, 5th Ed, 2000, Churchill Livingstone Inc, p 614

Weimann J, Toxicity of Nitrous Oxide, Best Practice and Research Clinical Anaesthesiology. 2003; 17: 47-
61.

Deacon R, Lumb M, Perry J et al. Inactivation of Methionine Synthetase by Nitrous Oxide. European Journal
of Biochemistry. 1980; 104: 419-423.

Chanarin I. Cobalamin and Nitrous Oxide: A Review. Journal of Clinical Pathology. 1980; 33: 909-916.

Danenberg PV. Malli H. Swenson S. Thymidylate synthase inhibitors. Seminars in Oncology. 1999; 26:621-
31

Axelrod FB, Donenfeld RF, Danzinger F, Turndorf M. Anesthesia in Familial Dysautonomia.
Anesthesiology. 1988; 62: 631.

Stubbig K, Schmidt H, SchreckenbergerR et al: Anaesthesia and Intensive Therapy in Autonomic
Dysfunction. 1993; 42: 316.

Miller, Ronald D, Anesthesia, Fifth Edition, Churchill Livingstone, Philadelphia, 2000, p. 471.

Flewellen EH, Bodensteiner JB: Anesthetic Experience in a Patient with Hyperkalemic Periodic Paralysis.
Aneth Rev 7: 44, 1980.

Mitchell MM, Ali HH, Savarese JJ. Myotonia and Neuromuscular Blocking Agents. Anesthesiology. 1978;
49: 44.

Barash Paul G, Cullen Bruce F, Stoelting Robert K, Clinical Anesthesia, Fourth Edition, Lippincott-Raven,
Philadelphia, 2001, p.492

Miller, Ronald D, Anesthesia, Fifth Edition, Churchill Livingstone, Philadelphia, 2000, p. 973.

Miller, Ronald D, Anesthesia, Fifth Edition, Churchill Livingstone, Philadelphia, 2000, p. 422.
Barash Paul G, Cullen Bruce F, Stoelting Robert K, Clinical Anesthesia, Fourth Edition, Lippincott-Raven,
Philadelphia, 2001, p.424.

Miller, Ronald D, Anesthesia, Fifth Edition, Churchill Livingstone, Philadelphia, 2000, p. 987.

Miller, Ronald D, Anesthesia, Fifth Edition, Churchill Livingstone, Philadelphia, 2000, p. 1987.

Engelfriet CP, Overbecke MA, Van Der Berne AE. Autoimmune hemolytic Anemia. Seminars.
Hematology. 1992; 29: 3

Barash Paul G, Cullen Bruce F, Stoelting Robert K, <u>Clinical Anesthesia, Fourth Edition</u>, Lippincott-Raven, Philadelphia, 2001, p.538.

Viby-Mogensen J. Succinylcholine Neuromuscular Blockade in Subjects Homozygous for Atypical Plasma Cholinesterase. Anesthesiology. 1981; 55: 429.

Barash Paul G, Cullen Bruce F, Stoelting Robert K, <u>Clinical Anesthesia, Fourth Edition</u>, Lippincott-Raven, Philadelphia, 2001, p.540.

Barash Paul G, Cullen Bruce F, Stoelting Robert K, <u>Clinical Anesthesia, Fourth Edition</u>, Lippincott-Raven, Philadelphia, 2001, p.539.

Miller, Ronald D, <u>Anesthesia, Fifth Edition,</u> Churchill Livingstone, Philadelphia, 2000, p. 557, 315, 316.

Hong R. The DiGeorge Anomaly. Clinical Reviews in Allergy & Immunology, 2001; 20: 43-60.

Murphy PC. Acute Intermittent Porphyria; The Anesthetic Problem and its Background. British Journal of Anesthesiology. 1964; 36: 801.

Barash Paul G, Cullen Bruce F, Stoelting Robert K, <u>Clinical Anesthesia, Fourth Edition</u>, Lippincott-Raven, Philadelphia, 2001, p.541.

Miller, Ronald D, <u>Anesthesia, Fifth Edition,</u> Churchill Livingstone, Philadelphia, 2000, p. 1263.

Miller, Ronald D, <u>Anesthesia, Fifth Edition,</u> Churchill Livingstone, Philadelphia, 2000, p. 2482.

Miller, Ronald D, <u>Anesthesia, Fifth Edition,</u> Churchill Livingstone, Philadelphia, 2000, p. 1266.

Hahh I. Hoffman RS. Nelson Ls. EMLA-induced methemoglobinemia and systemic topical anesthetic toxicity. Journal of Emergency Medicine. 2004; 26: 85-88.

Salamat A. Watson HG. Drug-induced methemoglobinemia presenting with angina following the use of dapsone. Clinical and Laboratory Hematology. 2003; 25: 327.

Miller, Ronald D, <u>Anesthesia, Fifth Edition,</u> Churchill Livingstone, Philadelphia, 2000, p. 2482.

Miller, Ronald D, <u>Anesthesia, Fifth Edition,</u> Churchill Livingstone, Philadelphia, 2000, p. 1033.

Miller, Ronald D, <u>Anesthesia, Fifth Edition,</u> Churchill Livingstone, Philadelphia, 2000, p. 1046.

Barash Paul G, Cullen Bruce F, Stoelting Robert K, <u>Clinical Anesthesia, Fourth Edition</u>, Lippincott-Raven, Philadelphia, 2001, p.491.

Barash Paul G, Cullen Bruce F, Stoelting Robert K, <u>Clinical Anesthesia, Fourth Edition</u>, Lippincott-Raven, Philadelphia, 2001, p.489.

Barash Paul G, Cullen Bruce F, Stoelting Robert K, <u>Clinical Anesthesia, Fourth Edition</u>, Lippincott-Raven, Philadelphia, 2001, p.490.

Miller, Ronald D, <u>Anesthesia, Fifth Edition,</u> Churchill Livingstone, Philadelphia, 2000, p. 1034.

Barash Paul G, Cullen Bruce F, Stoelting Robert K, <u>Clinical Anesthesia, Fourth Edition</u>, Lippincott-Raven, Philadelphia, 2001, p.497.

Miller, Ronald D, <u>Anesthesia, Fifth Edition,</u> Churchill Livingstone, Philadelphia, 2000, p. 1039.

Barash Paul G, Cullen Bruce F, Stoelting Robert K, <u>Clinical Anesthesia, Fourth Edition</u>, Lippincott-Raven, Philadelphia, 2001, p.498.

Barash Paul G, Cullen Bruce F, Stoelting Robert K, <u>Clinical Anesthesia, Fourth Edition</u>, Lippincott-Raven, Philadelphia, 2001, p.493.

Iohom G. Lyons B. Anaesthesia for children with epidermolysis bullosa: a review of 20 years' experience. European Journal of Anaesthesiology. 2001; 18: 745

Barash Paul G, Cullen Bruce F, Stoelting Robert K, <u>Clinical Anesthesia, Fourth Edition</u>, Lippincott-Raven, Philadelphia, 2001, p.481.

Bork K. Ressel N. Sudden upper airway obstruction in patients with hereditary angioedema. Transfusion and Apheresis Science. 2003; 29: 235-238.

Miller, Ronald D, <u>Anesthesia, Fifth Edition,</u> Churchill Livingstone, Philadelphia, 2000, p. 1046.

Hameed SM, et al: Oxygen Delivery. Crit Care Med (2003); 31: 12.

Gauthier PM, et al: Metabolic Acidosis in the Intensive Care Unit. Crit Care Clin (2002); 18: 289-308.

Cochrane Injuries Group Albumin Reviewers: Human Albumin Administration in Critically Ill Patients: Systematic Review of Randomized Controlled Trials. BMJ (1998); 317: 235-40.

Nunn JF. Nunn's Applied Respiratory Physiology. 4th Ed. Stoneham, MA: Butterworth, 1993.

Berne RM and Levy MN. Physiology. 4th Ed. St. Louis, MO: Mosby, 1998.

Marino PL. The ICU Book. 2nd Ed. Philadelphia, PA: Lippincott, Williams, and Wilkins, 1998.

Sabiston DC. Textbook of Surgery: The Biological Basis of Modern Surgical Practice. 15th Ed. Philadelphia, PA: W. B. Saunders, 1997.

Braunwald E. Harrison's Principles of Internal Medicine. 15th Ed. New York, NY: McGraw-Hill, 2001.

Obstetric Anesthesiology Web Page, University of Florida. Author Rex Williams.

Tobin M. Principles and Practice of Intensive Care Monitoring. McGraw-Hill, New York, 1998.

Porsche R, Brenner ZR. Allergy to protamine sulfate. *Heart Lung.* Nov-Dec 1999;28(6):418-428.

J Allergy Clin Immunol, Vol 101(6, Part 2) Supplement. June 1998. S507-S509

David L. Hepner and Mariana C. Castells. Anaphylaxis During the Perioperative Period. Anesth Analg 2003 97: 1381-1395.

Khay W. Toh, Sarah J. Deacock, and William J. Fawcett. Severe Anaphylactic Reaction to Cisatracurium. Anesth Analg 1999 88: 462

Anesthesiology Review, Ed Ronald Faust, "Anaphylactic and Anaphylactoid Reactions" pp178-179

Pharmacology and Physiology in Anesthetic Practice
Robert K.Stoelting, 15th Jan 1999.

Clinical Anesthesia
Paul G. Barash, Bruce F Cullen, Robert K. Stoelting 2001.

Anesthesia
Ronald D. Miller, Edward D. Jr Miller, J. Gerald Reves, Michael F. Roizen, John F. Savarese, Roy F. Cucchiara, Alan Ross. 15 Jan 2000.

Clinical Pharmacology of Opioids for Pain. Charles E Inturrisi in the The Clinical Journal of Pain 18: S3-S13 2002

Principles and Practice of Pharmacology for Anaesthetists Fourth edition 2001. T.N. Calvey and N.E. Williams. Blackwell science Ltd Oxford U.K.

Clinical Pharmacology of Opioids for Pain. Charles E Inturrisi in the The Clinical journal of pain 18: S3-S13 2002

Dreyfuss D, Saumon G. Ventioator-induced lung injury: lessons from experimental studies. Am J Respir Crit Care Med 1998; 157; 294-323

Slinger PD, Johnston MR. Preoperative assessment and management. In Kaplan JW, Slinger PD, eds. Thoracic anesthesia 3rd ed. Philadelphia: Churchhill Livingstone, 2003: 1-23

Reilly JJ. Evidence-based preoperative evaluation of candidates for thoractomoy. Chest 1999; 116:474s-6

Cerfolio RJ, Allen MS, Trastak VF, et. al. Lung resection in patients with compromised pulmonary function. Ann Thorac Surg 1996; 62:348-51

Schulman DS, Mathony RA. The right ventricle in pulmonary disease. Cardiol Clin 1992; 10:111-35

Ingrassia TE III, Ryu JH, Trasek VF, Rosenow ECIII. Oxygenexacerbated bleomycin pulmonary toxicity. Mayo Clin Proc 1991; 66:173-8

Pennefather SH, Russel GN. Placement of double-lumen tubes: time to shed light on an old problem. Br J Anaesth 2000;84:308-10

Slinger P, Kruger M, McRae K, Winton T. Relation of the static compliance curve and positive end-exprtiatory pressure to oxygenation during one-lung. Anesthesiology 2001;95:1096-102

Grichnik KP, Hill SE. The perioperative management of patients with severe emphysema. J Cardiothorac Vasc Anesth 2003; 17(3): 364-87

Sabision Textbook of Surgery; "The biological basis of modern surgical practice" 16th edition, editor Townsend

Atlas of Regional Anesthesia. 2nd Edition. Brown DL. W.B. Saunders Company 1999.

Textbook of regional anesthesia. Raj PP. Elsevier Science (USA) 2002.

Clinically oriented anatomy. 3rd Ed. Moore KL. Williams & Wilkins 1992.

Horlocker TT, Wedel DJ, Benzon H, et al. Regional anesthesia in the anticoagulated patient: defining the risks (the second ASRA Consensus Conference on Neuraxial Anesthesia and Anticoagulation). *Regional Anesthesia & Pain Medicine.* May-Jun 2003;28(3):172-197

Anesthesia
Ronald D. Miller, Edward D. Jr Miller, J. Gerald Reves, Michael F. Roizen, John F. Savarese, Roy F. Cucchiara, Alan Ross. 15 Jan 2000.

NOTES

NOTES

NOTES